Hemostasis in Head and Neck Surgery

Editors

HARSHITA PANT
CARL H. SNYDERMAN

OTOLARYNGOLOGIC CLINICS OF NORTH AMERICA

www.oto.theclinics.com

June 2016 • Volume 49 • Number 3

ELSEVIER

1600 John F. Kennedy Boulevard • Suite 1800 • Philadelphia, Pennsylvania, 19103-2899

http://www.oto.theclinics.com

OTOLARYNGOLOGIC CLINICS OF NORTH AMERICA Volume 49, Number 3
June 2016 ISSN 0030-6665, ISBN-13: 978-0-323-40260-6

Editor: Jessica McCool
Developmental Editor: Alison Swety

Otolaryngologic Clinics of North America (ISSN 0030-6665) is published bimonthly by Elsevier, Inc., 360 Park Avenue South, New York, NY 10010-1710. Months of issue are February, April, June, August, October, and December. Business and Editorial Offices: 1600 John F. Kennedy Blvd., Suite 1800, Philadelphia, PA 19103-2899. Customer Service Office: 6277 Sea Harbor Drive, Orlando, FL 32887-4800. Periodicals postage paid at New York, NY and additional mailing offices. Subscription prices are $370.00 per year (US individuals), $765.00 per year (US institutions), $100.00 per year (US student/resident), $485.00 per year (Canadian individuals), $969.00 per year (Canadian institutions), $540.00 per year (international individuals), $969.00 per year (international institutions), $270.00 per year (international & Canadian student/resident). Foreign air speed delivery is included in all *Clinics'* subscription prices. All prices are subject to change without notice. **POSTMASTER:** Send address changes to *Otolaryngologic Clinics of North America*, Elsevier Health Sciences Division, Subscription Customer Service, 3251 Riverport Lane, Maryland Heights, MO 63043. **Telephone: 1-800-654-2452 (U.S. and Canada); 314-447-8871 (outside U.S. and Canada). Fax: 314-447-8029. E-mail: journalscustomerservice-usa@elsevier.com (for print support); journalsonlinesupport-usa@elsevier.com (for online support).**

Reprints. For copies of 100 or more of articles in this publication, please contact the Commercial Reprints Department, Elsevier Inc., 360 Park Avenue South, New York, NY 10010-1710. Tel.: 212-633-3874; Fax: 212-633-3820; E-mail: reprints@elsevier.com.

Otolaryngologic Clinics of North America is also published in Spanish by McGraw-Hill Interamericana Editores S.A., P.O. Box 5-237, 06500 Mexico D.F., Mexico.

Otolaryngologic Clinics of North America is covered in *MEDLINE/PubMed (Index Medicus), Current Contents/Clinical Medicine, Excerpta Medica, BIOSIS, Science Citation Index,* and *ISI/BIOMED.*

PROGRAM OBJECTIVE

The goal of the *Otolaryngologic Clinics of North America* is to provide information on the latest trends in patient management, the newest advances; and provide a sound basis for choosing treatment options in the field of otolaryngology.

LEARNING OBJECTIVES

Upon completion of this activity, participants will be able to:

1. Review education, training, and preoperative assessment of risk factors for hemostasis in head and neck surgery.
2. Discuss surgical adhesives, simulation training, and other innovations in treating vascular emergencies in head and neck surgery.
3. Recognize management of injury and diseases related to hemostasis in head and neck surgery.

ACCREDITATION

The Elsevier Office of Continuing Medical Education (EOCME) is accredited by the Accreditation Council for Continuing Medical Education (ACCME) to provide continuing medical education for physicians.

The EOCME designates this enduring material for a maximum of 15 *AMA PRA Category 1 Credit*(s)™. Physicians should claim only the credit commensurate with the extent of their participation in the activity.

All other health care professionals requesting continuing education credit for this enduring material will be issued a certificate of participation.

DISCLOSURE OF CONFLICTS OF INTEREST

The EOCME assesses conflict of interest with its instructors, faculty, planners, and other individuals who are in a position to control the content of CME activities. All relevant conflicts of interest that are identified are thoroughly vetted by EOCME for fair balance, scientific objectivity, and patient care recommendations. EOCME is committed to providing its learners with CME activities that promote improvements or quality in healthcare and not a specific proprietary business or a commercial interest.

The planning committee, staff, authors and editors listed below have identified no financial relationships or relationships to products or devices they or their spouse/life partner have with commercial interest related to the content of this CME activity:

Amin Aghaebrahim, MD; Jacqui Allen, MBChB, FRACS; Abdullah Alobaid, MD, FRCSC; Martha Cordoba Amorocho, MD; Theodore Athanasiadis, MBBS, PhD, FRACS; Ahmed Yassin Bahgat, MD; Henry P. Barham, MD; Brad Bauer, BS; Jo-Lawrence Bigcas, MD; Benjamin Bleier, MD; Adrianne Brigido; Quintin M. Cappelle, MD; Shu-Hong Chang, MD; Victor K. Chung, MD; Daniel Clayburgh, MD, PhD; David M. Cognetti, MD, FACS; James Cohen, MD, PhD; Andrew Coughlin, MD; Julia A. Crawford, MBBS; Amir R. Dehdashti, MD, FACS, FMH; Iuliu Fat, MD; Juan C. Fernandez-Miranda, MD; Anjali Fortna; Paul A. Gardner, MD; John Gleysteen, MD; Christine Gourin, MD; Rebecca Harvey, MD; Brian T. Jankowitz, MD; Rachel Kaye, MD; Giant Lin, MD; Jessica McCool; Kelly Michelle Malloy, MD; Erin McKean, MD, MBA; Ryan M. Mitchell, MD, PhD; Kris S. Moe, MD, FACS; Premkumar Nandhakumar; Gurston G. Nyquist, MD; Vikram Padhye, MBBS, PhD; Harshita Pant, BMBS, PhD; Sanjay R. Parikh, MD; Diego A. Preciado, MD, PhD; Mindy R. Rabinowitz, MD; Pamela C. Roehm, MD, PhD; Soham Roy, MD, FACS; Raymond Sacks, MD; Asmi Sanghvi, DO; Nathan B. Sautter, MD; Cecelia E. Schmalbach, MD; Solomon S. Shaftel, MD, PhD; Susan Showalter; Russell B. Smith, MD; Timothy L. Smith, MD, MPH, FACS; Carl H. Snyderman, MD, MBA; Megan Suermann; Andrew Tassler, MD; Samuel A. Tisherman, MD, FACS, FCCM; Dean M. Toriumi, MD; Rowan Valentine, MBBS, FRACS, PhD; Laura Vandelaar, MD; Hilary N. White, MD.

The planning committee, staff, authors and editors listed below have identified financial relationships or relationships to products or devices they or their spouse/life partner have with commercial interest related to the content of this CME activity:

Richard J. Harvey, MD, PhD is on the speakers' bureau for Bayer AG, is a consultant/advisor for Olympus America; Medtronic; Neilmed Pharmaceuticals Inc; and Seqirus; and has research support from Medtronic; Neilmed Pharmaceuticals Inc; Stoneygenes, and ENT Technologies.

Tudor Jovin, MD is a consultant/advisor for Neuravi and Codman & Shurtleff, Inc., and has stock ownership in Blockade Medical, LLC and Silk Road Medical.

J. Scott Magnusson, MD is a consultant/advisor for Intuitive Surgical, Inc.

Peter-John Wormald, MD is a consultant/advisor for Neilmed Pharmaceuticals Inc, and receives royalties/patents from Medtronic; Integra LifeSciences Corporation; and Scopis GmbH.

UNAPPROVED/OFF-LABEL USE DISCLOSURE
The EOCME requires CME faculty to disclose to the participants:
1. When products or procedures being discussed are off-label, unlabelled, experimental, and/or investigational (not US Food and Drug Administration [FDA] approved); and
2. Any limitations on the information presented, such as data that are preliminary or that represent ongoing research, interim analyses, and/or unsupported opinions. Faculty may discuss information about pharmaceutical agents that is outside of FDA-approved labelling. This information is intended solely for CME and is not intended to promote off-label use of these medications. If you have any questions, contact the medical affairs department of the manufacturer for the most recent prescribing information.

TO ENROLL
To enroll in the *Otolaryngologic Clinics of North America* Continuing Medical Education program, call customer service at 1-800-654-2452 or sign up online at http://www.theclinics.com/home/cme. The CME program is available to subscribers for an additional annual fee of USD 260.

METHOD OF PARTICIPATION
In order to claim credit, participants must complete the following:
1. Complete enrolment as indicated above.
2. Read the activity.
3. Complete the CME Test and Evaluation. Participants must achieve a score of 70% on the test. All CME Tests and Evaluations must be completed online.

CME INQUIRIES/SPECIAL NEEDS
For all CME inquiries or special needs, please contact elsevierCME@elsevier.com.

Contributors

EDITORS

HARSHITA PANT, BMBS, PhD
Senior Lecturer, Department of Otolaryngology – Head and Neck Surgery, The University of Adelaide School of Medicine, Adelaide, South Australia, Australia

CARL H. SNYDERMAN, MD, MBA
Professor, Departments of Otolaryngology and Neurological Surgery, University of Pittsburgh School of Medicine; Co-Director, UPMC Center for Cranial Base Surgery, Pittsburgh, Pennsylvania

AUTHORS

AMIN AGHAEBRAHIM, MD
University of Pittsburgh Medical Center, Pittsburgh, Pennsylvania

JACQUI ALLEN, MBChB, FRACS
Laryngologist Auckland Voice and Swallow, Auckland, New Zealand

ABDULLAH ALOBAID, MD, FRCSC
Cerebrovascular/Skull Base Fellow, Department of Neurosurgery, Northshore University Hospital, Northwell Health, Manhasset, New York

MARTHA CORDOBA AMOROCHO, MD
Department of Anesthesiology, Massachusetts Eye and Ear Infirmary, Instructor in Anesthesia, Anesthesiologist, Harvard Medical School; Department of Anesthesiology and Critical Care, Brigham and Women's Hospital, Boston, Massachusetts

THEODORE ATHANASIADIS, MBBS, PhD, FRACS
Adelaide Voice Specialists, Adelaide, South Australia, Australia

AHMED YASSIN BAHGAT, MD
Department of Otorhinolaryngology, Faculty of Medicine, Alexandria Hospital, Alexandria, Egypt

HENRY P. BARHAM, MD
Department of Otolaryngology – Head and Neck Surgery, LSUHSC SOM, Louisiana State University, New Orleans, Louisiana; Rhinology and Skull Base Research Group, St Vincent's Centre for Applied Medical Research, University of New South Wales, Sydney, Australia

BRAD BAUER, BS
Department of Otolaryngology – Head and Neck Surgery, Temple University School of Medicine, Philadelphia, Pennsylvania

JO-LAWRENCE BIGCAS, MD
University of Texas at Houston, McGovern Medical School, Houston, Texas

BENJAMIN BLEIER, MD
Assistant Professor, Department of Otolaryngology – Harvard Medical School,
Massachusetts Eye and Ear Infirmary, Boston, Massachusetts

QUINTIN M. CAPPELLE, MD
University of Illinois at Chicago, Chicago, Illinois

SHU-HONG CHANG, MD
Division of Orbital and Ophthalmic Plastic Surgery, Department of Ophthalmology,
University of Washington, Seattle, Washington

VICTOR K. CHUNG, MD
La Jolla Facial Plastic Surgery, San Diego, California

DANIEL CLAYBURGH, MD, PhD
Assistant Professor, Department of Otolaryngology – Head and Neck Surgery, Portland
VA Medical Center, Oregon Health Sciences University, Portland, Oregon

DAVID M. COGNETTI, MD, FACS
Associate Professor, Co-Director, Jefferson Center for Head and Neck Surgery,
Department of Otolaryngology – Head and Neck Surgery, Thomas Jefferson University,
Philadelphia, Pennsylvania

JAMES COHEN, MD, PhD
Professor, Department of Otolaryngology – Head and Neck Surgery; Chief, ENT, Portland
VA Medical Center, Oregon Health Sciences University, Portland, Oregon

ANDREW COUGHLIN, MD
Assistant Professor, Department of Otolaryngology – Head and Neck Surgery, University
of Nebraska Medical Center; Nebraska Methodist Hospital, Estabrook Cancer Center,
Omaha, Nebraska

JULIA A. CRAWFORD, MBBS
Department of Otolaryngology – Head and Neck Surgery, St Vincent's Hospital Sydney,
Darlinghurst, New South Wales, Australia

AMIR R. DEHDASHTI, MD, FACS, FMH
Associate Professor, Department of Neurosurgery, Northshore University Hospital,
Northwell Health, Manhasset, New York

IULIU FAT, MD
Anesthesiologist, Department of Anesthesiology, Harbor Hospital, Baltimore, Maryland

JUAN C. FERNANDEZ-MIRANDA, MD
Associate Professor, Department of Neurological Surgery, University of Pittsburgh School
of Medicine, Pittsburgh, Pennsylvania

PAUL A. GARDNER, MD
Associate Professor, Department of Neurological Surgery, University of Pittsburgh School
of Medicine, Pittsburgh, Pennsylvania

JOHN GLEYSTEEN, MD
Resident, Department of Otolaryngology – Head and Neck Surgery, Portland VA Medical
Center, Oregon Health Sciences University, Portland, Oregon

CHRISTINE GOURIN, MD
Department of Otolaryngology – Head and Neck Surgery, Johns Hopkins University,
Baltimore, Maryland

REBECCA HARVEY, MD
Resident, Department of Otolaryngology – Head and Neck Surgery, University of
Michigan, Ann Arbor, Michigan

RICHARD J. HARVEY, MD, PhD
Rhinology and Skull Base Research Group, St Vincent's Centre for Applied Medical
Research, University of New South Wales; Australian School of Advanced Medicine,
Macquarie University, Sydney, Australia

BRIAN T. JANKOWITZ, MD
Department of Neurological Surgery, University of Pittsburgh School of Medicine,
Pittsburgh, Pennsylvania

TUDOR JOVIN, MD
University of Pittsburgh Medical Center, Pittsburgh, Pennsylvania

RACHEL KAYE, MD
House Staff, Department of Otorhinolaryngology – Head and Neck Surgery, Montefiore
Medical Center, Bronx, New York

GIANT LIN, MD
Advocare Aroesty Ear, Nose, and Throat Associates, Mount Arlington, New Jersey

J. SCOTT MAGNUSON, MD
Professor, Department of Otolaryngology – Head and Neck Surgery, University of Central
Florida College of Medicine, Orlando, Florida

KELLY MICHELE MALLOY, MD
Assistant Professor, Department of Otolaryngology – Head and Neck Surgery, University
of Michigan, Ann Arbor, Michigan

ERIN McKEAN, MD, MBA
Associate Professor, Otolaryngology – Head and Neck Surgery and Neurosurgery,
University of Michigan, Ann Arbor, Michigan

RYAN M. MITCHELL, MD, PhD
Resident, Department of Otolaryngology – Head and Neck Surgery, University of
Washington, Seattle, Washington

KRIS S. MOE, MD, FACS
Professor and Chief, Division of Facial Plastic and Reconstructive Surgery, Departments
of Otolaryngology and Neurological Surgery, University of Washington School of
Medicine, Seattle, Washington

GURSTON G. NYQUIST, MD
Associate Professor, Department of Otolaryngology – Head and Neck Surgery, Division of
Rhinology and Skull Base Surgery, Thomas Jefferson University, Philadelphia,
Pennsylvania

VIKRAM PADHYE, MBBS, PhD
Department of Surgery, Otorhinolaryngology, Head and Neck Surgery, The Queen
Elizabeth Hospital, University of Adelaide, Adelaide, South Australia, Australia

HARSHITA PANT, BMBS, PhD
Senior Lecturer, Department of Otolaryngology – Head and Neck Surgery, The University
of Adelaide School of Medicine, Adelaide, South Australia, Australia

SANJAY R. PARIKH, MD
Professor, Department of Otolaryngology – Head and Neck Surgery, University of Washington; Division of Pediatric Otolaryngology – Head and Neck Surgery, Seattle Children's Hospital, Seattle, Washington

DIEGO A. PRECIADO, MD, PhD
Associate Professor of Otolaryngology, Pediatrics, and Integrative Systems Biology, Children's National Health System, George Washington University School of Medicine, Washington, DC

MINDY R. RABINOWITZ, MD
Clinical Instructor, Department of Otolaryngology – Head and Neck Surgery, Division of Rhinology and Skull Base Surgery, Thomas Jefferson University, Philadelphia, Pennsylvania

PAMELA C. ROEHM, MD, PhD
Director, Division of Otology and Neurotology; Associate Professor, Department of Otolaryngology – Head and Neck Surgery, Temple University School of Medicine, Philadelphia, Pennsylvania

SOHAM ROY, MD, FACS
University of Texas at Houston, McGovern Medical School, Houston, Texas

RAYMOND SACKS, MD
Australian School of Advanced Medicine, Macquarie University; University of Sydney, Sydney, Australia

ASMI SANGHVI, DO
Department of Medicine, Crozer-Keystone Health System, Drexel Hill, Pennsylvania

NATHAN B. SAUTTER, MD
Department of Otolaryngology – Head and Neck Surgery, Oregon Sinus Center, Oregon Health and Science University, Portland, Oregon

CECELIA E. SCHMALBACH, MD
Department of Otolaryngology, University of Indiana, Indianapolis, Indiana

SOLOMON S. SHAFTEL, MD, PhD
Department of Ophthalmology, Southern California Permanente Medical Group, San Diego, California

RUSSELL B. SMITH, MD
Professor, Department of Otolaryngology – Head and Neck Surgery, University of Nebraska Medical Center; Nebraska Methodist Hospital, Estabrook Cancer Center, Omaha, Nebraska

TIMOTHY L. SMITH, MD, MPH, FACS
Professor, Department of Otolaryngology – Head and Neck Surgery, Oregon Sinus Center, Oregon Health and Science University, Portland, Oregon

CARL H. SNYDERMAN, MD, MBA
Professor, Departments of Otolaryngology and Neurological Surgery, University of Pittsburgh School of Medicine; Co-Director, UPMC Center for Cranial Base Surgery, Pittsburgh, Pennsylvania

ANDREW TASSLER, MD
Assistant Professor, Department of Otorhinolaryngology – Head and Neck Surgery, Montefiore Medical Center, Bronx, New York

SAMUEL A. TISHERMAN, MD, FACS, FCCM
RA Cowley Shock Trauma Center, Professor of Surgery, University of Maryland School of Medicine, Baltimore, Maryland

DEAN M. TORIUMI, MD
University of Illinois at Chicago, Chicago, Illinois

ROWAN VALENTINE, MBBS, FRACS, PhD
Department of Surgery, Otorhinolaryngology, Head and Neck Surgery, The Queen Elizabeth Hospital, University of Adelaide, Adelaide, South Australia, Australia

LAURA VANDELAAR, MD
University of Texas at Houston, McGovern Medical School, Houston, Texas

HILLIARY N. WHITE, MD
Head and Neck Surgery Center of Florida, Celebration, Florida

PETER-JOHN WORMALD, MD
Department of Surgery, Otorhinolaryngology, Head and Neck Surgery, The Queen Elizabeth Hospital, University of Adelaide, Adelaide, South Australia, Australia

Contents

Hemostasis is essential during endoscopic sinus and skull base surgery. Patients must be adequately assessed for bleeding risk to appropriately consent to surgery. The patient and the surgeon must be aware of the individual bleeding risk for a given procedure. A thorough history and physical examination is the best screening methodology available to determine whether a patient requires further hematologic work-up. Included in this assessment should be any medications and herbals that the patient consumes. This ensures a safe evaluation of the patient, streamlines appropriate consultation and testing when necessary, and confers accurate surgical risk assessment.

Endoscopic sinus approach has become one of the most common surgical techniques for endoscopic sinus and skull base surgery. Anesthetic management has an important impact on the overall patient management, from the preoperative assessment and management to the quality of the surgical field and the postoperative recovery. Hemostasis is critical for adequate anatomical endoscopic visualization. Mild controlled hypotension seems to improve the visibility of the surgical field. Reduction of intraoperative bleeding should be considered during the treatment planning. Preoperative preparations include the optimization of comorbidities and cessation of drugs that may inhibit coagulation.

Given the risks and potential complications of allogenic blood transfusion (ABT), as well as the expanding population of patients for whom ABT may not be an option, it is important for the treating physician, anesthesiologist, and surgeon to be well-versed in various alternatives. A good grasp of the concepts discussed in this article will help to customize a treatment plan that is specific to each patient's underlying disease and personal preferences without compromising appropriate medical care.

Quality can be defined by processes of care and by the characteristics of the care and its outcomes. In terms of blood loss and transfusion, otolaryngologists should be aware of available guidelines, standards for use of blood products, devices and hemostatic agents, outcomes metrics relevant to patients, and tools for implementing quality improvements. This article reviews the definition of health care quality, and discusses the data regarding anticoagulant medications (particularly new oral anticoagulants) and guidelines for blood product transfusion. A brief outline of quality tools is provided to help otolaryngologists create quality plans for themselves and their institutions/systems.

Numerous absorbable substances have been introduced to aid hemostasis in sinus and skull base surgery. Within the confines of the sinus and nasal cavities, ideal hemostatic agents must have several qualities. They must provide hemostasis, conform to an irregular wound bed, and enable healing of the traumatized mucosa without additional detriment to the epithelium. Traditional nasal packing has been substituted largely by absorbable materials designed to improve patient comfort and outcomes. Although many promising agents exist, none have become standard therapy.

In facial plastic surgery, attaining hemostasis may require adjuncts to traditional surgical techniques. Fibrin tissue adhesives have broad applications in surgery and are particularly useful when addressing the soft tissue encountered in facial plastic surgery. Beyond hemostasis, tissue adhesion and enhanced wound healing are reported benefits associated with a decrease in operating time, necessity for drains and pressure dressings, and incidence of wound healing complications. These products are clinically accessible to most physicians who perform facial plastic surgery, including skin grafts, flaps, rhytidectomy, and endoscopic forehead lift.

Hemostasis is an important concept in pediatric otolaryngologic surgery. This article details the considerations the otolaryngologist should take when it comes to clinical evaluation and surgical technique. It begins with the preoperative evaluation, and evolves into the use of different mechanical and chemical methods of operative hemostasis. We detail use of different hemostatic techniques in common pediatric procedures, and finally, we discuss indications for intraoperative and postoperative blood transfusion in pediatric patients if the surgeon encounters significant intraoperative hemorrhage. This article gives a comprehensive look into the hemostatic considerations for the pediatric patient through the preoperative to postoperative period.

Tonsillectomy is a commonly performed procedure with an accepted risk of posttonsillectomy hemorrhage (PTH) approaching 5%, but catastrophic effects of hemorrhage are exceedingly rare. A variety of surgical techniques and hemostatic agents have been used to reduce the rate of hemorrhage, although none eliminate the risk. Numerous patient, surgical, and postoperative care factors have been studied for an association with PTH. The most consistent risk factors for PTH seem to be patient age and coagulopathies. Surgeon skill and surgical technique are most consistently associated with primary PTH.

Many patients with severe epistaxis benefit from endoscopic intervention for control of bleeding. Critical maneuvers to improve endoscopic visualization during surgery include head-of-bed elevation, application of topical vasoconstrictors, and local injection of vasonstrictors. Controlled, hypotensive anesthesia may also decrease intraoperative blood loss and improve visualization during surgery. Intractable posterior epistaxis can be controlled with high rates of success with endoscopic sphenopalatine artery ligation. Although less common, intractable anterior epistaxis may be controlled by anterior ethmoid artery ligation once this artery is identified as the primary source. Less common sources of severe epistaxis are also discussed in this article.

 Video content accompanies this article at http://www.oto.theclinics.com

Hereditary hemorrhagic telangiectasia (HHT) is an autosomal dominant disease with an incidence of 1:5000. Recurrent, spontaneous epistaxis is the most common presenting symptom. Severity of epistaxis varies widely, from mild, self-limited nosebleeds to severe, life-threatening nasal hemorrhage. Treatment of HHT-related epistaxis presents a challenge to the otolaryngologist due to the recurrent, persistent nature of epistaxis often requiring multiple treatments. Treatment modalities range from conservative topical therapies to more aggressive surgical treatments.

Intraoperative bleeding during endoscopic sinus surgery poses an additional dimension to an already technically challenging surgical approach because of the narrow sinonasal surgical field, single working hand, and the use of endoscopic instruments. Poor visualization is one of the most important factors that increase the risk of intraoperative complications such as inadvertent injury to major vessels and nerves, and incomplete surgery. This article provides a logical approach to improving the surgical field, minimizing risk of inadvertent vascular injury, and managing intraoperative bleeding.

Having absolute hemostasis is crucial in skull base surgery, because bleeding decreases visualization and increases the risk of postoperative complications. Achieving hemostasis starts from the preoperative evaluation. A thorough clinical history and routine tests guide the surgeon to minimize bleeding risk preoperatively, and comprehensive study of preoperative images helps the surgeon to predict bleeding risk and to consider preoperative embolization in suitable cases. Many hemostatic agents are available to control intraoperative bleeding; understanding of their indications and properties is crucial to achieve hemostasis. Whether endoscopic or transcranial approach, microsurgical techniques to avoid and control bleeding are the same.

Surgical bleeding is an unlikely, but potentially devastating, event during the surgical management of pediatric and adult laryngotracheal disorders. Therefore, an intimate knowledge of the anatomy of the large vessels coursing in the vicinity of the airway is imperative. Anatomic variants in the position of the inominate artery or the superior thyroid artery can place individuals with these variations at particular risk in these cases. Delayed bleeding from an inominate artery fistula is a particularly devastating complication from open airway surgery. A high index of suspicion is necessary to allow for early identification and aggressive treatment of this potential complication.

The larynx is a highly vascularized organ supplied by the superior and inferior laryngeal arteries. Both microphonosurgery and external laryngeal surgery require excellent hemostasis. Topical agents including adrenalin and fibrin-based products as well as surgical instrumentation, such as coagulation devices or in some cases embolization, are in the surgeon's armamentarium and facilitate efficient and successful surgery.

Surgery with transoral robotic surgery (TORS) offers significant advantages compared with traditional open surgical approaches and potentially minimizes the long-term side effects of organ preservation therapy with chemoradiation. Angled telescopes and wristed instruments allow visualization and access to areas of the pharynx that are difficult to reach with line-of-sight instrumentation. Although the application of TORS in head and neck surgery has expanded considerably, there are still only limited data available on the postoperative complications and their management.

As further data become available, it is likely that further risk factors and treatment strategies will become available.

Total thyroidectomy has significantly changed over the years from a morbid procedure to one that is performed routinely on an outpatient basis. This article reviews the history of thyroid surgery with regard to hemostasis, discusses surgical vascular anatomy, and describes the methods of hemostasis. It compares traditional hemostatic surgical techniques with newer techniques such as the Harmonic Scalpel and LigaSure hand pieces. The use of adjunctive hemostatic agents and indications for a drain in thyroid are discussed.

Hemostasis is a critical component of otologic and neurotologic surgery. In these surgeries the surgical field is small; thus, even a small amount of bleeding can obstruct the view of critical and extremely small structures. Additionally, relatively large vascular structures traverse the area; if they are encroached on by trauma or disease, bleeding must be controlled within a very small space in a meticulous fashion that does not encroach on structures of the middle ear and mastoid. The authors discuss several hemostatic agents in the middle ear, mastoid, and lateral skull base, highlighting their origins, mechanisms, advantages, and complications.

This article highlights the major vascular supply of the orbit and structures supplied by these vessels. Key anatomic principles are then reviewed as they pertain to endoscopic orbital surgery in order to avoid serious orbital hemorrhages. Next, preoperative planning and patient education are outlined as well as description of orbital compartment syndrome. This is followed by discussion of various techniques for managing orbital hemorrhage in the intraoperative and postoperative setting.

The most common vascular tumors encountered by the otolaryngologist are rare chromaffin cell tumors termed paragangliomas. Within the head and neck region, they commonly arise from the carotid body, vagus nerve (glomus vagale), and jugular vein (glomus jugulare). Other vascular head and neck tumors include sinonasal malignancies, because of proximity to or involvement of the pterygoid plexus as well as the rich vascularity of the sinonasal mucosa; juvenile nasopharyngeal angiofibroma, a

diagnostic and therapeutic angiography can manage most of these patients in a safe and effective manner. Surgery has a limited role in acute management, although surgical techniques are useful both for prevention of this problem and for wound management after carotid blowout.

OTOLARYNGOLOGIC CLINICS
OF NORTH AMERICA

RELATED INTEREST

Hematology/Oncology Clinics of North America
December 2015 (Vol. 29, Issue 6)
Head and Neck Cancer
A. Dimitrios Colevas, *Editor*
Available at: http://www.hemonc.theclinics.com/

THE CLINICS ARE AVAILABLE ONLINE!
Access your subscription at:
www.theclinics.com

Preface

Hemostasis in Otolaryngology— Head and Neck Surgery

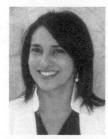 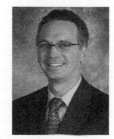

Harshita Pant, BMBS, PhD   Carl H. Snyderman, MD, MBA
Editors

The only weapon with which the unconscious patient can immediately retaliate upon the incompetent surgeon is haemorrhage.
> —*William Stewart Halstead, 1852-1922*

This issue of *Otolaryngologic Clinics of North America* addresses a matter of importance for every surgeon with every surgical encounter. In some circumstances, intraoperative hemorrhage is a life-threatening situation. In most cases, poorly controlled hemorrhage is a nuisance that slows the surgery and makes operating more difficult. Intraoperative bleeding impedes visualization and obscures normal anatomical landmarks. Poor visualization due to bleeding is probably the number one factor for avoidable complications such as injury of a nerve or major vessel. There is additional avoidable morbidity associated with perioperative anemia and hypovolemia, and their treatment. The hidden economic costs of operative bleeding are the management of complications, incomplete surgery, administration of blood products, decreased operative inefficiency, lost productivity of patients and families, and medicolegal issues.

The management of operative bleeding begins with prevention. Recognition of risk factors and stratification of patients into risk categories can help avoid many problems. With the increased use of long-acting irreversible antiplatelet drugs and other anticoagulants, patients are at greater risk for a bleeding complication. Common use of nonprescription drugs and herbal products contributes to the risk.

All of these topics are tackled in this issue of *Otolaryngologic Clinics of North America*, which starts with preoperative screening and preparation of patients and continues with discussions of hemostatic materials and techniques with specific recommendations for all types of otolaryngologic procedures and high-risk patient

Otolaryngol Clin N Am 49 (2016) xix–xx
http://dx.doi.org/10.1016/j.otc.2016.03.013
0030-6665/16/$ – see front matter © 2016 Published by Elsevier Inc.
oto.theclinics.com

populations. The authors are acknowledged experts in their areas and bring a global perspective to this topic. We hope that this issue of *Otolaryngologic Clinics of North America* will become an indispensable resource for you as you wage the battle against bleeding.

Harshita Pant, BMBS, PhD
Department of Otolaryngology
Head and Neck Surgery
The University of Adelaide
School of Medicine
Eleanor Harrald Building, Frome Road
Adelaide, South Australia 5005
Australia

Carl H. Snyderman, MD, MBA
Department of Otolaryngology
University of Pittsburgh Medical Center
200 Lothrop Street
Eye & Ear Institute, Suite 500
Pittsburgh, PA 15213, USA

E-mail addresses:
harshita.pant@adelaide.edu.au (H. Pant)
snydermanch@upmc.edu (C.H. Snyderman)

Preoperative Assessment of Risk Factors

Andrew Tassler, MD*, Rachel Kaye, MD

KEYWORDS

- Preoperative assessment • Coagulation disorders • High-risk populations
- Bleeding risk • Anticoagulants • Herbal medication

KEY LEARNING POINTS

At the end of this article, the reader will:

- Be able to identify patients who are in the high-risk category for bleeding during surgery.
- Be able to ask relevant questions to delineate a significant history of hemostatic deficits.
- Be able to recognize the common coagulation disorders.
- Be familiar with pertinent anticoagulant medications and their perioperative management.
- Be familiar with herbal medicines that confer bleeding risk.
- Be able to describe diagnostic tests for coagulation disorders.
- Be able to determine when a referral to a hematologist is required.

INTRODUCTION

Hemostasis is essential during endoscopic sinus and skull base surgery. Patients must be adequately assessed for bleeding risk to appropriately consent to surgery. The patient and the surgeon must be aware of the individual bleeding risk for a given procedure. A thorough history and physical examination is the best screening methodology available to determine whether a patient requires further hematologic work-up. Included in this assessment should be any medications and herbals that the patient consumes. This ensures a safe evaluation of the patient, streamlines appropriate consultation and testing when necessary, and confers accurate surgical risk assessment.

Disclosures: The authors have nothing to disclose.
Department of Otorhinolaryngology–Head and Neck Surgery, Montefiore Medical Center, Medical Arts Pavilion, 3400 Bainbridge Ave, 3rd Floor, Bronx, NY 10467, USA
* Corresponding author.
E-mail address: atassler@montefiore.org

Otolaryngol Clin N Am 49 (2016) 517–529
http://dx.doi.org/10.1016/j.otc.2016.01.002

DISCUSSION

What are the risk factors for perioperative bleeding?
• Hereditary bleeding tendency
• Personal or family history of predisposition to bleeding
• Abnormal coagulation testing results
• Coexisting medical conditions
• Medication use (including herbal)
• Need for antithrombotic therapy in the perioperative period

Patients at risk for bleeding during the perioperative period include those with a hereditary disorder, especially with a suggestive family history. Abnormal coagulation results can sometimes indicate an underlying hemostatic disorder, but the prevalence of inherited coagulopathies is low. Furthermore, some patients with inherited coagulopathies require specific testing to diagnose and have normal results on routine screening with prothrombin time, international normalized ratio, and partial thromboplastin time. Concomitant medical conditions, such as hepatic or renal dysfunction, medications, and herbal medications, significantly influence a patient's hemostatic tendencies. It is pertinent to determine whether patients are at increased bleeding risk before surgery to obtain the best possible outcomes (**Fig. 1**).

Hereditary bleeding tendency
• Adequate history
• Important to diagnose because
○ Appropriate precautions can be taken
○ Risk assessment can be outlined to patient
○ If hereditary disorder found, other family members can be screened (ie, hemophilia A)

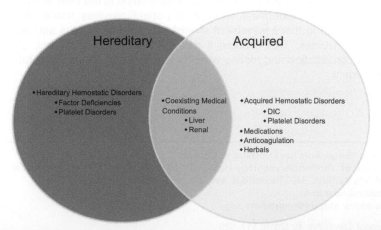

Fig. 1. Hereditary and acquired bleeding disorders. Hepatic and renal dysfunction can constitute either hereditary or acquired disorders. DIC, disseminated intravascular coagulation.

The most effective means of screening patients for potential surgical hemorrhage is an adequate and thorough patient history. Laboratory testing should not be used in lieu of a patient history because inconclusive testing results are common. The importance of diagnosing a hereditary bleeding disorder is of obvious importance for the patient, but also has potential impact on family members in the future.

Notable hereditary bleeding disorders

- Most common
  - Hemophilia A (factor VIII deficiency)
  - Hemophilia B (factor IX deficiency)
  - von Willebrand disorder (vWD)
    - Mild (prevalence is 0.8%–1.6%[1])
    - Overall prevalence is 1%

- Less common
  - Factor I
  - Factor II
  - Factor V
  - Factor X
  - Factor XI
  - Factor XII
  - Platelet disorders

- Rare
  - α_2-Antiplasmin deficiency
  - α_1-Antitrypsin Pittsburgh deficiency
  - Combined factor deficiencies

Notable and common factor/hereditary bleeding disorders include hemophilia A and B and vWD. Hemophilia A stems from a deficiency of factor VIII, which itself is activated by thrombin to become a cofactor for the synthesis of activated factor Xa, a major mediator of the common pathway. Hemophilia B is explained by a deficiency in factor IX, the activated form of which is also a cofactor in the production of activated factor Xa. vWD is the most prevalent coagulation disorder, where there is a deficiency in von Willebrand factor (vWF). vWF is important in platelet adhesion to the subendothelium and binding factor VIII. Consequently, the half-life of factor VIII is significantly shortened without vWF.

The extremely rare disorders listed have all been case reports with approximately 50 cases/families reported for all three deficiencies. **Fig. 2** shows the coagulation cascade with appropriate markings highlighting the physiology of hemophilia A, hemophilia B, and vWD.

Why obtain laboratory tests at all?

- Unreliable historian: patient does not recognize bleeding disorder
- Patient not exposed to significant bleeding risk, such as trauma, surgery, or dental extractions (ie, factor XI deficiency)
- Acquired hemostatic defects (ie, thrombocytopenia)

Laboratory tests for hemostasis are advisable if patients are undergoing high-risk surgery, even when adequate history is obtained that does not suggest a bleeding problem. A patient at risk for perioperative bleeding could still be detected on the basis of laboratory screening tests because the patient may not yet have been exposed to

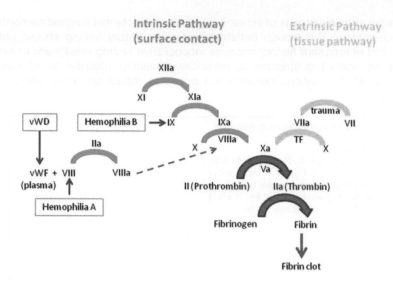

Fig. 2. Coagulation cascade with hemophilia A, hemophilia B, and von Willebrand disease. The intrinsic pathway is shown in green, the extrinsic pathway is highlighted in yellow, the common pathway is highlighted in blue. All factors are listed as roman numerals with the active form of the factor indicated by the suffix "a". vWD, von Willebrand disease; vWF, von Willebrand factor; TF, tissue factor.

surgical tests of hemostasis, such as dental extractions and trauma. In fact, factor XI deficiency results in significant bleeding only after major trauma or surgery. Furthermore, the patient could have acquired a hemostatic defect later in life that has been asymptomatic up until the point of consult.

Suggested questions to screen for a potential bleeding risk

- Have you ever bled for a long time? Specifically, have you had profuse menstrual bleeding, blood in the stool, or bleeding into a muscle or a joint?
- Have you had either immediate or delayed significant bleeding following a dental extraction?
- Do any of your immediate family members have a problem with unusual bruising or bleeding after surgery?
- Do you bruise without an inciting event?
- What operations/procedures have you undergone (including minor procedures, such as biopsies or endoscopies)? Have you ever developed significant bleeding or bruising afterward? Did you require blood transfusions?
- What pain medications do you take? Do you take over-the-counter supplements or herbal remedies?

This is a concise list of questions to screen patients for potential hemostatic bleeding disorders. This aims to be a supplement to a full interview consisting of past medical history, past surgical history, medications, and allergies. Asking specifically about patients and family members' reactions to surgery and dental extractions may help elucidate abnormal bleeding that the patient themselves does not recognize. Asking about bruising without an inciting event may help to identify patients with an acquired disorder or one that was previously undiagnosed. From the answers to these questions the surgeon can develop levels of increasing concern for surgical hemostatic risk and several risk categories have been described in the past.[2] A proposed stratification of surgical hemostatic risk is shown in **Table 1**.

Physical examination findings
• Petechiae
• Ecchymosis
• Telangiectasias
• Stigmata of prior hemarthroses (joint deformities)
• Hematomas
• Stigmata of Ehlers-Danlos syndrome: skin hyperelasticity and hyperextendable joints
• Stigmata of vitamin C deficiency: bleeding gums, poor wound healing
• Stigmata of Cushing syndrome: skin atrophy, striae, hyperpigmentation

Table 1
Surgical hemostatic risk classification

Significant Bleeding History	Prior Exposure to Hemostatic Risk	Major Surgery/Surgical Bleeding Risk	Concern Level	Suggested Testing
None	Yes	No	Minimal	None
None	None	No	Mild	None
None	None	Yes	Mild-moderate	Coagulation test (PTT/PT/INR)
Suspected but unclear	Yes or No	Yes or No	Moderate	Initial testing (platelet count, bleeding time, coagulation tests) vs hematology consultation
Yes	Yes or No	No	Moderate-severe	Initial testing (platelet count, bleeding time, coagulation) and hematology consultation counseling
Yes	Yes or No	Yes	Severe	As above with intensive counseling

Abbreviations: INR, international normalized ratio; PT, prothrombin time; PTT, partial thromboplastin time.

Several disorders are suggested based on physical examination, which mostly focuses on skin abnormalities, including petechiae, ecchymosis, telangiectasias, and hematomas. Petechiae and ecchymosis are suggestive of platelet dysfunction. Telangiectasias can either represent underlying liver dysfunction or a patient with hereditary hemorrhagic telangiectasia. Prior hemarthroses (joint deformities) can suggest severe factor deficiency. Hematomas can be secondary to factor deficiencies or clotting factor inhibitors (**Fig. 3**).

Selected laboratory testing for bleeding diathesis
• Prothrombin time (PT)/international normalized ratio
• Partial thromboplastin time (PTT)
• Bleeding time
• Platelet count
• Peripheral smear
• Thrombin time
• Factor deficiencies and inhibitors
• Fibrinogen

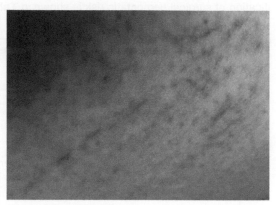

Fig. 3. Telangiectasias.

Originally, PT/international normalized ratio/PTT were used as a screening tool and routine laboratory testing for all patients undergoing surgery. However, based on retrospective reviews, these laboratory studies are now not recommended if physical examination and patient history are not suggestive of a bleeding disorder.[3] Bleeding time is a good screening tool for a bleeding diathesis, but not as a predictor of surgical bleeding. A peripheral smear is especially important when patients are diagnosed with thrombocytopenia to exclude a pseudothrombocytopenia caused by platelet agglutination. Furthermore, a blood smear allows for quantitative and qualitative platelet analysis. Further explanations of common screening tests are shown in **Table 2**.

Common medication classes affecting hemostasis
• Vitamin K antagonist (VKA)

• Antithrombus medication
  ◦ Unfractionated heparin (UFH)
  ◦ Low-molecular-weight heparin (LMWH)
  ◦ Direct thrombin inhibitors (DTIs)

• Antiplatelet medications
  ◦ Nonsteroidal anti-inflammatory drugs
  ◦ Cilostazol
  ◦ Thienopyridines
  ◦ Integrin/glycoprotein IIb/IIIa antagonists

Table 2
Common screening markers

Screening Test	Tested Pathway	Decreased Levels Effects	Dysfunctional Product Effects
Activated partial thromboplastin time	Intrinsic and common pathways	Deficiency of factor I, II, V, VIII, IX, X	vWD, certain lupus anticoagulants
PT	Extrinsic pathway	Factor VII, X, II, V, or fibrinogen deficiency	Vitamin K deficiency, liver disease, DIC, antiphospholipid antibodies, polycythemia (artificially prolongs PT)
Bleeding time	Platelet function (poor predictive value for significant operative bleeding)	Thrombocytopenia	vWD, Glanzmann thrombasthenia, DIC, liver failure, uremia, Bernard-Soulier syndrome
Thrombin clotting time	Abnormalities in the conversion of fibrinogen to fibrin	Rare congenital hypofibrinogemia (hepatic storage disease)	Anticoagulants, presence of fibrin/fibrinogen degredation products
Fibrinogen	Fibrin clot formation	Acquired disorders (DIC)	Rare, but can occur in hepatic or autoimmune disease

Abbreviation: DIC, disseminated intravascular coagulation.

Nonsteroidal anti-inflammatory drugs should be stopped before surgery. The remainder of common medications affecting hemostasis are anticoagulants and their effects range widely. Their effects and half-lives vary and must be discontinued or bridged appropriately as determined by the patient's primary physician, cardiologist, anesthesiologist, and surgeon. Bridging therapy is recommended in patients at moderate to high risk of thromboembolism, whereas it can be held in those patients at low risk. Risk determination is best elucidated by thrombophilia experts.[4] A summary of current bridging and antidote recommendations[5] is outlined in **Table 3**.

Common anticoagulants acting on the coagulation cascade

- VKA
  - Warfarin (Coumadin)
  - Acenocoumarol (Sintrom)
  - Phenprocoumon (Marcoumar)
- Antithrombus
  - UFH
  - LMWH
    - Dalteparin (Fragmin)
    - Enoxaparin (Lovenox)
    - Fondaparinux (Arixtra)
  - Direct factor Xa inhibitor
    - Rivaroxaban (Xarelto)
  - DTIs
    - Lepirudin (Refludan)
    - Bivalirudin (Angiomax)
    - Argatroban (Argatroban)
    - Dabigatran (Pradaxa)

Table 3
Common anticoagulants, bridging techniques, and antidotes

Anticoagulant Type	Name	Discontinuation Timeline	How to Bridge	Antidote
Vitamin K antagonist	Warfarin	5 d	Subcutaneous LMWH or intravenous UFH	Vitamin K reversal, may need FFP, PCC, or recombinant factor VIIA
Antiantithrombin III	UFH (bridging)	4–6 h	N/A	Protamine sulfate
Anti-factor Xa	LMWH (enoxaparin, dalteparin)	24 h	UFH	Protamine sulfate
	Apixaban, rivaroxaban	1 d (2 d if high bleeding risk)	UFH	None
Direct thrombin inhibitor	Argatroban, dabigatran	1–2 d (2–4 d if high bleeding risk)	UFH	None
Antiplatelet	ASA	7–10 d (if low cardiac risk)	Glycoprotein IIb/IIIa inhibitor	dDAVP and platelet transfusion
	Cilostazol	1–2 d	Glycoprotein IIb/IIIa inhibitor	dDAVP and platelet transfusion
	Clopidogrel (Plavix)	7–10 d (if low cardiac risk)	Glycoprotein IIb/IIIa inhibitor	dDAVP and platelet transfusion
	Dipyridamole (Persantine)	1–2 d	Glycoprotein IIb/IIIa inhibitor	dDAVP and platelet transfusion
	Prasugrel (Effient)	5–7 d	Glycoprotein IIb/IIIa inhibitor	dDAVP and platelet transfusion
NSAIDs	Celecoxib, diclofenac, ibuprofen, indomethacin, ketorolac, meloxicam, naproxen, sulindac	7 d	N/A	Unlikely, but if needed could use dDAVP and/or platelet transfusion

Abbreviations: ASA, aspirin; dDAVP, desmopressin; FFP, fresh frozen plasma; N/A, not applicable; NSAID, nonsteroidal anti-inflammatory drugs; PCC, prothrombin complex concentrate.

VKAs interfere with the conversion of vitamin K and inhibit proteins C, S, and Z. Consequently, VKA can also have procoagulant properties. Vitamin K is important in synthesizing mature factors II, VII, IX, and X. An antidote exists for VKA with prothrombin complex concentrates or recombinant factor VIIa and vitamin K. Several VKAs exist in the United States, but the most common in use is warfarin.

Heparins and DTIs are antithrombus medications. UFH binds to lysine residues on antithrombin that converts it to a rapid inhibitor. Antithrombin in turn inactivates factors IIa, IXa, Xa, and XIa. In contrast, LMWH is derived from UFH by depolymerization. It has a reduced ability to inactivate thrombin but is extremely capable of promoting factor Xa inactivation by antithrombin. The pentasaccharide sequence on LMWH interacts with antithrombin. Dalteparin and enoxaparin do undergo partial neutralization by protamine; however, fondaparinux does not. Instead, recombinant factor VIIa is proposed as an antidote for this particular medication.

DTIs are superior in inhibiting clot-bound thrombin; however, no antidote currently exists. In fact, only dialysis can be used to clear these medications or reverse the effects. Lepirudin is hiruden-based, whereas bivalirudin, argatroban, and dabigatran are all chemically derived from hiruden. **Fig. 4** shows these anticoagulants and their effect on the coagulation cascade.

Common antiplatelet anticoagulants

- Dipyridamole (Persantine or Aggrenox)

- Cilostazol (Pletal)

- Aspirin

- Thienopyridines
  - Ticlopidine (Ticlid)
  - Clopidogrel (Plavix)
  - Prasugrel (Effient)
  - Ticagrelor (Brilique)

- Integrin/glycoprotein IIb/IIIa antagonists
  - Abciximab (ReoPro)
  - Eptifibatide (Integrilin)
  - Tirofiban (Aggrastat)

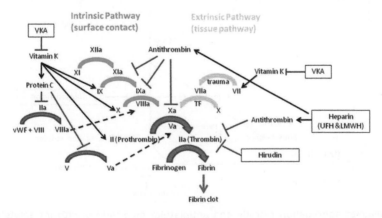

Common Pathway

Fig. 4. Coagulation cascade and common anticoagulants. The intrinsic pathway is shown in green, the extrinsic pathway in yellow, and the common pathway in blue. LMWH, low-molecular-weight heparin; UFH, unfractionated heparin; VKA, vitamin K antagonists.

Common antiplatelet medications include dipyridamole and cilostazol, which both increase intracellular cyclic adenosine monophosphate, which in turn inhibits platelet aggregation via increased protein kinase A. Aspirin is well-known to cause a permanent inhibition of the cyclooxygenase activity of prostaglandin H synthase. Conversely, thienopyridines selectively inhibit adenosine diphosphate–induced platelet aggregation without a direct effect on the arachidonic acid/cyclooxygenase pathway. Glycoprotein antagonists are novel in their inhibition of the final common pathway of platelet aggregation. Abciximab is a murine monoclonal antibody that blocks the glycoprotein IIb/IIIa receptor, whereas Eptifibatide is a synthetic heptapeptide patterned after snake venom. These antiplatelet medications and their interaction with platelet aggregation are shown in **Fig. 5**.

Herbal medicines

- Known bleeding risk
  - Garlic
  - Ginkgo biloba
  - Ginseng
  - Ginger
  - Feverfew

- Possible bleeding risk
  - Fish oil
  - Dong quai
  - Omega-3
  - Vitamin E
  - Chondroitin
  - Saw palmetto
  - Bromelain

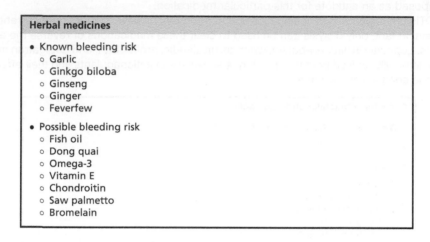

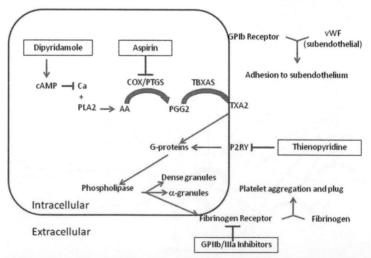

Fig. 5. Platelet aggregation cascade and antiplatelet medications with intraplatelet and extracellular reactions shown. COX/PTGS, cyclooxyenase; GP IIb/IIIa inhibitor, glycoprotein IIb/IIIa inhibitors; P2RY, P2Y receptor; PGG2, prostaglandin G$_2$; PLA2, phospholipase A$_2$; TBXAS, thromboxane synthase; TXA2, thromboxane A$_2$.

Table 4
Common herbal medications with recommended discontinuation timeline

Herbal	Hemostatic Effect	Recommended Discontinuation
Garlic	Inhibits platelet aggregation, possible irreversible antiplatelet activity	1 wk
Ginger	Antiplatelet activity	1 wk
Ginkgo biloba	Inhibition of platelet-activating factor	36 h
Ginseng	Inhibits platelet aggregation, possible irreversible antiplatelet activity	1 wk

Herbal medication use is prevalent in the population and knowledge of known side effects is important to the surgeon in properly counseling the patient. Garlic has been associated with postoperative bleeding in case reports by irreversibly inhibiting platelet function for 7 days (via its constituent, ajoene) in a dose-dependent fashion, and garlic extracts can reduce platelet adhesion to fibrinogen by 30%.[6] Ginkgolides (found in Ginkgo biloba) inhibit platelet activating factor and thus have antiplatelet properties causing several case reports of spontaneous and surgical bleeding. Ginkgo terpenoids have an elimination half-life between 3 and 10 hours, and so it is advised to discontinue at least 36 hour before surgery.[7] Ginger inhibits thromboxane synthetase activity in vitro, and is thus purported to impair platelet function, although in vivo studies have not shown a significant effect.[8] Ginsenosides (ginseng constituents) inhibit in vitro platelet aggregation while causing coagulation testing abnormalities (prolonged coagulation time and activated PTT) in rats. Furthermore, the constituent panaxynol may have irreversible antiplatelet activity. Because the elimination half-life is between 1 and 7 hours, ginseng should be discontinued at least 24 hours before surgery. However, given the potential irreversible platelet inhibition many recommend discontinuing ginseng at least 1 week before surgery.[7] Feverfew may potentiate platelet inhibitors although its significance is unclear. Dong Quai contains coumarins that can possibly cause hemorrhagic complications (especially potentiating warfarin), but no perioperative bleeding risk has been described as of yet. Omega-3 fatty acids have potential antiplatelet effects and increased activation of protein S. **Table 4** summarizes some of the discontinuation timelines as discussed previously.

SUMMARY

An accurate preoperative assessment of patients with potential hemostatic risk is imperative to the surgeon for patient safety and optimal surgical outcome. An awareness of common coagulation disorders is important in perioperative management. Finally, familiarity with anticoagulants and understanding appropriate bridging techniques and antidotes is vital information for surgeons. Herbal supplement use in society is increasing, and likewise, should not be overlooked because they can have a significant impact on perioperative hemostasis.

Post-Test Questions (Correct answers are in italics)

1. In which of the following scenarios is coagulation testing required? (Select all that apply)
   a. 18 year old with no past surgical history who is to undergo dental extraction
   b. *40 year old with no past surgical history who is to undergo a maxillectomy*
   c. 40 year old with prior uncomplicated skin biopsies who is to undergo direct laryngoscopy with biopsy
   d. *25 year old scheduled to undergo tonsillectomy that is found on examination to have two moderate-sized hematomas on his upper extremity and one on his trunk*
2. Which of the following is false about tests for hemostasis?
   a. Activated PTT tests the intrinsic pathway, whereas PT tests the extrinsic pathway
   b. Polycythemia can artificially prolong PT results
   c. *Bleeding time is an excellent predictor of significant operative bleeding*
   d. Thrombin clotting time tests for abnormalities in the conversion of fibrinogen to fibrin
3. Which of the following is true about antidotes?
   a. Protamine sulfate can be used as an antidote for UFH but not for LMWH
   b. *There is no antidote for DTIs*
   c. dDAVP is used as the antidote for direct factor Xa inhibitors, such as rivaroxaban.
4. A patient presents to your outpatient office for necessary ambulatory surgery. He has a history of severe coronary artery disease and is on Clopidogrel. What can be used to bridge him in preparation for his ambulatory surgery?
   a. Subcutaneous low molecular weight heparin
   b. Ultrafractionated heparin
   c. *Glycoprotein IIb/IIIa inhibitor*
   d. Protamine sulfate
5. Which of the following medications can be discontinued 36 hours before surgery rather than 1 week before surgery to minimize risk of surgical bleeding?
   a. Garlic
   b. Ginger
   c. *Ginkgo biloba*
   d. Ginseng

SUPPLEMENTARY DATA

Supplementary PDF slides related to this article can be found online at http://www.oto.theclinics.com/.

REFERENCES

1. Rodeghiero F, Castaman G, Dini E. Epidemiological investigation of the prevalence of von Willebrand disease. Blood 1987;69(2):454–9.

2. Rapaport SI. Preoperative hemostatic evaluation: which tests, if any? Blood 1983; 61(2):229–31.
3. Chee YL, Crawford JC, Watson HG, et al. Guidelines on the assessment of bleeding risk prior to surgery or invasive procedures. British Committee for Standards in Haematology. Br J Haematol 2008;140(5):496–504.
4. Horlocker TT, Wedel DJ, Rowlingson JC, et al. Regional anesthesia in the patient receiving antithrombotic or thrombolytic therapy: American Society of Regional Anesthesia and Pain Medicine Evidence-Based Guidelines (Third Edition). Reg Anesth Pain Med 2010;35(1):64–101.
5. Douketis JD, Berger PB, Dunn AS, et al. The perioperative management of antithrombotic therapy: American College of Chest Physicians Evidence-Based Clinical Practice Guidelines (8th Edition). Chest 2008;133(6 Suppl):299S–339S.
6. Fessenden JM, Wittenborn W, Clarke L. Gingko biloba: a case report of herbal medicine and bleeding postoperatively from a laparoscopic cholecystectomy. Am Surg 2001;67(1):33–5.
7. Ang-Lee MK, Moss J, Yuan CS. Herbal medicines and perioperative care. JAMA 2001;286(2):208–16.
8. Hodges PJ, Kam PC. The peri-operative implications of herbal medicines. Anaesthesia 2002;57(9):889–99.

SUGGESTED READINGS

Ang-Lee MK, Moss J, Yuan CS. Herbal medicines and perioperative care. JAMA 2001;286(2):208–16.

This article summarizes the practice guidelines for neuraxial anesthesia in patients receiving anticoagulation as determined by the American Society of Regional Anesthesia and Pain Medicine. It provides a good review of anticoagulation methods and physiology and risk factors for surgical bleeding.

Douketis JD, Berger PB, Dunn AS, et al. The perioperative management of antithrombotic therapy: American College of Chest Physicians Evidence-Based Clinical Practice Guidelines (8th Edition). Chest 2008;133(6 Suppl):299S–339S.

This article discusses the guidelines for perioperative management of antithrombotic therapy as determined by the American College of Chest Physicians. It primarily focuses on perioperative management of oral anticoagulants, bridging anticoagulation, and management of patients who have received anticoagulation and require urgent surgery.

Horlocker TT, Wedel DJ, Rowlingson JC, et al. Regional anesthesia in the patient receiving antithrombotic or thrombolytic therapy: American Society of Regional Anesthesia and Pain Medicine Evidence-Based Guidelines (Third Edition). Reg Anesth Pain Med 2010;35(1):64–101.

Using selected studies and case reports this article reviews eight common herbal medications and their safety profile. It also reviews the pharmacology of those herbal medications including (when indicated) associated bleeding risk.

Anesthetic Techniques in Endoscopic Sinus and Skull Base Surgery

Martha Cordoba Amorocho, MD[a,b,*], Iuliu Fat, MD[c]

KEYWORDS

- Anesthesia for endoscopic sinus and skull base surgery • Anesthetic techniques
- Anesthesia review • Endoscopic sinus surgery • Endoscopic skull base surgery
- Endoscopic surgery

KEY LEARNING POINTS

At the end of this article, the reader will:

- Understand specific areas of concern involved in preoperative evaluation for these surgeries.
- Become familiar the anesthetic goals for endoscopic sinus and skull base surgery.
- Understand the steps that can be performed preoperatively to prepare the patient for the surgery and to facilitate anesthesia and recovery.
- Recognize important considerations during and immediately after induction of anesthesia.
- Be able to discuss the effects of maintenance anesthesia techniques on blood loss and surgical field.
- Become familiar with some specific challenges during emergence of anesthesia for those surgeries.
- Describe some postoperative problems that can affect recovery after surgery and how to best treat them.

The authors have nothing to disclose.
[a] Department of Anesthesiology, Massachusetts Eye and Ear Infirmary, Harvard Medical School, 243 Charles Street, Boston, MA 02114, USA; [b] Department of Anesthesiology and Critical Care, Brigham and Women's Hospital, 75 Francis Street, Boston, MA 02115, USA; [c] Department of Anesthesiology, Harbor Hospital, 3001 South Hanover Street, Baltimore, MD 21225, USA
* Corresponding author. Department of Anesthesiology and Critical Care, Brigham and Women's Hospital, 75 Francis Street, Boston, MA 02115.
E-mail address: mcordoba-amorocho@partners.org

Otolaryngol Clin N Am 49 (2016) 531–547
http://dx.doi.org/10.1016/j.otc.2016.03.004
0030-6665/16/$ – see front matter © 2016 Elsevier Inc. All rights reserved.
oto.theclinics.com

INTRODUCTION
Role of the Anesthesiologist in Endoscopic Sinus and Skull Base Surgery

Role of anesthetist
• Preoperative assessment
• Perioperative management
• Anesthetic management
• Quality of the surgical field
• Postoperative recovery

Endoscopic approach to the sinuses has become one of the most common surgical techniques not just for sinus surgery but also for skull base surgery (**Table 1**). The anesthesiologist has a vital role in the overall management of the patient, from the preoperative assessment and management to the quality of the surgical field and the postoperative recovery. Most of the principles of anesthetic care discussed in this review come from studies done in endoscopic sinus surgery. Mild controlled hypotension, with remifentanil and either propofol or an inhaled anesthetic, can improve the visibility of the surgical field. However, if there is concern regarding intracranial pressure and cerebral perfusion, it would be more appropriate to manage the patient following the basic principles of neuroanesthesia. Some patients may be at increased risk for postoperative respiratory depression, given comorbidities such as obstructive sleep apnea (OSA), obesity, acromegaly, and nasal packing. Pain and control of postoperative nausea and vomiting (PONV) are crucial, and their management starts in the preoperative period.

PREOPERATIVE EVALUATION OF PITUITARY AND SKULL BASE SURGICAL PATIENTS

Specific areas of concern include
• Coexisting medical manifestations of operative disease
• Staged surgery
• Risk of excessive intraoperative blood loss and transfusion
• Risk of prolonged intubation
• Risk of perioperative respiratory depression
• Cardiovascular status

Endoscopic pituitary resection
• Evaluate neurologic deficits and endocrine function
• Adenomas secreting adrenocorticotrophic hormone (ACTH): obesity, hypertension, osteopenia, fluid retention, and hyperglycemia
• Growth hormone (GH) secreting adenomas: careful evaluation of the airway

Table 1	
Some indications for endoscopic sinus and skull base surgery	
Sinonasal surgery	Sinusitis, nasal polyposis, epistaxis, sinus mucoceles, tumors, turbinate reduction, septoplasty
Skull base surgery	CSF leak closure, pituitary surgery, encephaloceles/meningoceles, tumors
Orbital surgery	Orbital decompression, dacryocystorhinostomy, optic nerve decompression

ENDOSCOPIC SKULL BASE SURGERY

Patients undergoing endoscopic pituitary resection can present with manifestations of the disease for which they are having surgery. It is necessary to assess and document any neurologic deficits and to evaluate the endocrine function. Perioperative testing should include measurement of glucose and electrolytes. Prolactin-secreting adenomas are the most common lesions, but for the anesthesiologist, ACTH and GH are cause for greater concern.

GH excess causes acromegaly. Careful evaluation of the airway is important for these patients.[1] They can have an enlarged tongue causing difficult intubation, and cartilaginous hypertrophy of the arytenoids and narrowing of the tracheal rings require the use of small size endotracheal tubes (ETTs). ACTH excess causes Cushing disease, leading to obesity, hypertension, osteopenia, fluid retention, and hyperglycemia. Patients with pituitary hypofunction are usually receiving hormone replacement therapy that must be continued perioperatively.

For patients with vascular tumors, preoperative embolization of the tumor reduces bleeding and the need for transfusion as well as improves the visualization of intraoperative surgical field.

LOCAL VERSUS GENERAL ANESTHESIA IN SINUS AND SKULL BASE SURGERY

Advantages of local anesthesia

- Patient able to signal pain should minimize surgical complications
- Less blood loss with better surgical field has been described for local anesthesia
- Better recovery profile with fewer incidences of nausea and faster discharge

Advantages of general anesthesia

- Less anxiety and discomfort
- Total immobility should provide a better surgical field and minimize surgical complications
- Improved control of airway with increased safety for the patient
- Decreased fire risk

When endoscopic sinus surgery was introduced, patients were often operated totally under local anesthesia with combined sedation. However, surgical techniques have evolved, and many of the currently performed surgical procedures require general anesthesia. Surgery under local anesthesia alone is still considered appropriate for minor sinus procedures in selected patients.[2–4] However, presently, local anesthesia is used to complement general anesthesia.

Goals of anesthesia for endoscopic sinus and skull base surgery

- Provide a still and bloodless surgical field to minimize surgical complications
- Prevent cerebral ischemia
- Protect the patient's airway during and after surgery from contamination by blood and gastric fluid and from respiratory depression and obstruction
- Facilitate early recovery, by optimizing pain and nausea control

---

Increased risk of perioperative respiratory depression

- Acromegaly
- Moderate to severe OSA
- STOPBANG 5 or greater
- Body mass index (BMI) of 45 or greater

STOPBANG is an acronym for a series of questions that can be asked to patients to screen for OSA, which increases a patient's risk for postoperative respiratory depression. STOPBANG stands for: Snoring? Tired? Observed (observed apnea during sleep)? Pressure (high blood pressure)? BMI (>35 kg/m^2), Age (>50 years old), Neck circumference (>16 inches), Gender (male). If the patient answers "yes" to 5 to 8 of the questions, there is a high risk of having OSA.

There is an increased risk of respiratory complications during the perioperative period for patients undergoing endoscopic surgery. Patients should be routinely screened for OSA and obesity.[5] The severity of previously diagnosed OSA should be documented as well as the home use of continuous positive airway pressure (CPAP) devices. Patients without a formal diagnosis of OSA should be screened with instruments such as the STOPBANG scale,[6,7] and scores of 5 or more should be noted, because they correlate with a likelihood of moderate to severe OSA. Patient's height and weight should be documented and their BMI calculated, because obese patients are at higher risk for respiratory depression **(Table 2)**.

Table 2 Recommendations for patients at risk for perioperative respiratory depression	
Preoperative	Use nonopioid analgesics: acetaminophen, COX-2 inhibitors
Induction of anesthesia	Careful positioning and prolonged preoxygenation of obese patients; use muscle relaxants to facilitate intubation; availability of additional tools for intubation such as videoscopes; consider use of ETT over LMA
Maintenance of anesthesia	Consider use of desflurane, remifentanil, dexmedetomidine; try to avoid long-acting medications such as isoflurane, morphine, hydromorphone
Emergence of anesthesia	Verify complete reversal of muscle relaxation; consider awake extubation

> **Cardiovascular evaluation for endoscopic sinus and skull base surgery**
>
> - Formulate a perioperative plan for antiplatelet and anticoagulant therapy, in consultation with cardiologist and primary care physician
> - Evaluate patient's ability to tolerate local vasoconstrictors
> - Evaluate patient's ability to tolerate hypotension

Patients should be evaluated for a history of coronary artery disease (CAD) and arrhythmias. Cessation of anticoagulants and antiplatelet agents is ideal, but at the same time, the risks of stopping these medications must be considered. If the patient has CAD, has a history of cardiac stents, or is chronically on anticoagulants, care should be coordinated with the cardiologist and the primary care physician in order to prevent perioperative cardiac ischemia, pulmonary embolism, or ischemic strokes.

The ability to tolerate locally applied vasoconstrictors should be evaluated, because there is a risk of these medications producing cardiac arrhythmias or cardiac ischemia. However, if used appropriately, the risk is significantly reduced (see Pant H: Hemostasis in Endoscopic Sinus Surgery, in this issue). Relative hypotension with controlled heart rate provides a better surgical field for endoscopic surgery. A cardiovascular evaluation should also take into consideration the ability of the patient to tolerate mild hypotension. Acromegaly is associated with increased risk of cardiovascular disease ranging from cardiomyopathy to CAD and arrhythmias; proper evaluation of these potential complications should be made preoperatively.

> **Preoperative preparation**
>
> - Glucocorticosteroids (steroids)
> - Antibiotics
> - Topical vasoconstrictors and local anesthesia
> - Pain medications: acetaminophen and cyclooxygenase-2 (COX-2) selective inhibitors
> - Inhaled bronchodilators if indicated
> - Invasive monitoring, such as arterial line, if required
> - For cerebrospinal fluid (CSF) leak repair: intrathecal fluorescein injection; consider lumbar drain

Many patients undergoing endoscopic sinus and skull base surgery may be on steroids chronically. These patients do not routinely need a stress dose of steroids as long as they receive their usual daily maintenance steroid dose, orally preoperatively or the equivalent intravenous dose intraoperatively.

A short course of antibiotics is used preoperatively in some patients where indicated, to decrease inflammation and risk of infection. However, there is no good evidence for their routine use in prevention of infections or improving the surgical field. Most surgeons request one dose of intravenous antibiotics for infection prophylaxis before surgical incision.

Many patients undergoing sinus surgery have concomitant asthma; preoperative use of inhaled bronchodilators is indicated in these patients. Concerns exist about the probability of life-threatening bronchospasm with the triad of nonsteroidal anti-inflammatory drugs (NSAIDs), asthma, and nasal polyps.

Local vasoconstrictors and local anesthesia are typically applied topically and via mucosal injections to improve the surgical field by providing mucosal decongestion, and perioperative pain management. Longer-acting local anesthetics such as ropivacaine should be considered for their longer lasting benefit.

Pain management can start in the preoperative period. Acetaminophen and COX-2 inhibitors can improve pain management and reduce narcotic requirements.[8]

In patients undergoing skull base surgery, depending on the approach and the operative lesion, the anesthesiologist should be prepared to resuscitate the patient in the rare event of a vascular injury. The anesthesiologist may choose to have blood products readily available and to place additional monitors, such as an arterial line, depending on the patient and the surgical plan.

In some patients undergoing repair of a CSF leak, fluorescein administration through a lumbar spinal puncture may be needed. Anesthesiologists usually assist the surgeon by performing the procedure in the preoperative area under sterile technique. The fluorescein helps localize the site of the CSF leak during surgery. The surgeon may also request a lumbar drain to be placed to drain CSF in cases where increases in intracerebral pressure (ICP) are expected.

Induction of anesthesia

- Anxiolytics: midazolam, lorazepam
- Analgesics: fentanyl, remifentanil
- Hypnotics: inhaled anesthetics, propofol, etomidate
- Muscle relaxants: succinylcholine, nondepolarizing muscle relaxants (NMBDs)
- Other medications
  - Dexamethasone
  - Tranexemic acid

An anxiolytic medication such as midazolam may be administered in the preoperative area. Patients also benefit from opioids, like fentanyl or remifentanil, to reduce the sympathetic response to intubation. In children, anesthesia is usually induced by inhaled agents such as sevoflurane and nitrous oxide. In adults, anesthesia is usually induced by intravenous agents such as propofol or etomidate. Once the patient is unconscious, the airway is secured with either an ETT or laryngeal mask (LMA). If an ETT is placed, a muscle relaxant is often administered to facilitate the laryngoscopy.

Dexamethasone may be administered to reduce PONV. Antithrombolytic therapy, with tranexamic acid, has been used with success in endoscopic sinus surgery and craniofacial procedures and may be of benefit in endoscopic skull base surgeries in which extensive blood loss is anticipated. However, there are just a few studies, limited in size, with not enough data regarding complications associated with its use.[9]

Muscle relaxation

- Used to facilitate intubation
- Not needed if LMA used
- Measure neuromuscular function at the end of the case
- Reverse residual effect of muscle relaxant in all patients
- Need special consideration if cranial nerves are being monitored

In some patients, cranial nerves (III, IV, V, VI, XII) may be at risk for injury and are monitored intraoperatively. During these procedures, it is necessary to avoid paralysis, so that the cranial nerve may be periodically stimulated to verify its integrity. In other procedures, any patient movement carries the risk of injury, and it is recommended to discuss the use of muscle relaxants with the surgical team.

Whenever muscle relaxants are used, there is a risk of residual muscle relaxation at the end of the case that may lead to increased complications during emergence of anesthesia or in the recovery unit. Avoiding the use of muscle relaxants will eliminate the risk of residual paralysis. LMA is used without muscle relaxation. However, if an ETT is used to manage the airway, most anesthesiologists would use a muscle relaxant for intubation. The response of individual patients to muscle relaxants can be variable. It is recommended to measure neuromuscular function at the end of the surgery and to reverse the residual effect of NMBDs in all patients.[10] Reversal is accomplished by giving acetylcholinesterase inhibitors such as neostigmine and an anticholinergic agent such as glycopyrrolate.

ENDOTRACHEAL TUBE VERSUS LARYNGEAL MASK

The cuff of an ETT provides a seal around the trachea that protects the lower airways. The advantages of using an ETT are familiarity, ability to secure the airway for a prolonged period of time, protection of lower airways from contamination with blood, secretions, and gastric fluid, and ability to provide positive pressure ventilation at high pressures. However, the vocal cords and subglottis are located above the cuff of the ETT, and blood can still pass along the outer surface of the ETT and reach their level. Using an ETT has some disadvantages, compared with using an LMA, such as increased incidence of coughing, bucking, and desaturation during awake extubation (Table 3).

LMA can be adequate for endoscopic sinus surgery in carefully selected patients. It is counterintuitive, but LMA provides an equivalent protection from contamination of the lower airways and better protection of the glottis.[11] The LMA sits like an umbrella and protects the glottis. Incorrect placement, dislodgement during surgery, or suboptimal recovery, however, creates the potential for airway obstruction and contamination of the airways with blood, secretions, or gastric fluid. The advantages of using LMA are less stimulation of the trachea with decreased risk of bronchospasm, smoother emergence from anesthesia compared with awake extubation using an ETT,[12] ability to avoid muscle relaxant use, and decreased depth of anesthesia, with faster emergence after surgery.

Ultimately, the choice between an ETT and LMA for endoscopic sinus surgery depends on the level of comfort and experience of the anesthesiologist and surgeon, duration of the surgery, need of muscle relaxation, and patient factors, such as history of obesity, asthma, gastroesophageal reflux disease, and previous gastric surgery.

Table 3 Endotracheal tube versus laryngeal mask	
LMA advantages	Smoother emergence; faster recovery; avoidance of muscle relaxants; protection of glottis; less airway stimulation
ETT advantages	Secure airway for long surgery; ability to provide positive pressure ventilation at high pressures; proven protection of lower airways

There is not enough literature to guide the decision between LMA and ETT for endo-scopic skull base surgery. For these procedures, ETT is likely the best choice, because surgeries usually are long, and many of them may require muscle relaxation.

PREPARATION OF THE PATIENT FOR SURGERY

Preparation of the patient for surgery
• Elevate surgical field (reverse Trendelenburg position): risk of air embolism; blood pressure at the head lower than blood pressure measure at the level of the heart
• Patient's eyes should be accessible to the surgeon during the procedure
• Secure ETT or LMA in the midline
• Place stereotactic navigation system
• Use local anesthetics and vasoconstrictors

It is common for surgeons to elevate the head of the operating table by 10°, and some of them also put the table in mild reverse Trendelenburg position.[13] Patients are posi-tioned this way to allow venous decongestion of the head, by increasing blood pooling in the lower extremities. This position reduces blood loss and improves the operating conditions. However, every time that the surgical field is elevated, with relation to the position of the heart, there is an increased risk of air embolism. The overall low morbidity and mortality of endoscopic surgery seem to indicate that the risk of air em-bolism is low, but there are no studies measuring the specific risk of air embolism for these surgeries. Also, in the context of deliberate hypotension, it is important to remember that blood pressure measurements at the level of the heart do not reflect the real and lower values of the most elevated body parts, such as the brain.

After intubation, the ETT or the LMA is usually positioned midline and secured to the chin. The eyes are taped shut, but in a way that allows the surgeon to palpate and eval-uate them during the surgery, as a means to evaluate possible surgical complications. Before starting the surgery, for complex cases or for teaching purposes, a localizing headset is placed on the patient's forehead. A stereotactic navigation system allows the surgeon to map out the surgical field, using a previously obtained computed tomo-graphic or MRI scan.

Injected and topical local anesthetics combined with vasoconstrictors are applied to the nasal mucosa to decrease surgical stimulation, reduce mucosal congestion, decrease blood loss, and enhance surgical visibility. The surgeon may place pledgets soaked in vasoconstrictors drugs such as cocaine, epinephrine, oxymetazoline, or phenylephrine before starting the operation.[14] The nasal walls are also infiltrated before starting the case. Additional pledgets may be placed in the operative field dur-ing the procedure.

Systemic absorption of local anesthetics, cocaine, and vasoconstrictors occurs, so it is important to monitor patients carefully during the infiltration with these agents and during surgery. Cocaine has both vasoconstrictor and local anesthetic properties.

Local anesthetic systemic toxicity (LAST) can occur, if used in excessive doses or administered improperly, and the anesthesiologist should be prepared to manage this rare complication. Treatment of LAST includes getting additional help, making sure that the airway is secured, managing any seizure activity with benzodiazepines, using lipid emulsion therapy, and alerting the nearest facility having cardiopulmonary bypass capabilities.

Systemic absorption of cocaine and other vasoconstrictors can produce hemodynamic instability with hypertension, hypotension, and cardiac arrhythmias. These medications should be used with great caution, or avoided altogether, in patients with a history of CAD, congestive heart failure, arrhythmias, or poorly controlled hypertension and in those taking monoamine oxidase inhibitors. Appropriate patient selection and good communication between surgeon and anesthesiologist are imperative. The use of β-blocking agents to treat hypertension seems to be particularly dangerous. Most anesthesiologists try to allow blood pressure values to return to normal levels without treatment, and if needed, direct vasodilator agents or α-antagonists are preferred for treatment of vasoconstrictor-induced hypertension.

MAINTENANCE OF ANESTHESIA
Controlled Hypotension

Controlled hypotension is advocated in endoscopic sinus surgery mainly to improve surgical conditions (**Table 4**). Whether hypotension actually reduces blood loss for endoscopic sinus surgery is controversial.[15] It is important to keep in mind that blood loss in endoscopic sinus surgery is low and the need for transfusion is very rare. Also, hypotension carries the risk of increased morbidity and mortality because of ischemic organ failure. Taking all these factors into consideration, it seems reasonable to aim for a mild to moderate (15%–20%) reduction in blood pressure, avoiding any profound hypotension (mean arterial pressure, MAP, <60–65 mm Hg).

Remifentanil infusion, combined with propofol or an inhaled anesthetic, is the current preferred method to produce hemodynamic stability and hypotension.[16] The assumed mechanism is thought to be the result of bradycardia and a reduction in cardiac output.[17] It has the advantage of an extremely short context-sensitive half-life (the time required for the plasma drug concentration to decline by 50% after terminating an infusion), quick metabolism through sterum esterases, and fast postoperative recovery time.

Other medications have been tried, but not enough evidence could be found to support their use in endoscopic sinus surgery. β-Blocker drugs, such as esmolol or metoprolol, have proven to be effective, but their impact on morbidity and mortality is not clear.[18] When vasodilating agents such as sodium nitroprusside,[19] or nitroglycerin are used, only profound hypotension has been proven to be effective. Magnesium infusion is effective, but it has significant side effects, such as drowsiness and potentiation of muscle relaxants.[20] Clonidine seems to be effective, but it has a long duration of action. Dexmedetomidine is a medication that deserves future research, because it seems it could be at least as effective as remifentanil.[21]

Table 4 Controlled hypotension in endoscopic sinus and skull base surgery	
Risks	Severe hypotension (MAP <60–65 mm Hg) can cause ischemic organ failure
	If ICP is elevated, decreased blood pressure will compromise cerebral perfusion
Advantage	Improved surgical conditions
Remifentanil infusion	Short half-life, quick metabolism through sterum esterases, fast recovery time

The impact of controlled hypotension in endoscopic skull base surgery is not clear, and more studies are needed.[22] The authors recommend making a distinction between approaches that do not impact ICP, and any other approaches that have the potential to affect ICP, or that involve intradural contents or brain vasculature. Making this distinction requires communication between the surgeon and the anesthesiologist.

If there is any concern about increased ICP, or involvement of intradural contents or brain vasculature, the anesthesiologist should follow the principles of neuroanesthetic management. Hypotension would likely be contraindicated, and the blood pressure should be adjusted to ensure adequate cerebral perfusion. Direct vasodilating drugs (nitroglycerin, nitroprusside, hydralazine, calcium channel blockers) lower the blood pressure but cause an increase in cerebral blood flow and ICP, so use of these drugs should likely be avoided, if possible.

TOTAL INTRAVENOUS ANESTHESIA VERSUS INHALATIONAL ANESTHESIA

To achieve good surgical conditions, what is most pertinent: (1) to achieve controlled hypotension or (2) the anesthetic method used to achieve controlled hypotension?

In other words, in the presence of controlled hypotension, are there good data that indicates total intravenous anesthesia (TIVA) with propofol alone provides a better surgical field? The authors' understanding is that there are no data currently to answer this question, and studies suggesting these have low patient numbers and study groups are not comparable (systemic disease and sinus disease). In addition, there is no prospective comparison with combined anesthesia (such as Propofol/remifentanil), without other confounding factors (clonidine, metoprololol).

To reduce the incidence of surgical complications during endoscopic sinus surgery, it is important to have the best possible visualization with a surgical field as free of blood as possible. TIVA, a technique of general anesthesia using a combination of agents given solely by the intravenous route and in the absence of inhalational agents, based on propofol and remifentanil infusions, has been shown to provide the best operating conditions, making it the preferred anesthetic technique for many surgeons **(Table 5)**.[23] TIVA also has the potential to decrease coughing on emergence and PONV.

However, there are some challenges inherent to the use of TIVA for endoscopic sinus surgery. During endoscopic surgery, there is frequently a need to keep the patient deeply anesthetized until the last minutes of surgery, and given the context sensitive half-life of propofol, emergence can be delayed. Monitors of electroencephalographic activity, such as the bispectral index (BIS) monitor, although of controversial usefulness, are often used to indicate depth of anesthesia. However, if the BIS monitor is used, consideration must be given to the position of the localizing headset. Last, there are concerns regarding the cost of propofol and the recent shortage of this medication in the United States.

Table 5	
Total intravenous anesthesia versus inhalational anesthesia in endoscopic sinus surgery	
Agents of choice	Propofol and remifentanil
Advantages	Less blood loss, better surgical field, smoother emergence, less PONV
Disadvantages	Potential for delayed emergence, inability to use BIS monitors, propofol shortage, cost

Given these challenges, many anesthesiologists continue using a mixed technique, combining an inhalational agent, such as sevoflurane, with remifentanil. This technique can be considered acceptable,[24] unless there is severe sinus disease, wherein TIVA might reduce the blood loss and improve the surgical field.[25]

Regarding endoscopic skull base surgery, there is just not enough literature to make a recommendation regarding anesthetic technique of TIVA versus inhaled anesthesia. Volatile anesthetics are cerebral vasodilators and can increase ICP. However, low concentrations (<0.5 MAC) are mostly safe and are useful to reduce the hemodynamic response to the surgical stimulation, in combination with remifentanil.[26]

SPONTANEOUS VERSUS POSITIVE PRESSURE VENTILATION

- CO_2 has not been proven to influence surgery
- Remifentanil inhibits spontaneous ventilation

As during neuroanesthesia, manipulation of CO_2 has been suggested as another mechanism to decrease blood loss and to improve visibility during endoscopic surgery; however, this has not been proven effective.[27]

Remifentanil is currently a cornerstone of anesthetic care in endoscopic sinus surgery, combined either with propofol or with an inhalational agent. As remifentanil strongly inhibits spontaneous ventilation, the use of positive pressure ventilation becomes mandatory, through either an ETT or an LMA. To use an LMA for positive pressure ventilation, it is important to have a good seal and to keep the inspiratory pressure below 20 cm of water.

EMERGENCE OF ANESTHESIA

One of the anesthetic goals during endoscopic sinus and skull base surgery is to achieve a smooth emergence and to keep the patient's airway safe.

- Sphenopalatine ganglion block might help with pain control, but current data are not sufficient to recommend it as routine practice.[28]
- Remove throat packing.
- Suction and inspect throat and postnasal space.
- Perform awake or deep extubation.

At the end of the surgery, some surgeons may perform a sphenopalatine ganglion block, to provide postoperative pain relief. As preparation for emergence from anesthesia, it is imperative than any pharyngeal or throat packing is removed, and to carefully suction the oral cavity and postnasal space. Any clot left behind can lead to airway obstruction or even death. Extubation can be done, either in an awake patient or under deep anesthesia.

The advantage of awake extubation is the return of laryngeal reflexes with airway protection from further contamination from blood and secretions. The disadvantage is that awake extubation, while using an ETT, is associated with coughing, bucking, and laryngospasm with an increased risk of bleeding. LMA removal is usually performed once the patient is awake and is able to open the mouth on command. LMA removal, however, has a better profile than ETT, with decreased incidence of coughing, bucking, and laryngospasm.

The advantage of deep extubation is the belief that it can produce a smoother emergence than awake extubation. However, deep extubation leaves an unprotected airway. Deep extubation during endoscopic surgery has additional risks of the presence of nasal packing, further obstructing the airway at the nasal level, and the presence of blood and even clots in the airway. If deep extubation is performed, careful consideration should be given to patient selection, and patients at risk for postoperative respiratory depression, or patients with a difficult airway during induction, should likely not have a deep extubation (**Table 6**).

Table 6
Awake and deep extubation

Awake extubation	
Advantages	Return of laryngeal reflexes allowing lower airway protection; smooth LMA removal
Disadvantages	ETT removal can cause significant coughing, bucking, and laryngospasm
Deep extubation	
Advantages	Smooth ETT removal
Disadvantages	Leaves an unprotected airway; presence of nasal packing exacerbates obstruction; not indicated in high-risk patients

Postoperative recommendations for patients at high risk for respiratory depression

- Consider nonopioid analgesics: acetaminophen, NSAIDs, COX-2 inhibitors
- Consider shorter-acting narcotics, such as fentanyl, as rescue pain medications
- Consider avoidance of home narcotic prescriptions
- Consider prolonged postanesthesia recovery unit (PACU) observation if patient is to be discharged home the same day of surgery with a narcotic prescription
- Admit patient overnight if patient has signs of persistent respiratory depression
- Use CPAP as needed

POSTOPERATIVE CARE

The goals of postoperative care in endoscopic sinus and skull base surgery include the recovery of the patient from surgery and anesthesia to an awake and comfortable state of health, so that the patient can be safely discharged home or admitted to an inpatient unit. Most endoscopic sinus procedures are performed on an outpatient basis. Endoscopic skull base surgeries usually require admission, because they are more complex procedures.

Postoperative care

- Pain management: acetaminophen, COX-2 selective inhibitors, fentanyl, oxycodone
- PONV management: scopolamine, dexamethasone, ondansetron
- Patients with increased risk of postoperative respiratory depression need prolonged observation and may require overnight admission
- Patients who undergo endoscopic pituitary resection are at risk of developing diabetes insipidus

Pain experienced after endoscopic surgery ranges from mild to moderate and is related to both surgical trauma and nasal packing. The effect of preoperative local anesthetics seems to be insignificant by the time surgery is completed. Remifentanil can unfortunately produce unintended hyperalgesia in the postoperative period.

Acetaminophen is a safe and effective option, but it is usually not enough to control pain. NSAIDs, such as ketorolac and ibuprofen, are not usually used for pain control, because most surgeons have concerns regarding bleeding risk. They may also cause life-threatening bronchospasm with the triad of NSAIDs, asthma, and nasal polyps.

COX-2 selective inhibitor NSAIDs,[29] such celecoxib, may provide analgesia without increasing the risk of perioperative bleeding. However, caution should be taken in patients at risk of thrombotic complications, because COX-2 selective inhibitors have been associated with an increased risk of thrombotic cardiovascular complications such as myocardial infarctions and strokes. Rofecoxib was withdrawn from the market because of these concerns.

Patients are usually discharged home with a narcotic prescription. Patients with moderate to severe OSA, an STOPBANG of 5 or greater, or a BMI of 45 or greater are at high risk of having perioperative respiratory depression from sedatives and narcotics given during the surgery. This increased risk continues, at least for the first 24 hours postoperatively, for patients who take narcotics at home.

If these high-risk patients are scheduled to be discharged home on the same day of surgery, with a narcotic prescription, the anesthesiologist should request the surgeon consider admitting these patients. If the surgeon declines, these patients should have a prolonged observation time in the PACU. If patients have signs of persistent respiratory depression, obstruction, or oxygen desaturation, they should be monitored for an even longer period of time. A prudent option to be considered at that time would be to admit the patient for overnight observation.[30]

Early discharge requires adequate control of PONV. The presence of blood in the stomach, inflammation of the uvula and throat, and the use of opioids may all be contributing factors. Decompressing the stomach with an orogastric tube before extubation may be helpful, if possible. Other standard treatments for PONV are scopolamine patch, ondansetron, and dexamethasone.

Patients undergoing endoscopic pituitary resection are at risk for perioperative antidiuretic hormone deficiency, which presents as diabetes insipidus. These patients produce large volumes of urine and can develop high serum osmolality. Serum and urine osmolalities should be measured, and vasopressin replacement maybe indicated.

LOOKING INTO THE FUTURE

The surgical literature contains hundreds of articles, ranging from case reports, case series, prospective and retrospective studies, and review articles, covering the recent advances in endoscopic sinus and skull base surgery. These articles cover recent advances in the surgical technique, technological advances, surgical approaches, new applications of the surgery, and complications. However, the anesthesia literature lags behind the surgical literature for this field.

The next years will surely bring new studies exploring many areas of the anesthetic care in endoscopic skull base surgery. The impact of blood pressure, CO_2, and fluid interventions, use of TIVA versus other techniques, use of new medications such as dexmedetomidine, risk of air embolism, and specific anesthetic complications are some areas in which research could be advanced.

Post-Test Questions (Correct answers are in italics)

1. Which one of the following statements is CORRECT, regarding the preoperative evaluation of patients for endoscopic sinus and skull base surgery?
   a. The enlarged size of mouth, mandible, and trachea in patients with acromegaly facilitates the intubation.
   b. Patients started on steroids by the surgeon, days before the surgery, require an intraoperative stress dose of steroids to prevent adrenal insufficiency.
   c. *STOPBANG scores higher than 5 correlate with risk of moderate to severe OSA.*
   d. To prevent intraoperative bleeding, antiplatelet drugs and anticoagulants should be stopped 5 to 7 days before the surgery, regardless of patient's comorbidities.
2. Which one of the following steps is INCORRECT while preparing patients for endoscopic sinus and skull base surgery?
   a. Elevation of the head of the bed and reverse Trendelenburg position increase the risk of air embolism.
   b. Preoperative intrathecal injection of fluorescein facilitates localization of CSF leaks for repair during surgery.
   c. Acetaminophen and COX-2 inhibitors can be started preoperatively to assist pain management.
   d. *If blood pressure rises after infiltration with vasoconstrictor agents, immediate treatment should be given with β-blocker medications.*
3. Regarding the maintenance of anesthesia for endoscopic sinus and skull base surgery, which one of the following statements is CORRECT?
   a. If a nondepolarizing muscle relaxant was used just for intubation, there is no need to use reversal medications at the end of the case.
   b. *Total intravenous technique (TIVA), using propofol and remifentanil, improves the visibility of the surgical field in endoscopic sinus surgery.*
   c. Laryngeal mask use is contraindicated for endoscopic sinus surgery, due to concerns of blood contamination of the glottis and lower airways.
   d. If the intracranial pressure is elevated, it is necessary to lower the patient's blood pressure to increase cerebral perfusion and to prevent ischemia.
4. Which one of the following statements is CORRECT regarding emergence of anesthesia and postoperative management?
   a. Discharging patients home with a narcotic prescription is a completely safe practice that ensures adequate pain control without significant complications.
   b. Deep extubation should be performed in all patients, because it guarantees a smooth emergence with less coughing, bucking, and oxygen desaturation.
   c. *Remifentanil has been shown to produce postoperative hyperalgesia.*
   d. Patients undergoing endoscopic pituitary resection are not at increased risk for diabetes insipidus.

SUPPLEMENTARY DATA

Supplementary PDF slides related to this article can be found online at http://www.oto.theclinics.com/.

REFERENCES

1. Friedel M, Rosen MR, Nyquist GG, et al. Airway management and perioperative concerns in acromegaly patients undergoing endoscopic surgery for pituitary tumors. J Neurol Surg B Skull Base 2013;74(S 01):A032.
2. Oostra A, van Furth W, Georgalas C. Extended endoscopic endonasal skull base surgery: from the sella to the anterior and posterior cranial fossa. ANZ J Surg 2012;82(3):122–30.
3. Baker AR, Baker AB. Anaesthesia for endoscopic sinus surgery. Acta Anaesthesiol Scand 2010;54(7):795–803.
4. Amorocho MRC, Sordillo A. Anesthesia for functional endoscopic sinus surgery: a review. Anesthesiol Clin 2010;28(3):497–504.
5. Joshi GP, Ankichetty SP, Gan TJ, et al. Society for Ambulatory Anesthesia consensus statement on preoperative selection of adult patients with obstructive sleep apnea scheduled for ambulatory surgery. Anesth Analg 2012;115(5): 1060–8.
6. Chung F, Subramanyam R, Liao P, et al. High STOP-BANG score indicates a high probability of obstructive sleep apnoea. Br J Anaesth 2012;108(5):768–75.
7. Wright ED, Agrawal S. Impact of perioperative systemic steroids on surgical outcomes in patients with chronic rhinosinusitis with polyposis: evaluation with the novel Perioperative Sinus Endoscopy (POSE) scoring system. Laryngoscope 2007;117(S115):1–28.
8. Issioui T, Klein KW, White PF, et al. The efficacy of premedication with celecoxib and acetaminophen in preventing pain after otolaryngologic surgery. Anesth Analg 2002;94(5):1188–93.
9. Abbasi H, Behdad S, Ayatollahi V, et al. Comparison of two doses of tranexamic acid on bleeding and surgery site quality during sinus endoscopy surgery. Adv Clin Exp Med 2012;21(6):773–80.
10. Debaene B, Plaud B, Dilly M-P, et al. Residual paralysis in the PACU after a single intubating dose of nondepolarizing muscle relaxant with an intermediate duration of action. Anesthesiology 2003;98(5):1042–8.
11. Kaplan A, Crosby GJ, Bhattacharyya N. Airway protection and the laryngeal mask airway in sinus and nasal surgery. Laryngoscope 2004;114(4):652–5.
12. Webster AC, Morley-Forster PK, Janzen V, et al. Anesthesia for intranasal surgery: a comparison between tracheal intubation and the flexible reinforced laryngeal mask airway. Anesth Analg 1999;88(2):421–5.
13. Ko MT, Chuang KC, Su CY. Multiple analyses of factors related to intraoperative blood loss and the role of reverse Trendelenburg position in endoscopic sinus surgery. Laryngoscope 2008;118(9):1687–91.
14. Lee T-J, Huang C-C, Chang P-H, et al. Hemostasis during functional endoscopic sinus surgery: the effect of local infiltration with adrenaline. Otolaryngol Head Neck Surg 2009;140(2):209–14.
15. Boonmak S, Boonmak P, Laopaiboon M. Deliberate hypotension with propofol under anaesthesia for functional endoscopic sinus surgery (FESS). Cochrane Database Syst Rev 2013;(6):CD006623.
16. Ragab SM, Hassanin MZ. Optimizing the surgical field in pediatric functional endoscopic sinus surgery: a new evidence-based approach. Otolaryngol Head Neck Surg 2010;142(1):48–54.
17. Eberhart LH, Folz BJ, Wulf H, et al. Intravenous anesthesia provides optimal surgical conditions during microscopic and endoscopic sinus surgery. Laryngoscope 2003;113(8):1369–73.

18. Nair S, Collins M, Hung P, et al. The effect of beta-blocker premedication on the surgical field during endoscopic sinus surgery. Laryngoscope 2004;114(6): 1042–6.

19. Boezaart AP, van der Merwe J, Coetzee A. Comparison of sodium nitroprusside-and esmolol-induced controlled hypotension for functional endoscopic sinus surgery. Can J Anaesth 1995;42(5):373–6.

20. Elsharnouby N, Elsharnouby M. Magnesium sulphate as a technique of hypotensive anaesthesia. Br J Anaesth 2006;96(6):727–31.

21. Lee J, Kim Y, Park C, et al. Comparison between dexmedetomidine and remifentanil for controlled hypotension and recovery in endoscopic sinus surgery. Ann Otol Rhinol Laryngol 2013;122:421–6.

22. Sieskiewicz A, Lyson T, Drozdowski A, et al. Blood flow velocity in the middle cerebral artery during transnasal endoscopic skull base surgery performed in controlled hypotension. Neurol Neurochir Pol 2014;48(3):181–7.

23. Pavlin JD, Colley PS, Weymuller EA Jr, et al. Propofol versus isoflurane for endoscopic sinus surgery. Am J Otolaryngol 1999;20(2):96–101.

24. Beule AG, Wilhelmi F, Kühnel TS, et al. Propofol versus sevoflurane: bleeding in endoscopic sinus surgery. Otolaryngol Head Neck Surg 2007;136(1):45–50.

25. Ahn H, Chung S-K, Dhong H-J, et al. Comparison of surgical conditions during propofol or sevoflurane anaesthesia for endoscopic sinus surgery. Br J Anaesth 2008;100(1):50–4.

26. Cafiero T, Cavallo L, Frangiosa A, et al. Clinical comparison of remifentanil-sevoflurane vs. remifentanil-propofol for endoscopic endonasal transphenoidal surgery. Eur J Anaesthesiol 2007;24(05):441–6.

27. Nekhendzy V, Lemmens HJ, Vaughan WC, et al. The effect of deliberate hypercapnia and hypocapnia on intraoperative blood loss and quality of surgical field during functional endoscopic sinus surgery. Anesth Analg 2007;105(5):1404–9.

28. Ismail SA, Anwar HM. Bilateral sphenopalatine ganglion block in functional endoscopic sinus surgery under general anaesthesia. AJAIC 2005;8(4):45–53.

29. Church CA, Stewart C, O-Lee TJ, et al. Rofecoxib versus hydrocodone/acetaminophen for postoperative analgesia in functional endoscopic sinus surgery. Laryngoscope 2006;116(4):602–6.

30. Adesanya AO, Lee W, Greilich NB, et al. Perioperative management of obstructive sleep apnea. Chest 2010;138(6):1489–98.

SUGGESTED READINGS

Boonmak S, Boonmak P, Laopaiboon M. Deliberate hypotension with propofol under anaesthesia for functional endoscopic sinus surgery (FESS). Cochrane Database Syst Rev 2013;(6):CD006623.

A Cochrane analysis compared the use of propofol versus other techniques for deliberate hypotension during functional endoscopic sinus surgery with regard to blood loss and operative conditions. After searching all randomized controlled trials available, 4 studies with 278 participants were reviewed. The analysis found that deliberate hypotension with propofol did not decrease total blood loss when compared with inhalation anesthetics. Propofol improved the quality of the surgical field by one category, on a scale from 0 (no bleeding) to 5 (severe bleeding). The conclusion was that using propofol to achieve deliberate hypotension may improve the surgical field, but the effect is small.

Chung F, Subramanyam R, Liao P, et al. High STOP-Bang score indicates a high probability of obstructive sleep apnoea. Br J Anaesth 2012;108(5):768–75.

The authors investigated the value of the STOP-Bang score in predicting OSA in surgical patients. S: snoring: do you snore loudly (loud enough to be heard through a closed door)? T: tired: do you often feel tired, fatigued, or sleepy during daytime? O: observed: has anyone observed you stop breathing during your sleep? P: blood pressure: do you have or are you being treated for high blood pressure? B: BMI: BMI more than 35? A: age > 50 years? N: neck circumference >40 cm? G: gender: Male? Results from 746 patients were analyzed. The odds ratio of moderate to severe OSA increased with an increase in the score. The study concluded that, in the surgical population, a STOP-Bang score of 5–8 identified patients with high probability of moderate to severe OSA.

Kaplan A, Crosby GJ, Bhattacharyya N. Airway protection and the laryngeal mask airway in sinus and nasal surgery. Laryngoscope 2004;114(4):652–5.

The authors compared the LMA and ETT for airway protection from blood during sinonasal surgery. Results from 74 patients were analyzed. Patients with an LMA were less likely to have staining of the glottis or trachea than patients managed with an ETT. However, the ETT provided better protection than LMA against distal tracheal blood contamination. The study concluded that LMA provided better protection of the upper airway, but with a higher incidence of lower airway contamination. Another conclusion was that the LMA was a reasonable alternative to ETT in sinonasal surgery.

Blood-Sparing Techniques in Head and Neck Surgery

Mindy R. Rabinowitz, MD*, David M. Cognetti, MD, Gurston G. Nyquist, MD

KEYWORDS

- Blood sparing • Jehovah's witness • Allogenic blood transfusion
- Bloodless medicine • Acute normovolemic hemodilution
- Preoperative autologous donation • Controlled hypotension • Cell saver

KEY LEARNING POINTS

At the end of this article, the reader will:

- Understand why we need blood-sparing techniques.
- Know which kinds of blood products are and are not acceptable to Jehovah's Witnesses.
- Know the preoperative, intraoperative, and postoperative techniques that can be used to decrease blood loss/reduce the need for allogenic blood transfusion.

INTRODUCTION

> **Why do we need blood-sparing techniques?**
>
> - Risk of perioperative anemia in head and neck patients is high.
> - Consequences of anemia include increased morbidity and mortality perioperatively, particularly for cancer patients.
> - Patients for whom blood transfusion not an option:
>   - Religious beliefs.
>   - Fear of the risks or complications of transfusion.
>   - Medical contraindications.
>   - Logistical issues.
> - This has led to the development of bloodless surgery programs.

Anemia frequently complicates the treatment of surgical patients. The high vascularity of the head and neck can foster significant blood loss during surgery. For example, allogenic blood transfusion (ABT) rates are quoted as high as 84% in head and neck cancer patients perioperatively.[1,2] Noteworthy factors that may predict the

Department of Otolaryngology - Head and Neck Surgery, Thomas Jefferson University, Philadelphia, PA 19107, USA
* Corresponding author. 925 Chestnut Street, 6th Floor, Philadelphia, PA 19107.
E-mail address: mfigures@gmail.com

Otolaryngol Clin N Am 49 (2016) 549–562
http://dx.doi.org/10.1016/j.otc.2016.02.008
0030-6665/16/$ – see front matter © 2016 Elsevier Inc. All rights reserved.

need for blood transfusion in head and neck oncologic surgery include the preoperative hemoglobin (Hb) level, patient age, the site and extent of the primary tumor, the need for flap reconstruction, and prior chemotherapy.[1] In addition to tumor location and stage, anemia of chronic disease, nutritional factors, and chemotherapy are all major contributors to preoperative anemia and should be monitored and corrected when possible.[3] The effects of anemia on the surgical patient are wide-ranging and serve not only as a major risk factor for transfusion, but also as an independent predictor of morbidity and mortality.[4]

Traditionally, correction of anemia took place via ABTs. However, for a variety of reasons there remain populations unable to receive this option. For example, religious beliefs (Jehovah's Witnesses), fear of the risks and complications of transfusion, medical contraindications (ie, presence of autoantibodies), or logistical issues (ie, rare blood groups, unavailability of blood components) may preclude a patient from accepting a blood transfusion.[5] Additionally, ABTs are not without complication, and may result in transfusion reactions, fever, hemolysis, lung injury, and immunodeficiency.[6]

Bloodless medicine and surgery programs have developed out of a need to find alternative means to treat acute and chronic anemia in patients who cannot receive ABTs. The goal of this article is to acquaint the otolaryngologist with alternative methods of managing blood loss and anemia in their surgical patients who cannot or should not receive ABTs.

JEHOVAH'S WITNESSES

- Aversion to ABT is rooted in their literal interpretation of the Bible.
- Refuse allogenic whole blood and its major components:
  - Red cells
  - White cells
  - Platelets
  - Plasma
  - Predonation of autologous blood
- Acceptance of "minor" blood components decided on individual basis:
  - Albumin
  - Immunoglobulin
  - Vaccines
  - Clotting factors
  - Prothrombin complex concentrates
- Reinfusion of autologous blood kept linked to the patient is usually acceptable:
  - Cardiopulmonary bypass
  - Hemodialysis
  - Cell salvage
  - Acute normovolemic hemodilution

The Jehovah's Witness faith began in Philadelphia, Pennsylvania, in the 1870s as a Bible study group.[7] A cornerstone of this religion is the literal interpretation of Bible passages. Passages such as "Every moving animal that is, alive may serve as food for you...Only flesh with its soul—its blood—you must not eat" from Genesis 9:3,4 are taken literally as a ban of blood via any route.[7] As such, a refusal of blood transfusions is a core value of their faith.[8] Disobeying this ban taints the recipient's immortal soul leading to shunning by friends, family, and the entire Jehovah's Witness community.[7]

Over the last 20 years, the Jehovah's Witness faith and prohibitions have evolved with a broader interpretation of what components, techniques, and kinds of blood and blood products are acceptable. As a rule, Jehovah's Witnesses refuse transfusion of allogenic blood and its major components—red cells, white cells, platelets, and plasma. However, acceptance of "minor" fractions such as albumin, immunoglobulin, vaccines, clotting factors, and prothrombin complex concentrates are considered a "matter of conscience" and is often left to be decided by the individual (**Table 1**).

With regard to perioperative planning, banking of the patient's own blood for later reinfusion (ie, preoperative autologous donation [PAD]) is not allowed; however, blood left connected to the patient as in cell salvage, hemodialysis, or cardiopulmonary bypass is acceptable for reinfusion. Additionally, acute normovolemic hemodilution (see "Intraoperative Techniques: Acute Normovolemic Hemodilution") and many of the pharmaceutical agents that promote hematopoiesis or hemostasis (ie, iron, topical hemostatic agents, antifibrinolytics, and erythropoiesis stimulating agents) are also accepted by most Jehovah's Witnesses.[5]

It was the refusal of ABTs in this population that served as one of the impetuses to develop alternative means for treating anemia and decreasing surgical blood loss, which can be applied to a plethora of other populations and medical and surgical conditions.

COMPLICATIONS OF BLOOD TRANSFUSIONS

Risks of ABT

- Infection
- Acute and chronic hemolytic reactions
- Transfusion-related acute lung injury
- Immunosuppression

Although safer than ever before, ABT is not without risk. Although infectious complications, such as human immunodeficiency virus and hepatitis B and C are dwindling in number owing to better screening techniques, risks of ABT remain. Furthermore, new threats, such as variants of Creutzfeldt-Jakob disease and West Nile virus have been reported in the blood supply.[4]

Human error may lead to acute hemolytic reactions, often owing to ABO incompatibility, which is characterized by fevers, chills, nausea, vomiting, hypotension, renal failure, disseminated intravascular coagulation, and death in up to 40% of cases.[4]

Table 1
Blood components that are/are not acceptable to Jehovah's witnesses

Refuse	Individual Decision	Usually Acceptable
Whole blood and its major components	Minor blood products	Reinfusion of autologous blood kept linked to the patient
• Red cells	• Albumin	• Cardiopulmonary bypass
• White cells	• Immunoglobulin	• Hemodialysis
• Platelets	• Vaccines	• Cell salvage
• Plasma	• Clotting factors	• Acute normovolemic hemodilution
• Predonation of autologous blood	• Prothrombin complex concentrates	

Delayed hemolytic reactions, owing to extravascular hemolysis caused by antibodies to red blood cells (RBCs), occur about 3 days to 2 weeks after a transfusion and display symptoms of inability to maintain Hb levels, fever, chills, dyspnea, and jaundice. These hemolytic reactions are particularly problematic in the surgical patient where it may be difficult to parse out whether these symptoms are related to infection or the transfusion.

Transfusion-related acute lung injury is another well-recognized complication of ABT. The underlying mechanism is poorly understood but it seems to involve localization of antibody-coated leukocytes to the pulmonary vasculature resulting in increased permeability and edema.[4] Usually during or shortly after transfusion, patients present with dyspnea, hypotension, fever, and bilateral pulmonary infiltrates without evidence of cardiac compromise or fluid overload. It develops fully within 1 to 6 hours of transfusion and is fatal in 5% to 10% of cases.[4] Treatment of transfusion-related acute lung injury includes prompt recognition, cessation of the ABT, and oxygen therapy. The blood in question should be returned to the blood center for testing.

Finally, another untoward result of ABT is immunosuppression. The immunosuppressive effects of ABT were first noted in 1978 when renal transplant patients undergoing multiple ABT showed improved graft survival.[1] McRae and colleagues examined the immune profiles of 20 head and neck cancer patients treated with surgery, one-half of whom received blood transfusions. In patients who received transfused blood, total lymphocyte, T cell, helper T4 cells, and interleukin-2 receptor–positive T4 cell counts were significantly decreased.[1,9] This immunosuppressive effect leads some to fear the risk of cancer recurrence in those patients who undergo multiple transfusions. However, some authors have failed to find this relationship and counter that patients with advanced disease require more extensive surgery and have a worse prognosis regardless of the number of transfusions.[1] Nonetheless, a possible immunosuppressive effect and therefore increased risk of recurrence should at least be considered when treating perioperative anemia, particularly in oncologic patients.

PREOPERATIVE TECHNIQUES

What techniques can be used preoperatively to prevent blood loss?
• Pharmacotherapy
• PAD

As with any surgery, careful preoperative planning is crucial for successful outcomes and this is especially true in those patients in whom blood transfusion is not an option. For these patients, the preoperative period should be viewed as a golden opportunity to intervene or prevent blood loss thereby minimizing the chance that a blood transfusion would be necessary.[5]

Pharmacotherapy
• Anticoagulation
• Erythropoietin (EPO)
• Iron, vitamin B_{12}, folate

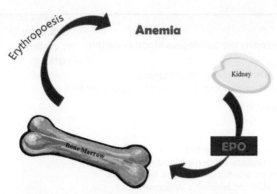

Fig. 1. Erythropoietin (EPO) is a glycoprotein produced by the kidneys that stimulates the production and differentiation of erythroid progenitors in the bone marrow to treat anemia.

Anticoagulants have been shown to cause increased bleeding during surgery; however, the clinical significance of such bleeding has yet to be determined.[5] Nonetheless, in patients who cannot undergo blood transfusions, anticoagulants should be discontinued preoperatively, if possible, to decrease bleeding risk. In the emergent setting, reversal may be an option for certain anticoagulants (ie, vitamin K for warfarin).[5]

EPO is a glycoprotein produced by the kidneys that stimulates the production and differentiation of erythroid progenitors in the bone marrow (**Fig. 1**). Epoetin alfa is a recombinant form of EPO manufactured to be functionally indistinguishable from endogenous EPO. It is capable of stimulating erythropoiesis and, therefore, increasing Hb and hematocrit levels and can produce the equivalent of 1 U of blood per week of treatment.[2,3,10]

Recombinant human EPO has been used to successfully manage perioperative Hb and decrease transfusion requirements and is most effective when used before elective procedures.[8] Despite a small about of albumin present in the commercially available formulations (individuals who refuse blood products should be forewarned), most Jehovah's Witnesses will accept recombinant human EPO.[8]

EPO, however, is not without its risks. Increased mortality, and cardiovascular and thromboembolic events have been reported with the use of EPO; therefore, patients should receive thromboembolic prophylaxis while on this therapy.[4,11] Additionally, EPO has been associated with increased recurrence in head and neck cancer patients possibly owing to thrombogenesis and tumor hypoxia.[12,13]

Iron is the fuel for EPO and in some studies has been shown to significantly reduce transfusion requirements when given in combination with EPO preoperatively.[11,14] Adverse events associated with intravenous iron are usually mild. Anaphylaxis is the most feared complication but this reaction is increasingly rare with newer intravenous formulations.[3]

Perioperative deficiency of vitamin B_{12} is also common, particularly among cancer patients. Therefore, supplementation of vitamin B_{12} as well as folate should be considered as part of the routine pre and perioperative care of cancer patients.[4]

PAD

- Weekly preoperative autologous blood donation.

- Indications:
  ○ 500 to 1000 mL blood loss anticipated
  ○ Estimated transfusion pro-bability of greater than 50%

- Contraindications:
  ○ High cardiac risk

- Limitations:
  ○ High rate of blood wasted
  ○ May still require allogenic blood
  ○ May render anemic and require hematinics
  ○ Not suitable for Jehovah's Witnesses

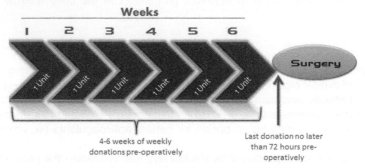

4-6 weeks of weekly
donations pre-operatively

Last donation no later
than 72 hours pre-
operatively

Fig. 2. Preoperative autologous donation (PAD). The usual algorithm entails weekly donation of 1 unit of blood within 4 to 6 weeks before surgery. The final donation must not be performed later than 72 hours before surgery.

PAD is a technique whereby patients donate a few units of blood several weeks preoperatively, to be stored and used perioperatively when transfusion needs arise.[5] This method allows for the patient's own blood to be transfused as a first line treatment against intraoperative or postoperative anemia. The usual algorithm entails weekly donation of 1 U of blood within 4 to 6 weeks before surgery. The final donation must not be performed later than 72 hours before surgery (**Fig. 2**).[15]

PAD is suitable when blood loss is estimated to be between 500 to 1000 mL (mL) in at least 5% to 10% of cases, or when the probability of transfusion exceeds 50%. The minimum acceptable Hb concentration for PAD is 11 g/dL.[15] Contraindications to PAD include, most notably, those patients with increased cardiac risks—unstable angina, myocardial infarction within the previous 3 months, coronary artery main stem stenosis, congestive heart failure, and significant aortic valve stenosis.[15]

Despite the potential upsides of this technique, there are some marked limitations to PAD. First, PAD is not typically cost effective because wastage rates approach 40%.[16] Stored blood has a limited lifespan, likely shorter than the 42 days allowable by most United States blood banks leading to significant waste of predonated blood that is not used within this time period (given that most blood is donated about 4–6 weeks preoperatively). In fact, it has been estimated that for every 2 U donated, on average, only 1 U is ultimately used.[5,8]

Second, under physiologic conditions, it takes 21 to 30 days from the first appearance of erythroid progenitor cells within the bone marrow to the appearance of mature RBCs in the circulating blood.[17] As such, patients are typically unable to regenerate all of the RBC volume lost in the period between self-donation and surgery and therefore many still require ABT.[8] About 10% to 20% of patients who predonate blood also require allogenic blood, mitigating the positive effects of autologous blood transfusion.[16] Furthermore, the effect of PAD is akin to chronic hemodilution, rendering the patient anemic without the help from hematinic agents such as EPO and iron.[5]

Finally, given the complete removal of blood from the patient's circulation and its storage, PAD is not acceptable to Jehovah's Witnesses.

INTRAOPERATIVE TECHNIQUES

What techniques can be used intraoperatively to prevent/mitigate blood loss?
• Surgical techniques/equipment
• Controlled hypotension
• Temperature control
• Medical therapy
• Hb-like substitutes
• Acute normovolemic hemodilution
• Cell Saver

The sine qua non of reducing transfusion need in surgical patients is to prevent blood loss.[18]

Surgical techniques/equipment
• Equipment: ○ Electrocautery, ultrasonic dissector, tourniquets
• Patient positioning
• Staged procedures

Efforts to decrease intraoperative blood loss begin with meticulous surgical technique. Electrocautery, either monopolar or bipolar, hemostat clamps, tourniquets, and infiltration of local vasoconstrictors may help to decrease blood loss. New modifications to electrocautery such as argon beam-enhanced devices can coagulate vessels up to 3 mm in diameter while minimizing surrounding tissue trauma.[18] Other devices that rely on water, gas, sound, and microwaves have been developed in the past few years and have allowed other means of obtaining hemostasis. The harmonic scalpel is an ultrasonic coagulator dissector (Ethicon, Cincinnati, OH) that simultaneously cuts and coagulates tissue. It operates at significantly lower temperature than traditional electrocautery thereby causing less adjacent thermal injury and smoke.[13,18]

Patient positioning is a simple measure that can lessen blood loss. Elevating the surgical site may help to reduce arterial pressure and venous congestion, and facilitate venous drainage away from the surgical wound. Care must be taken to avoid introducing air into the venous circulation.[18]

Finally, if able, performing complex procedures in a staged fashion may minimize blood loss in certain clinical situations. Furthermore, it may also allow for appropriate time to reoptimize the patient medically or allow them to recover from any acute blood loss experienced during the first procedure before moving forward with the next.

Controlled hypotension

- Limits blood loss
- Provides clear surgical field
- Multiple agents
- Side effects

Controlled hypotension is an anesthetic technique that may help to decrease intraoperative blood loss and provide a clearer surgical field. Various agents are available including magnesium sulfate, sodium nitroprusside, nicardipine, nitroglycerine, esmolol, α_2-agonists, labetolol and high-dose potent inhalational anesthetics (ie, sevoflurane)[19] (see Cordoba Amorocho M, Fat I: Anesthetic Techniques in Endoscopic Sinus and Skull Base Surgery, in this issue).

Some of the drawbacks of these drugs include resistance to vasodilators, tachyphylaxis, and cyanide toxicity with sodium nitroprusside, the possibility of myocardial depression with esmolol and magnesium sulfate and a long postanesthetic recovery period with isoflurane.[19]

Temperature control

- Avoid hypothermia:
  - Platelet dysfunction

Hypothermia has been shown to adversely affect platelet functioning and result in increased blood loss. Therefore, avoidance of unnecessary hypothermia may help to reduce some of the intraoperative blood loss.[5] Even mild perioperative hypothermia has been reported to be associated with increased blood loss and risk of transfusion.[3] On the other hand, in some experimental models mild hypothermia was shown to increase anemia tolerance by decreasing total body oxygen demand.[15]

Medical therapy

- Oxygen
- Artificial oxygen carriers (AOCs):
  - Stroma-free Hb solutions
  - Perfluorocarbon emulsions
- Topical hemostatic agents:
  - Thrombin, fibrinogen, collagen, gelatin, and cellulose
- Systemic hemostatic agents:
  - Lysine analogues
  - Coagulation factors

One approach to increasing the physiologic tolerance to anemia and avoiding critically low Hb levels is to increase the oxygen content of the blood. In its simplest form, this can be accomplished by increasing the partial pressure of oxygen delivered to the lungs. Although the plasma-dissolved oxygen is usually less than the Hb-bound oxygen, it does not face the same saturation plateau seen when all of the oxygen binding sites are filled on a given Hb molecule. The plasma-dissolved oxygen increases linearly with increasing partial pressure of oxygen.[5] Therefore, in a severely anemic patient, providing increased oxygen can lead to an increased dissolved oxygen concentration in the blood and end-organs, resulting in at least some ability to compensate for a low Hb.[5] Most commonly, this can be accomplished via 100% nasal oxygen or by providing 100% oxygen through a ventilator.[5]

Traditionally, treatment of anemia has been accomplished with blood transfusions; however, in its absence other avenues must be explored. AOCs are currently under investigation and are generally based on the Hb molecule (ie, stroma-free Hb solutions) or chemicals (ie, perfluorocarbon emulsions) that are capable of dissolving large amounts of oxygen. They are often acceptable to Jehovah's Witnesses.[5]

AOCs provide the benefit of a long shelf-life at room temperature and a lack of immunogenic cell membranes. Additionally, AOCs can act as a replacement fluid during blood loss.[18] Disadvantages include a relatively short circulation time (24–48 hours), methemoglobin production, nitric oxide-mediated vasoconstriction, and gastrointestinal discomfort.[18]

Stroma-free Hb solutions are derived either from human Hb (either extracted from outdated RBCs or genetically engineered) or bovine Hb.[20] Stroma-free Hb solutions have a lower oxygen affinity than native Hb, and facilitate offloading of oxygen in tissues.[15] Owing to their oncotic properties, they serve as oxygen-carrying volume expanders suitable for the treatment of surgical blood loss. Furthermore, they inherently possess vasoconstrictive effects which can contribute to hemodynamic stabilization and blood preservation during resuscitation or surgery.[15,20]

Perfluorocarbon emulsions are another form of AOCs derived from cyclic or straight-chain hydrocarbons with hydrogen atoms replaced by halogens.[15] With perfluorocarbons there is a linear relationship between the partial pressure of arterial oxygen and oxygen content; therefore high partial pressures of arterial oxygen are required to maximize the amount of oxygen transported by the perfluorocarbons.[15] Given that these AOCs are not derived from any human products, some patients may find them more acceptable than stroma-free Hb solutions. Unfortunately, however, despite the potential benefit of these products over ABT, none of the AOCs are currently approved for human use in the United States.

Other pharmacologic agents that can be instituted intraoperatively to assist with hemostasis includes topicals such as those that contain thrombin, fibrinogen, collagen, gelatin and cellulose and act by promoting coagulation at the site of application.[3] Alternatively, systemic hemostatic agents are available and most commonly include the lysine analogues (tranexamic acid and epsilon aminocaproic acid) that act by inhibiting plasmin and preserving blood clots formed at sites of bleeding. In appropriate patient populations, repletion of coagulation factors may also help to decrease bleeding and, in turn, decrease the need for blood transfusions.[3]

Acute normovolemic hemodilution

- Technique:
  - Immediate preoperative removal of blood replaced by crystalloid/colloid
- Mechanism of action:
  - Allows lower Hb and hematocrit
- Rationale:
  - Reduces RBC mass lost
  - Preserves clotting factors
- Benefits:
  - More economical than PAD
- Disadvantages:
  - Acute kidney injury, longer operating time
- Contraindications:
  - Cardiac disease, renal disease, and bacteremia

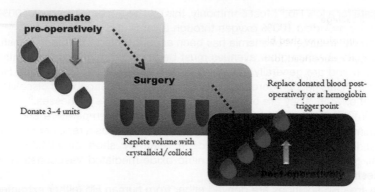

Fig. 3. Acute normovolemic hemodilution involves removing a volume of blood (usually 3–4 units) immediately before the start of the surgical procedure, which is then stored at bedside in the operating room. The removed blood is replaced with an equivalent amount of crystalloid or colloid to maintain normovolemia. At the conclusion of the case, or at the hemoglobin level at which transfusion is determined to be necessary, the collected blood is returned to the patient.

Acute normovolemic dilution (ANH) involves removing a volume of blood (usually 3–4 U) immediately before the start of the surgical procedure, which is then stored at bedside in the operating room. The removed blood is replaced with an equivalent amount of crystalloid or colloid (AOCs are potentially a newer option) to maintain normovolemia.[8,15] At the conclusion of the case, or at the Hb level at which transfusion is determined to be necessary, the collected blood is returned to the patient (**Fig. 3**).[18] Given that oxygen delivery to tissue begins to decrease at hematocrit levels of less than 25% (corresponds with a Hb concentration around 8 g/dL), hemodilution can usually safely occur down to this level.[15]

The rationale behind ANH is that the more diluted the patient—that is, the lower the intravascular Hb concentration—the less RBC mass lost per milliliter of blood loss while preserving clotting factors. Additionally, postponing transfusion until the completion of surgical hemostasis increases the percentage of RBCs that are maintained in the vasculature rather than being spilled out during surgical blood loss.[8,15]

The benefits of ANH are often compared with PAD and are associated with less waste and need for storage, less transfusion mishaps, reduced cost, and obviating the need for prescreening for infectious agents.[8] Additionally, other potential benefits include improvement in tissue oxygenation owing to decreased blood viscosity, reduction in the need for ABT, and a decrease in exposure to blood-borne pathogens and transfusion reactions and finally, the ready availability of whole blood containing clotting factors and fresh platelets for reinfusion after their removal during the dilutional process.[21]

The downside to ANH is that the technique is labor intensive and requires special preparation and staff experienced in its use. Furthermore, it has been associated with longer anesthesia and operative times as well as an increase in the need for vasopressor support.[22]

ANH is contraindicated with unstable angina, coronary artery disease with significant main-stem stenosis or myocardial infarction within the past 6 months, high-grade aortic valve and carotid artery stenosis, renal insufficiency, and gross bacteremia.[15]

Cell salvage
• Reinfusion of shed blood
• Can reduce need for transfusion
• Effective when high blood loss expected
• Risks: reintroduction of tumor cells, infection, and loss of coagulation factors

Intraoperative autologous blood cell salvage involves recovery of the patient's own shed blood, washing or filtering, and returning it back to the patient, often continuously during surgery.[18] Often used in cardiac and orthopedic surgery where high blood loss is expected, it can reduce the need for ABT.[23] It is also effective for patients whose religious beliefs preclude them from receiving allogenic blood and it has been shown to be cost effective in cases where at least 2 U of blood are recovered and reinfused.[4,18]

Cell salvage procedures have been associated with infection, loss of coagulation factors (if washed), hemolysis and reintroduction of tumor cells. However, these limitations notwithstanding, cell salvage techniques overall appear safe and effective.[8]

Postoperative techniques
• Reduce the transfusion trigger
• Decrease blood draws
• Postoperative pharmacologic options

Intraoperative hemostasis has arguably one of the largest impacts on postoperative Hb concentration. However, careful attention to detail in the postoperative period can help to decrease further blood loss and delay the necessity for blood transfusion.

Studies have shown that better outcomes are associated with a restrictive transfusion policy (Hb $\leq$ 7 g/dL) compared with more liberal transfusion policies ($\leq$10 g/dL) in most patients, except in those with severe cardiac disease.[8] Reducing the transfusion trigger requires institution-wide education and commitment but the efforts may be well worth the risk reduction associated with ABT.[8]

Frequent blood draws can lead to cumulative effects on Hb concentrations; therefore, postoperative standing laboratory orders should be avoided. Laboratory tests should only be ordered when a clear indication exists.[3]

Finally, if anemia does occur postoperatively, it can be treated in combination with erythropoietic support, proper nutrition, iron, folate and vitamin B_{12} (see "Preoperative Techniques: Pharmacotherapy").[3] Additionally, holding nonsteroidal antiinflammatory drugs and prophylactic antithrombotic drugs may help to decrease the risk of postsurgical bleeding.[24]

SUMMARY

Given the risks and potential complications of ABT, as well as the rising population of patients for whom ABT may not be an option, it is important for the treating physician, anesthesiologist and surgeon to be well versed in various alternatives. A good grasp of the concepts discussed in this article will help to customize a treatment plan that is specific to each patient's underlying disease and personal preferences without sacrificing appropriate medical care.

Post-Test Questions (Correct answers are in italics)

1. Jehovah's Witnesses uniformly refuse all of the following, *except*:
   a. Red blood cells
   b. White blood cells
   c. Plasma
   d. *Albumin*
2. Preoperative autologous donation (PAD) usually entails:
   a. Biweekly donation of 1 U of blood within 4 to 6 weeks of surgery
   b. *Weekly donation of 1 U of blood within 4 to 6 weeks of surgery*
   c. Weekly donation of 1 U of blood within 2 weeks of surgery
   d. Weekly donation of 2 U of blood within 2 weeks of surgery.
3. All of the following agents can be used to induce controlled hypotension *except*:
   a. Esmolol
   b. Labetolol
   c. *Succinylcholine*
   d. Nitroglycerine
4. Which of the following is *true* about stroma-free hemoglobin (SFH) solution?
   a. *They are derived from human or bovine hemoglobin*
   b. They possess vasodilatory effects
   c. They behave more like a crystalloid than a colloid
   d. They have a higher oxygen affinity than native hemoglobin
5. Which of the following is *incorrect* regarding acute normovolemic hemodilution (ANH)?
   a. It involves removing blood immediately before the procedure
   b. Most patients can tolerate a hematocrit of 25%
   c. It leads to reduced red blood cell mass lost during surgical blood loss
   d. *Reinfusion usually occurs continuously throughout the case*

SUPPLEMENTARY DATA

Supplementary PDF slides related to this article can be found online at http://www.oto.theclinics.com/.

REFERENCES

1. Weber RS. A model for predicting transfusion requirements in head and neck surgery. Laryngoscope 1995;105(8 Pt 2 Suppl 73):1–17 [review].

2. Scott SN, Boeve TJ, McCulloch TM, et al. The effects of epoetin alfa on transfusion requirements in head and neck cancer patients: a prospective, randomized, placebo-controlled study. Laryngoscope 2002;112(7 Pt 1):1221–9.

3. Weber RS, Jabbour N, Martin RC 2nd. Anemia and transfusions in patients undergoing surgery for cancer. Ann Surg Oncol 2008;15(1):34–45 [review].

4. Shander A, Javidroozi M, Perelman S, et al. From bloodless surgery to patient blood management. Mt Sinai J Med 2012;79(1):56–65.

5. Shander A, Javidroozi M. The approach to patients with bleeding disorders who do not accept blood-derived products. Semin Thromb Hemost 2013;39(2): 182–90.

6. Pérez Ferrer A, Ferrazza V, Gredilla E, et al. Bloodless surgery in a patient with thalassemia minor. Usefulness of erythropoietin, preoperative blood donation and intraoperative blood salvage. Minerva Anestesiol 2007;73(5):323–6.
7. Allison G, Feeney C. Successful use of a polymerized hemoglobin blood substitute in a critically anemic Jehovah's Witness. South Med J 2004;97(12):1257–8.
8. Shander A, Goodnough LT. Objectives and limitations of bloodless medical care. Curr Opin Hematol 2006;13(6):462–70.
9. McRae JD, Lampe H, Banerjee D. Blood transfusions and phenotypic immune profile in head and neck cancer patients undergoing surgical resection. J Otolaryngol 1991;105:293–4.
10. Lynn S, McDaniel J. Managing severe anemia when the patient is a Jehovah's Witness. JAAPA 2013;26(4):24, 27–9.
11. Lin DM, Lin ES, Tran MH. Efficacy and safety of erythropoietin and intravenous iron in perioperative blood management: a systematic review. Transfus Med Rev 2013;27(4):221–34.
12. Henke M, Laszig R, Rübe C, et al. Erythropoietin to treat head and neck cancer patient with anaemia undergoing radiotherapy: randomize, double-blind, placebo-controlled trial. Lancet 2003;362(9392):1255–60.
13. Kullar PJ, Sorenson K, Weerakkody R, et al. Case report: the management of advanced oral cancer in a Jehovah's Witness using the Ultracision Harmonic Scalpel. World J Surg Oncol 2011;9:115.
14. Bacuzzi A, Dionigi G, Piffaretti G, et al. Preoperative methods to improve erythropoiesis. Transplant Proc 2011;43(1):324–6.
15. Pape A, Habler O. Alternatives to allogeneic blood transfusions. Best Pract Res Clin Anaesthesiol 2007;21(2):221–39.
16. Monk TG, Goodnough LT, Brecher ME, et al. A prospective randomized comparison of three blood conservation strategies for radical prostatectomy. Anesthesiology 1999;91(1):24–33.
17. Singbartl G, Held AL, Singbartl K. Ranking the effectiveness of autologous blood conservation measures through validated modeling of independent clinical data. Transfusion 2013;53(12):3060–79.
18. Goodnough LT, Shander A, Spence R. Bloodless medicine: clinical care without allogeneic blood transfusion. Transfusion 2003;43(5):668–76 [review].
19. Kol IO, Kaygusuz K, Yildirim A, et al. Controlled hypotension with desflurane combined with esmolol or dexmedetomidine during tympanoplasty in adults: a double-blind, randomized, controlled trial. Curr Ther Res Clin Exp 2009;70(3):197–208.
20. Habler OP, Messmer KF. Tissue perfusion and oxygenation with blood substitutes. Adv Drug Deliv Rev 2000;40(3):171–84.
21. Segal JB, Blasco-Colmenares E, Norris EJ, et al. Preoperative acute normovolemic hemodilution: a meta-analysis. Transfusion 2004;44(5):632–44.
22. Habib AS, Moul JW, Polascik TJ, et al, Duke Perioperative Outcome Study Group. Low central venous pressure versus acute normovolemic hemodilution versus conventional fluid management for reducing blood loss in radical retropubic prostatectomy: a randomized controlled trial. Curr Med Res Opin 2014;30(5):937–43.
23. Carless PA, Henry DA, Moxey AJ, et al. Cell salvage for minimising perioperative allogeneic blood transfusion. Cochrane Database Syst Rev 2010;(4):CD001888. [review].
24. Cooper L, Ford K, Miller E. Preparing a Jehovah's Witness for major elective surgery. BMJ 2013;346:f1588.

SUGGESTED READINGS

Goodnough LT, Shander A, Spence R. Bloodless medicine: clinical care without allogeneic blood transfusion. Transfusion 2003;43(5):668–76 [review].

Bloodless medicine refers to medical treatment without ABT. General principles of bloodless medicine include: Formulate a clear care plan under the umbrella of a multidisciplinary team; Proactive management, decisive and prudent clinical judgment with consultation when necessary; Decrease blood draws or anticoagulants where able.

Weber RS, Jabbour N, Martin RC 2nd. Anemia and transfusions in patients undergoing surgery for cancer. Ann Surg Oncol 2008;15(1):34–45 [review].

Peri-operative factors may lead to patient anemia. Anemia may be associated with increased morbidity and mortality, particularly in oncology patients. ABT are associated with several risks from infection to cancer recurrence. Blood conserving strategies are numerous and include preoperative donation, acute normovolemic dilution, blood salvage, preoperative epotin and nutritional supplements.

Quality Control Approach to Anticoagulants and Transfusion

Erin McKean, MD, MBA[a,b,*]

KEYWORDS

- Hemostasis • Blood transfusion • New oral anticoagulants • Anticoagulation
- Quality

KEY LEARNING POINTS

At the end of this article, the reader will:

- Be able to define quality.
- Understand how new anticoagulant medications can be reversed or managed in the acute setting.
- Know the indications for transfusion of red blood cells.
- Know the indications for transfusion of platelets, fresh frozen plasma, and cryoprecipitate.
- Know the possible metrics and tools for developing a quality plan for hemostasis and transfusion.

INTRODUCTION

Quality can be defined by processes of care and by the characteristics of the care and its outcomes. In terms of blood loss and transfusion, otolaryngologists should be aware of available guidelines, standards for use of blood products, devices and hemostatic agents, outcomes metrics relevant to patients, and tools for implementing quality improvements.

Disclosure: The author has nothing to disclose.
[a] University of Michigan, Department of Otolaryngology - Head and Neck Surgery, 1904 Taubman Center, 1500 East Medical Center Drive, Ann Arbor, MI 48109, USA; [b] University of Michigan, Department of Neurosurgery, 1500 East Medical Center Drive, Ann Arbor, MI 48109, USA
* University of Michigan, Department of Otolaryngology - Head and Neck Surgery, 1904 Taubman Center, 1500 East Medical Center Drive, Ann Arbor, MI 48109.
E-mail address: elmk@med.umich.edu

http://dx.doi.org/10.1016/j.otc.2016.02.005
oto.theclinics.com
0030-6665/16/$ – see front matter © 2016 Elsevier Inc. All rights reserved.

Definition and measures of health care quality

- Institute of Medicine (IOM) 2001 "Crossing the Quality Chasm" report:
  - ○ "The degree to which Health Services... increase the likelihood of desired health outcomes and are consistent with current professional knowledge."[1]
  - ○ IOM components of quality:
    - Safe
    - Effective
    - Patient centered
    - Timely
    - Efficient
    - Equitable
- Agency for Healthcare Research and Quality
  - ○ Doing the right thing (getting the health care services you need) at the right time (when you need them) in the right way (using the appropriate test or procedure) to achieve the best possible results, avoiding underuse, avoiding overuse, and eliminating misuse.[2]

Best practices in hemostasis have been developed individually and institutionally, but there are no national guidelines for the use of specific techniques, tools, devices, or hemostatic agents. In addition, newer anticoagulant medications have brought challenges in managing acute blood loss situations, creating the opportunity and obligation for otolaryngologists to be involved in developing personal and systems-based plans surrounding these challenges.

MANAGING ANTICOAGULANTS IN THE ACUTE AND PERIOPERATIVE SETTINGS

Otolaryngologists manage epistaxis, hemorrhage from the oral cavity and pharynx, maxillofacial trauma in the acute clinical setting, and intraoperative and perioperative bleeding. To better devise institutional plans and guidelines to best manage these problems, an understanding of current practices and medications for anticoagulant therapy is imperative (**Fig. 1**).

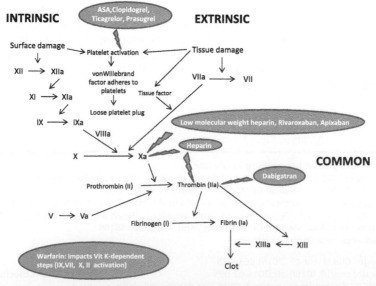

Fig. 1. Coagulation cascade and site of impact of anticoagulant medications.

Older Anticoagulant Medications

- Heparin: inactivates IIa (thrombin) and Xa via an antithrombin mechanism, binds to platelets
  - Indications: prevention and treatment of venous thromboembolism (VTE) and pulmonary embolus (PE); prevention of mural thrombus formation after myocardial infarction (MI); treatment of patients with unstable angina and MI; perioperative bridge
  - No gastrointestinal absorption; must be given intravenously or subcutaneously
  - Onset is immediate (intravenous) and 20 to 60 minutes (subcutaneous)
  - Half-life 1.5 hours (dose dependent and nonlinear)
  - Downsides: variable anticoagulant response, possible heparin resistance, heparin-induced thrombocytopenia (HIT), and osteopenia
  - HIT occurs within 2 days (type 1 immune response) or 4 to 10 days (type 2 immune response); suspect if platelet count decreases more than 50% from baseline; characterized by skin lesions at injection site, possible systemic response (fevers, chills, dyspnea, chest pain), and possible venous thromboembolism; 0.2% of all heparin-exposed patients
  - Dose is adjusted and therapeutic effect is monitored by activated partial thromboplastin time (aPTT)
  - Most institutions have nomograms for dosing
  - Main advantages: quick onset, short half-life, easy to monitor therapeutic effectiveness (as well as normalization before operating room)
- Low-molecular-weight heparin (Lovenox; Sanofi, and others): inactivates factor Xa
  - Indications: prevention of VTE, treatment of VTE
  - Time to peak effect 3 to 5 hours
  - Half-life 4.5 hours after subcutaneous administration
  - Laboratory monitoring is not generally required; anti–factor Xa level should be checked in patients with renal insufficiency, morbidly obese patients, and pregnant women; platelet count is generally checked throughout therapy if prolonged; platelet aggregation test should be done if patient has had HIT with unfractionated heparin
- Warfarin (Coumadin; Bristol-Myers Squibb)
  - Vitamin K antagonist
  - Hepatic metabolism, renal elimination
  - Narrow therapeutic index
  - Multiple drug and diet interactions
  - Slow onset of action (peak activity at 72–96 hours)
  - Half-life 40 hours
  - Antidote is vitamin K
  - If severe bleeding or intracranial bleeding and International Normalized Ratio (INR) greater than 1.5, treatment with vitamin K and prothrombin complex concentrate (discussed later) or fresh frozen plasma (FFP) is recommended, followed by repeat INR

Oral Antiplatelet Agents

- For patients on antiplatelet agents with severe bleeding or intracranial bleeding, reversal protocol may include desmopressin and platelet transfusion.
- Aspirin (acetylsalicylic acid [ASA]): irreversible cyclooxygenase (COX) inhibitor, affects COX-1 more than COX-2
  - Broad, well-known indications and variable dosing

- Primary and secondary prevention of stroke and MI
  - Recent studies have questioned utility in primary prevention
- Acute coronary syndrome (ACS)
- Percutaneous coronary intervention (PCI)
- Peripheral vascular disease (PVD)
  ○ Half-life 2 to 4.5 hours with small doses (<250 mg), 15 to 30 hours if greater than 4 g
  ○ Recommend holding 7 days before elective major surgery (unless contraindicated in patient with stent)
- Clopidogrel (Plavix; Bristol-Myers Squibb): irreversible inhibition of ADP receptor, preventing ADP binding and activation of platelets
  ○ Indications: ASA intolerance or failure, primary and secondary prevention of stroke and MI, ACS, PCI, PVD
  ○ Often used in addition to ASA
  ○ Peak effect 6 hours
  ○ Half-life 0.5 hours
  ○ Hold 5 to 7 days before elective procedure or surgery
- Ticagrelor (Brilinta; AstraZeneca): reversible inhibition of ADP receptor, preventing ADP binding and activation of platelets
  ○ Indications: treatment of ACS along with ASA
  ○ Peak effect 2 hours
  ○ Half-life 6 to 9 hours
  ○ Hold 5 days before elective procedure or surgery
- Prasugrel (Effient; Eli Lilly): irreversible inhibition of ADP receptor, preventing ADP binding and activation of platelets
  ○ Indications: treatment of ACS along with ASA for patients undergoing PCI
  ○ Contraindicated in advanced age or history of stroke
  ○ Peak effect 4 hours
  ○ Half-life 2 to 15 hours
  ○ Hold 7 days before elective procedure or surgery
- Ticlopidine (Ticlid): discontinued because of higher risk of thrombotic thrombocytopenic purpura and neutropenia

New Oral Anticoagulants: Target Xa and Thrombin

- More rapid onset of action than warfarin (**Table 1**)[3]
- No diet interactions
- All have drug interactions with P-glycoprotein inducers and inhibitors; rivaroxaban and apixaban additionally interact with drugs affecting cytochrome P 3A4
- Hepatic metabolism, renal and fecal elimination to varying degrees
- High cost
- No specific antidotes
- No long-term safety data
- Some institutions have restricted prescribing authority to select physician groups
- No monitoring required; downside is there is no direct ability to assess therapeutic effect
  ○ Dabigatran causes variable prolongation of the aPTT, variable increase of the INR (not sensitive), and increase in thrombin time (determines whether dabigatran is present but does not help with emergency monitoring)
  ○ Rivaroxaban prolongs aPTT in a dose-dependent fashion (but there is no standard calibration) and increases prothrombin time (PT), although INR is variably affected and not adequate
  ○ Apixaban may prolong aPTT (data are limited) and increases the INR

Table 1
Summary of new oral anticoagulant medications

NOA	Indication	Dosing Frequency	Peak Activity (h)	Half-life (h)
Dabigatran (Pradaxa; Boehringer Ingelheim)	Nonvalvular afib, prevention of VTE in THA, TKA	Twice daily	2–4	12–17
Rivaroxaban (Xarelto; Bayer and Janssen R&D LLC)	Prevention of VTE in THA, TKA, nonvalvular afib, tx of DVT/PE, risk reduction of recurrent VTE	Once daily	2–4	5–9 (9–13 elderly pts)
Apixaban (Eliquis; Pfizer and Bristol-Myers Squibb)	Nonvalvular afib, prevention of VTE in THA, TKA	Twice daily	3–4	10–14

Abbreviations: afib, atrial fibrillation; DVT, deep venous thrombosis; NOA, new oral anticoagulant; pts, patients; THA, total hip arthroplasty; TKA, total knee arthroplasty; tx, treatment.

- Dabigatran (Pradaxa; Boehringer Ingelheim): direct thrombin inhibitor
  - Indications: nonvalvular atrial fibrillation for stroke prevention, primary prevention of venous thromboembolic events in adults after total hip arthroplasty (THA) or total knee arthroplasty (TKA)
  - Patients with unstable INR on warfarin benefit most from dabigatran
  - Recommended dosage is 150 mg twice daily
  - Peak activity at 2 to 4 hours
  - Half-life 12 to 17 hours
  - Rates of major bleeding similar to warfarin; lower overall rate of bleeding events with dabigatran
  - No specific antidote but is reversible via hemodialysis
  - Activated charcoal impairs its absorption if taken within 2 hours of ingestion
- Rivaroxaban (Xarelto; Bayer and Janssen R&D LLC of Johnson & Johnson): inhibits Xa
  - Indications: primary prevention of venous thromboembolic events in adults after THA or TKA, nonvalvular atrial fibrillation for stroke prevention, treatment of deep vein thrombosis (DVT) and PE, reduction of risk of recurrent DVT and PE after initial treatment
  - Recommended dosage is 10 to 20 mg once daily (depending on indication)
  - Peak activity at 2 to 4 hours
  - Half-life 5 to 9 hours (9–13 hours in the elderly)
  - Bleeding rates similar to warfarin
  - No antidote, no reversibility via hemodialysis
- Apixaban (Eliquis; Pfizer and Bristol-Myers Squibb): inhibits Xa
  - Indications: nonvalvular atrial fibrillation for stroke prevention and primary prevention of venous thromboembolic events in adults after THA or TKA
  - Recommended dosage is 5 mg twice daily (less in elderly, low body weight, increased creatinine level)
  - Peak activity at 3 to 4 hours
  - Half-life 10 to 14 hours
  - Bleeding rates similar to aspirin, lower than warfarin
  - No antidote, no reversibility via hemodialysis

Stopping New Oral Anticoagulants Before Elective Surgery

- If possible, most surgeons request new oral anticoagulants to be stopped 1 week before elective procedures. Otherwise, based on creatinine clearance, medications should be stopped 1 to 4 days before the procedure, depending on risk for bleeding complications (**Table 2**).

Nonspecific Reversal Products and Agents May Increase the Risk of Thrombosis

- Recombinant factor VIIa (NovoSeven; Novo Nordisk BDI Pharma)
  - ○ Initiates thrombin formation by activation of factor X
  - ○ Decreases bleeding time in animal models
  - ○ No randomized controlled trials (RCTs), only anecdotal reports
- Activated prothrombin complex concentrate (factor 8 inhibitor bypassing activity; Baxter)
  - ○ Contains nonactivated factors II, IX, and X, and activated factor VII to stimulate thrombin formation
  - ○ No RCTs
- Four-factor prothrombin complex concentrate (Beriplex; CSL Behring)
  - ○ Contains 4 nonactive procoagulant factors (II, IX, X, VII) to stimulate thrombin generation
  - ○ RCT showed normalization of the PT alone for rivaroxaban
- Three-factor prothrombin complex concentrates (Bebulin VH; Baxter and Profilnine SD; Grifols BDI Pharma)
  - ○ Contain 3 nonactive factors (II, IX, X) to stimulate thrombin generation
- FFP
  - ○ 2011 American heart association guidelines recommend this for supportive therapy for patients on dabigatran with severe hemorrhage
  - ○ No evidence to support its use (does not effectively reverse inhibition of coagulation factors)

Developing a Care Pathway

- Consider the team: otolaryngologist, anesthesiologist, pharmacist, nurses, emergency medicine physicians, intensivists, hematologists, or prescribing physicians.
- Value stream mapping: draw out the process for managing patients with critical bleeding who are on anticoagulant medications; identify opportunities for standardization and improvements.
- Consider minor bleeding (symptomatic treatment and short-term withdrawal) versus life-threatening bleeding (aggressive intensive care unit [ICU] treatment, withdrawal of medication, reversal if possible, and blood transfusion as needed).

Table 2
When to discontinue new oral anticoagulant medications before elective procedures

NOA	Cr Cl (mL/min)	Low-risk Procedure	Major Operation (d)
Dabigatran	>50	24 h	2
	31–50	2 d	4
	≤30	4 d	6
Rivaroxaban, apixaban	>30	24 h	2
	≤30	2 d	4

- An example of a clinical pathway for critical bleeding in patients on oral anticoagulants comes from the University of Kentucky and may be found online at: http://www.hosp.uky.edu/pharmacy/formulary/criteria/Critical%20Bleeding%20Reversal%20Protocol.pdf. This pathway is also shown in **Fig. 2**.

QUALITY IN BLOOD TRANSFUSION

Blood is a valuable resource, and cost per unit of blood transfused is high (both in dollar amount and society costs).[4] In addition, the vein-to-vein value stream of blood donation and transfusion is complex and resource intensive. Given these factors, a great deal of attention has been paid to streamlining processes, as well as defining clear indications for the use of valuable blood products. Otolaryngologists have a role in appropriately ordering blood products and understanding the risks and costs associated with transfusion.

The World Health Organization (WHO) has stated that "a quality system [for blood transfusion] should cover all aspects for its activities and ensure traceability... it should also reflect the structure, needs and capabilities of the blood transfusion service, as well as the needs of the hospitals and patients that it serves."[5]

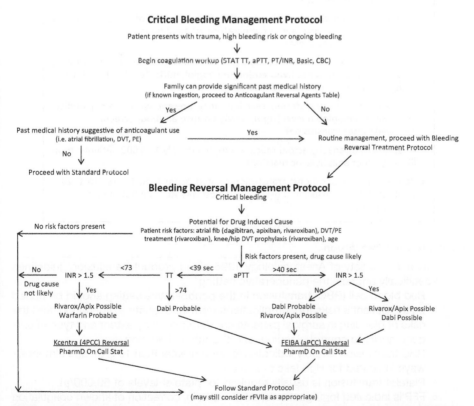

Fig. 2. University of Kentucky critical bleeding reversal protocol. (*Courtesy of* Jeremy Flynn, PharmD, Lexington, KY.)

WHO key elements of quality systems

- Organizational management
- Standards
- Documentation
- Training
- Assessment

Infectious risks of transfusion related to quality of blood product preparation[6]:

- Risk of hepatitis (Hep) B 1 in 282,000
- Risk of Hep C 1 in 1.15 million
- Risk of human immunodeficiency virus 1 in 1.5 million

Noninfectious risks of transfusion

- Urticarial reactions (seen in 1%–3% of patients; presents with rash, pruritus, flushing, mild wheezing)
- Febrile nonhemolytic transfusion reaction (less than 1% of patients; greater than or equal to 2°F increase in temperature within 2 hours; pretreat with acetaminophen if recurrent)
- Acute hemolytic transfusion reaction (1 in 12,000–35,000 per unit transfused; presents with chills, fever, hypotension, hemoglobinuria, renal failure, back pain, disseminated intravascular coagulopathy)
- Delayed hemolytic transfusion reaction (may present with fever, jaundice, decreasing hemoglobin level [Hgb], newly positive antibody screen; 1–2 weeks after transfusion)
- Anaphylaxis or anaphylactoid reaction (approximately 1:50,000 patients; treat like any other anaphylactic reaction)
- Rare severe complications: transfusion-related acute lung injury (10%–20% fatal), transfusion-associated graft-versus-host disease (rare but almost routinely fatal)

Indications for Transfusion

- American Society of Anesthesiology 1996 blood product transfusion guidelines specifically address the perioperative setting[7]
  - Red blood cell (RBC) transfusion in the perioperative setting should be based on the patient's risks for complications from inadequate oxygenation, and the risks of bleeding in surgical patients are determined by extent and type of surgery, ability to control bleeding, and the rate of bleeding
  - RBC transfusion is rarely indicated for Hgb greater than 10 g/dL and almost always indicated for Hgb less than 6 g/dL
  - Platelet transfusion is usually required for platelet levels of 50,000/μL
  - FFP is indicated for urgent reversal of warfarin, correction of known coagulation deficiencies for which specific treatment is not available, and correction of microvascular bleeding when PT and prothrombin time are greater than 1.5 times normal

- o Cryoprecipitate may be indicated in von Willebrand disease (VWD) unresponsive to DDAVP, patients with VWD actively bleeding, and bleeding patients with fibrinogen levels less than 80 to 100 mg/dL
- American Association of Blood Banks guidelines:
  - o Indications for RBC transfusion in adult hemodynamically stable patients[8]
    - ICU patients: Hgb less than or equal to 7 g/dL (high quality of evidence, strong recommendation)
    - Postoperative: Hgb less than or equal to 8 g/dL or for symptoms (high quality of evidence, strong recommendation)
    - Cardiovascular disease: Hgb less than or equal to 8 g/dL or symptoms (moderate quality of evidence, weak recommendation)
  - o Indications for platelet transfusion
    - Neurosurgery or ocular surgery: 100,000/μL
    - Other major surgery: 50,000/μL
    - Endoscopy: 50,000/μL therapeutic procedures; 20,000/μL for low-risk diagnostic procedures
    - Lumbar puncture: 10,000 to 20,000/μL in patients with hematologic malignancies and greater than 40,000 to 50,000/μL in patients without hematologic malignancies
    - Consideration in hematologic malignancies, extracorporeal membrane oxygenation, massive transfusion
  - o Indications for FFP
    - Management of bleeding in patients who require replacement of multiple coagulation factors (eg, disseminated intravascular coagulation, liver disease)
    - Part of massive transfusion protocol
    - Reversal of warfarin
    - Management of patients with rare specific plasma protein deficiencies
  - o Indications for cryoprecipitate
    - Fibrinogen deficiency
    - Factor XIII deficiency when FFP or specific proteins not available
    - Second line for VWD
  - o Special requirements: leukocyte poor, irradiated, cytomegalovirus (CMV) negative
    - Certain populations remain high risk for transfusion-related infectious and noninfectious complications, and blood bank and medical consultants should make recommendations regarding the transfusion of specially prepared blood components for these patients
      - Immunocompromised patients
      - Patients who have recently undergone bone marrow transplantation
      - Patients with congenital immunodeficiency syndromes
      - CMV-seronegative pregnant women
      - Premature infants
- American College of Physicians 2013 guidelines for RBC transfusion for patients with coronary disease[9]
  - o Restrictive transfusion strategy: 7 to 8 g/dL in hospitalized patients with coronary heart disease (low-quality evidence, weak recommendation)
- Transfusion in pediatric patients
  - o Hgb 7 g/dL was shown to be an optimal transfusion threshold for stable, critically ill children[10]
  - o A pediatric specialist can best evaluate a child's overall status and comorbidities to determine individual need for transfusion, as well as volume, rate, and possible alternatives to transfusion

- Transfusion in patients undergoing free tissue reconstruction
  - Consistent with other recommendations, for patients undergoing free flap surgery, a postoperative transfusion threshold of hematocrit less than 25 results in fewer transfusions and no increase in complications[11]
- With regard to wound complications in head and neck surgery, blood loss and blood transfusion were not significant factors on multivariate analysis[12]
- Alternatives to transfusion and blood-sparing techniques are considered elsewhere (see Rabinowitz MR, Cognetti DM, Nyquist GG: Blood-sparing techniques, in this issue).

DEVELOPING A QUALITY PLAN FOR HEMOSTASIS AND TRANSFUSION

Quality improvement plans may take place at the individual surgeon level, group practice level, or systems-based level. When considering quality, surgeons should consider the ability to measure a meaningful outcome and the ability to implement change. There is no single approach to developing a quality system or plan, but there are tools and processes that are easily accessible that may help in the endeavor.

- Lean thinking: maximize value for the patient while minimizing waste
  - A systems-based quality improvement strategy with a proven track record in health care[13]
    - Emphasizes purpose, process, and people
    - Requires a culture of innovation and improvement
    - Requires accountability but not blame
    - Gemba: leaders must go to the site where activity occurs, see the work, and empower those involved in the process to solve problems
    - Define value from the perspective of the end user (the patient)
    - Map the value stream (all activities of a process) and then the ideal state (without the existing waste)
    - Define the gap between actual and ideal and then set a measurable goal
    - Pilot the changes (test the hypothesis) on a small scale
    - Engage in the PDSA (Plan, Do, Study, Act) iterative process
      - Accept failure but analyze, revise, try again
      - Expand scope with successes (link improvements to further change opportunities)
- Possible metrics for individuals or systems: blood loss in specific cases, rates of transfusion for specific cases, rates of preoperative type and screen and complete blood count tests, number of critical bleeding events and success in management (define success), use of hemostatic agents, units of blood or supplies wasted (expired or other), number of steps in the transfusion process, numbers of errors in ordering products, number of unindicated transfusions
- Analysis tools: visualize the data
  - Time series plots (show results over time)
  - Box plots (help to identify outliers)
  - Control charts (help to visualize patterns of variation in results)
  - Bar graphs and pie charts (show relative percentages, results in quartiles or larger groupings of time)
  - Flow charts (visually show the steps in a process)
  - Root cause analysis
    - Fishbone (cause and effect) diagrams
      - Take into account multiple possible contributors to a problem
        - Environment

- ○ Equipment
- ○ People
- ○ Measurement
- ○ Methods
- ○ Materials
- ■ Five Whys
  - • Requires asking "why" until the root cause is identified
- • Implementation tools
  - ○ Checklists: useful for complex critical processes
  - ○ Gantt charts: allow visualization of implementation activities in bar chart format over time (including start date, duration, and end date); helps with accountability
  - ○ Outcomes: results must be measured and displayed/shared
  - ○ Communication tools
    - ■ Understand your audience/team and their motivations
    - ■ Respect the knowledge and skills of team members, acknowledging these out loud
    - ■ Ask open-ended questions (no leading questions)
    - ■ Set clear expectations
      - • Clearly define the timeline for implementation and the metrics that will be used
    - ■ Standard A3 (11.7 × 16.5 inch) paper is used in lean thinking to depict a problem with its associated background, analysis, goal statement, and possible and recommended countermeasures (interventions for improvement); often handwritten and meant to be shared with others during the problem definition, analysis, and intervention process

SUMMARY

This article reviews the definition of health care quality, and discusses the data regarding anticoagulant medications (particularly new oral anticoagulants) and guidelines for blood product transfusion. A brief outline of quality tools is provided to help otolaryngologists create quality plans for themselves and their institutions/systems.

Post-Test Questions (Correct answers are in italics)

1. What is health care quality?
   a. *Doing the right thing at the right time in the right way to achieve the best possible results, avoiding underuse, avoiding overuse, and eliminating misuse*
   b. Doing procedures that you think could be right, using available resources
   c. Keeping current standards because they have been working well all along
2. What can be done for reversal of dabigatran (Pradaxa) taken 4 hours earlier?
   a. Vitamin K
   b. Nothing
   c. *Hemodialysis*
   d. Activated charcoal
3. Which of the following is an indication for RBC transfusion?
   a. Hgb of 7.5 g/dL in a stable, otherwise healthy postoperative patient with no ongoing bleeding
   b. Hgb of 7.5 g/dL in a stable pediatric ICU patient
   c. *Hgb of 7.5 g/dL in a postoperative patient with known coronary disease and chest pain who continues to have epistaxis*

4. Which of the following is an indication for transfusion of platelets?
   a. Platelet count of 80,000/μL in a patient undergoing maxillary antrostomy and ethmoidectomy
   b. *Platelet count of 80,000/μL in a patient undergoing resection of a sinonasal malignancy via an expanded endonasal approach including dural resection*
   c. Platelet count of 80,000/μL in a patient undergoing thyroidectomy
5. Which of the following is an implementation tool for quality improvement projects, allowing visualization of the timeline of all steps in the project?
   a. Box plot
   b. *Gantt chart*
   c. Gemba
   d. Five Whys

SUPPLEMENTARY DATA

Supplementary PDF slides related to this article can be found online at http://www.oto.theclinics.com/.

REFERENCES

1. Committee on the Quality of Health Care in America. Crossing the quality chasm: a new health system for the 21st century. Washington, DC: National Academy Press; 2001.
2. AHRQ Web site: http://www.ahrq.gov/. Accessed December 3, 2014.
3. Gonsalves WI, Pruthi RK, Patnaik MM. The new oral anticoagulants in clinical practice. Mayo Clin Proc 2013;88(5):495–511. Available at: http://www.mayoclinicproceedings.org/article/S0025-6196(13)00222-X/pdf.
4. Shander A, Hofmann A, Gombotz H, et al. Estimating the cost of blood: past, present, and future directions. Best Pract Res Clin Anaesthesiol 2007;21(2):271–89.
5. World Health Organization Web site. http://www.who.int/bloodsafety/quality/en/.
6. Weinstein R. Red blood cell transfusion pocket guide. Washington, DC: American Society of Hematology; 2012. Available at: www.hematology.org/practiceguidelines.
7. Practice guidelines for blood component therapy: a report by the American Society of Anesthesiologists Task Force on Blood Component Therapy. Anesthesiology 1996;84(3):732.
8. Carson JL, Grossman BJ, Kleinman S, et al. Red blood cell transfusion: a clinical practice guideline from the AABB. Ann Intern Med 2012;157(1):49–58.
9. Qaseem A, Humphrey LL, Fitterman N, et al. Treatment of anemia in patients with heart disease: a clinical practice guideline from the American College of Physicians. Ann Intern Med 2013;159(11):770–9.
10. Lacroix J, Hebert PC, Hutchison JS, et al. Transfusion strategies for patients in pediatric intensive care units. N Engl J Med 2007;356(16):1609–19.
11. Rossmiller SR, Cannady SB, Ghanem TA, et al. Transfusion criteria in free flap surgery. Otolaryngol Head Neck Surg 2010;142(3):359–64.
12. Chaukar DA, Deshmukh AD, Majeed T, et al. Factors affecting wound complications in head and neck surgery: a prospective study. Indian J Med Paediatr Oncol 2013;34(4):247–51.
13. Going Lean in Health Care. IHI Innovation Series white paper. Cambridge, MA: Institute for Healthcare Improvement; 2005. Available at: www.IHI.org.

SUGGESTED READINGS

Gonsalves WI, Pruthi RK, Patnaik MM. The New Oral Anticoagulants in Clinical Practice. Mayo Clin Proc 2013;88(5):495–511.

This article concisely reviews the new oral anticoagulants (NOAs), summarizing the indications for NOAs, the results of large clinical trials, issues of bleeding management, and overall recommendations for use.

Shander A, Hofmann A, Gombotz H, et al. Estimating the cost of blood: past, present, and future directions. Best Pract Res Clin Anaesthesiol 2007;21(2):271–89.

This article discusses the complexity of estimating the cost of blood transfusion, and though this more relates to value than directly to quality, it provokes thoughts about the blood value stream and possible metrics for improvement.

Weinstein R. Red Blood Cell Transfusion Pocket Guide. American Society of Hematology; 2012. Available at: www.hematology.org/practiceguidelines.

This is a concise, easy to read, 3-page reference guide for red blood cell transfusion.

Institute for Healthcare Improvement. Going lean in healthcare. Institute for Healthcare Improvement White Paper; 2005.

This is a brief introduction to Lean and a description of its success in healthcare.

Hemostatic Materials and Devices

Henry P. Barham, MD[a,b,*], Raymond Sacks, MD[c,d], Richard J. Harvey, MD, PhD[b,c,e]

KEYWORDS

- Hemostatic • Sinus • Skull base • Materials • Vasoconstrictors • Topical • Agents

KEY LEARNING POINTS

At the end of this article, the reader will:

- Appreciate why bleeding is a problem in endoscopic sinus and skull base surgery.
- Understand the reasons for avoiding traditional nasal packing after endoscopic nasal surgery.
- Be familiar with the evolution of materials and devices in endoscopic sinus and skull base surgery.
- Be able to discuss the benefits and drawbacks of topical materials in use today.
- Be able to apply appropriate mechanisms to avoid bleeding in sinus and skull base surgery.

INTRODUCTION

Functional endoscopic sinus and skull base surgery has become an effective part of the management of chronic rhinosinusitis and tumors of the sinuses and anterior skull base. Technologic advances have been critical in advancing endoscopic surgical procedures, with the introduction of improved optics and lighting, advanced instrumentation, and image-guided surgical navigation. Hemostatic materials and devices have similarly evolved to assist in the management of the surgical field and the postoperative cavity.

[a] Department of Otolaryngology Head and Neck Surgery, LSUHSC SOM, Louisiana State University, 533 Bolivar Street, Suite 566, New Orleans, LA 70112, USA; [b] Rhinology and Skull Base Research Group, St Vincent's Centre for Applied Medical Research, University of New South Wales, Sydney, Australia; [c] Department of Otolaryngology, Australian School of Advanced Medicine, Macquarie University, Sydney, Australia; [d] Department of Otolaryngology, University of Sydney, Sydney, Australia; [e] Department of Otolaryngology, St Vincent's Centre for Applied Medical Research, University of New South Wales, Sydney, Australia
* Corresponding author. Department of Otolaryngology, LSUHSC SOM, 533 Bolivar Street, Suite 566, New Orleans, LA 70112.
E-mail address: hpbarham@hotmail.com

Otolaryngol Clin N Am 49 (2016) 577–584
http://dx.doi.org/10.1016/j.otc.2016.02.002
0030-6665/16/$ – see front matter © 2016 Elsevier Inc. All rights reserved.

oto.theclinics.com

DISCUSSION

Why is bleeding a problem in endoscopic sinus and skull base surgery?
• Decreased visualization can increase the risk of injury
• Early termination of surgery secondary to poor visualization
• Readmission or reoperation for the treatment of epistaxis

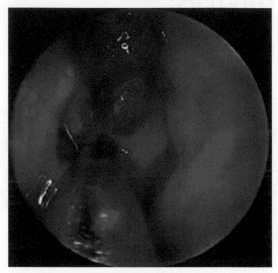

Fig. 1. Endoscopic bloody field.

Hemostasis, both during and after endoscopic procedures, is critical for successful outcomes.[1,2] Intraoperative bleeding, especially in the setting of highly vascular sinonasal tumors and polyposis, remains a common pitfall in performing endoscopic sinus and skull base surgery (**Fig. 1**). Although endoscopic bipolar forceps; suction cautery; and newer technologies, such as radiofrequency coblation, are indispensable for producing intraoperative hemostasis, various topical agents are also effective in controlling diffuse bleeding and, in some cases, also provide postoperative benefits.

Bleeding prevention
• Patient positioning
• Proper surgical technique
• Vasoconstriction

The primary modality to achieve hemostasis in surgery is the prevention of bleeding. The 3 steps to improve the ability to prevent bleeding are patient positioning, proper surgical technique with avoidance of stripped mucosa, and vasoconstriction. The patient's head should be placed in the neutral anatomic position and the operative bed placed in 15° to 20° reverse Trendelenburg with total intravenous anesthesia.[3] Proper surgical technique cannot be overemphasized to avoid nuisance bleeding. The stripping of mucosa causes oozing, which decreases visualization and is not amenable to topical vasoconstrictors. If persistent bleeding occurs in the absence of mucosal stripping, vasoconstrictors have an important role in endoscopic sinus and skull base surgery.

Adrenaline

- Topical and injectable preparations
- Excellent hemostatic ability
- Potential for cardiac complications

Epinephrine has been used as a hemostatic agent in various surgical procedures for many years both in topical and injectable preparations. It is inexpensive and has excellent hemostatic properties.[4] The major drawback to its use is the potential for cardiac complications, including tachycardia, arrhythmias, hypotension, or hypertension.[5] Hypertension and tachycardia historically are the most commonly observed complications.[6] Recently, use of topical epinephrine in endoscopic sinus and skull base surgery has experienced resurgence because topical preparations provide excellent hemostasis and greatly decrease the potential for cardiac complications.

The authors' practice routinely uses epinephrine with Naropin (anesthetic benefit)-soaked cotton pledgets to aid with hemostasis. Our preferred concentration is 1:2000, which provides excellent hemostasis with limited side effects. A prospective study evaluating varying concentrations of topical adrenaline, including 1:2000, 1:10,000, and 1:50,000, showed that the 1:2000 group had a statistically significant decrease in blood loss and shorter operative times.[7]

Why should traditional nasal packing be avoided after endoscopic nasal surgery?

- Immediate problems include pain, rhinorrhea, infection, sensation of pressure, alar necrosis, and nasal obstruction
- Packing removal caries a risk of epistaxis
- Significant subjective decrease in surgical experience for the patient

Nasal packing with gauze was routinely used in the postoperative care of the nasal cavity but carries significant drawbacks. Packing can result in pain, rhinorrhea, infection, nasal obstruction, sensation of pressure, alar necrosis, and epistaxis on removal.[8–12] Packing and the removal thereof has been reported as the most uncomfortable portion of the perioperative experience.[11]

HOW HAVE MATERIALS AND DEVICES IN ENDOSCOPIC SINUS AND SKULL BASE SURGERY EVOLVED?

Nasal packing was historically the workhorse of hemostasis control in the postoperative cavity but caries significant risks. To move away from these inherent risks, topical materials that have absorbable properties or aid with hemostasis have become increasingly popular to help improve patient comfort, avoid the need for removal, and assist with healing. Although there are multiple products available (**Table 1**), no single product provides a perfect solution to assist in postoperative care.[13]

Table 1
Absorbable hemostatic agents

Name	Composition	Hemostatic Ability	Scar Potential	Stent Ability
Tranexamic acid (Cyklokapron)	NA	Fair	Low	NA
Epsilon-aminocaproic acid (Amicar)	NA	Poor	Low	NA
FloSeal	Bovine gelatin + thrombin	Excellent	High	Fair
Surgiflo	Porcine gelatin	Good	Moderate	Fair
Sepragel	Cross-linked hyaluronic acid molecule	Fair	Low	Good
MeroGel	Hyaluronic acid ester	Fair	Low–high	Good
Seprapack	Hyaluron and carboxymethylcellulose	Fair	Low	Good
Microporous polysaccharide hemospheres (MPH)	Purified potato starch	Good	Low	Fair

Abbreviation: NA, not applicable.
Data from Virgin FW, Bleier BS, Woodworth BA. Evolving materials and techniques for endoscopic sinus surgery. Otolaryngol Clin North Am 2010;43(3):653–72, xi.

WHAT ARE THE BENEFITS AND DRAWBACKS OF TOPICAL MATERIALS IN USE TODAY?

Antifibrinolytics

- Tranexamic acid (TA; Cyklokapron) and epsilon-aminocaproic acid (EACA; Amicar)
- TA has fair hemostatic ability with improved surgical field
- Prevent the stabilization of blood clots

EACA (Amicar, Lederle Parenterals, Inc, Caroline, Puerto Rico) and TA; (Cyklokapron, Pfizer, Puurs, Belgium) are antifibrinolytics that competitively bind to lysine-binding sites on plasminogen, prevent the binding of plasminogen to fibrin, and prevent the transformation to plasmin. This action prevents fibrinolysis and stabilization of blood clots.

The hemostatic effects of EACA and TA have been evaluated during endoscopic sinus surgery, using standardized videoendoscopy and grading scales.[14] The use of topical TA resulted in improved surgical field bleeding, whereas no significant improvements were found with EACA.

Floseal

- Bovine gelatin particles plus thrombin
- Excellent hemostatic ability
- High risk of adhesions/scarring

FloSeal (Baxter Healthcare Corporation, Fremont, CA) is composed of bovine gelatin particles and thrombin, and can be injected topically to assist in hemostasis with essentially no risk of patient discomfort.[15] The major drawback to its use is increased risk of adhesions potentially causing obstruction of sinus outflow tracts and the need for revision surgery.[16–18]

Surgiflo

- Porcine gelatin plus thrombin
- Good hemostatic ability
- Low to moderate risk of adhesions/scarring

Surgiflo hemostatic matrix (Ethicon, Inc, West Sommerville, NJ) is composed of porcine gelatin combined with Thrombin-JMI (King Pharmaceuticals, Inc, Bristol, TN) and can also be injected topically to conform to an irregular wound bed. It provides good hemostasis with only moderate risk of adhesions. One multicenter, prospective study showed no evidence of synechiae, adhesions, or infections.[19]

Sepragel

- Cross-linked hyaluronic acid molecule
- Fair hemostatic ability
- Decrease in adhesions

Sepragel (Genzyme Biosurgery, Cambridge, MA) is a hylan B gel composed of a cross-linked hyaluronic acid molecule that can be injected topically into the nasal cavity after endoscopic sinus surgery. Hemostatic ability is considered fair, whereas significant evidence of its hemostatic properties is not available. Its benefits include a decrease in middle meatal stenosis and synechiae formation, and that it requires no postoperative removal.[20]

MeroGel

- Polyvinyl acetal sponge that is composed of hyaluronic acid ester derivative
- Fair hemostatic ability but standard for comparison
- Nonabsorbable

MeroGel (Medtronic-Xomed, Jacksonville, FL) is a nonabsorbable, porous, polyvinyl acetal sponge that is composed of hyaluronic acid ester derivative. It was one of the first absorbable materials used as a hemostatic agent and middle meatal stent and is often considered a standard against which newer materials are compared. When compared with traditional packing, MeroGel is associated with an improved postoperative endoscopic appearance, fewer adhesions, and improved patient comfort.[21]

Seprapack

- Hyaluronic acid and carboxymethyl cellulose
- Fair hemostasis ability, primary use as spacer
- Reduces postoperative debridement

Seprapack (Genzyme, Cambridge, MA) is composed of hyaluronic acid and carboxymethyl cellulose. It is packaged as a solid wafer that is inserted into the middle meatus and converted into a gel with saline irrigation. Its major advantage is as a spacer, because it carries only fair hemostatic ability. Fewer adhesions are seen at 2 weeks postoperatively compared with traditional packing, reducing the need for postoperative debridement.[22]

Microporous polysaccharide hemospheres (MPH)

- Product of purified potato starch
- Good hemostatic ability
- Decreases duration of healing and return to baseline

MPH (Medafor, Inc, Minneapolis, MN) are fully resorbable particles produced from purified potato starch that act as a sieve to extract fluids from blood. The absorption of fluid causes the particles to swell and concentrate serum proteins and platelets on their surfaces, creating a scaffolding for fibrin clot formation. In an animal model (rabbit) comparing MPH with FloSeal, at 2 weeks postoperatively the MPH group showed no residual substance and a return to baseline healing state, whereas the FloSeal group showed cilia loss, inflammation, and fibrosis.[23]

AUTHORS' INSIGHTS

Although a magnitude of absorbable materials have been created and are readily used to assist in hemostasis, no single product currently provides a perfect solution. In the event of postoperative bleeding, a low threshold for early evaluation and intervention should be used. There is no evidence that topical cooling devices or dietary modification affect the regional distribution of the external carotid artery and alter the course of bleeding. Appropriate surgical mucosal sparing techniques and simplicity of the material used seem to be current answers to improve patient comfort, avoid the need for removal, and assist with healing and postoperative care.

SUMMARY

Numerous absorbable substances have been introduced to aid hemostasis in sinus and skull base surgery. Within the confines of the sinus and nasal cavities, ideal hemostatic agents must have several qualities. They must provide hemostasis, conform to an irregular wound bed, and enable healing of the traumatized mucosa without additional detriment to the epithelium. Traditional nasal packing has been substituted largely by absorbable materials designed to improve patient comfort and outcomes. Although many promising agents exist, none have become standard therapy.

Post-Test Questions (Correct answers are in italics)

1. Which of the following is not a risk of bleeding in endoscopic sinus surgery?
   a. Early termination of surgery secondary to poor visualization
   b. *Improved visualization with the endoscope*
   c. Increased risk of injury secondary to decreased visualization
   d. Readmission secondary to epistaxis
2. Routine postoperative nasal packing with gauze can:
   a. Decrease postoperative pain
   b. *Cause rhinorrhea, infection, and alar necrosis*
   c. Improve the overall patient experience
   d. Decrease postoperative adhesions
   e. Reduce the risk of bleeding
3. Which of the following is correct regarding the use of FloSeal in the postoperative nasal cavity?
   a. It is composed of porcine gelatin
   b. It is associated with fair hemostatic abilities
   c. *It is associated with a high scarring/synechia potential*
   d. It is delivered via a nonabsorbable pack
   e. It can be used effectively in patients with platelet dysfunction
4. Which of the following is not a technique to prevent bleeding?
   a. Mucosa-sparing surgery
   b. Topical vasoconstrictors (epinephrine)
   c. *Topical ice packs on the neck perioperatively*
   d. Head positioning of 15° to 20° reverse Trendelenburg

REFERENCES

1. Kennedy DW. Technical innovations and the evolution of endoscopic sinus surgery. Ann Otol Rhinol Laryngol Suppl 2006;196:3–12.
2. Senior BA, Kennedy DW, Tanabodee J, et al. Long-term results of functional endoscopic sinus surgery. Laryngoscope 1998;108(2):151–7.
3. Gan EC, Habib AR, Rajwani A, et al. Five-degree, 10-degree, and 20-degree reverse Trendelenburg position during functional endoscopic sinus surgery: a double-blind randomized controlled trial. Int Forum Allergy Rhinol 2014;4(1): 61–8.
4. Valdes CJ, Bogado M, Rammal A, et al. Topical cocaine vs adrenaline in endoscopic sinus surgery: a blinded randomized controlled study. Int Forum Allergy Rhinol 2014;4(8):646–50.
5. Anderhuber W, Walch C, Nemeth E, et al. Plasma adrenaline concentrations during functional endoscopic sinus surgery. Laryngoscope 1999;109(2 Pt 1):204–7.
6. O'Malley TP, Postma GN, Holtel M, et al. Effect of local epinephrine on cutaneous bloodflow in the human neck. Laryngoscope 1995;105(2):140–3.
7. Sarmento Junior KM, Tomita S, Kós AO. Topical use of adrenaline in different concentrations for endoscopic sinus surgery. Braz J Otorhinolaryngol 2009;75(2): 280–9.
8. Civelek B, Kargi AE, Sensoz O, et al. Rare complication of nasal packing: alar region necrosis. Otolaryngol Head Neck Surg 2000;123(5):656–7.

9. Johannessen N, Jensen PF, Kristensen S, et al. Nasal packing and nocturnal oxygen desaturation. Acta Otolaryngol Suppl 1992;492:6–8.
10. Vaiman M, Eviatar E, Shlamkovich N, et al. Use of fibrin glue as a hemostatic in endoscopic sinus surgery. Ann Otol Rhinol Laryngol 2005;114(3):237–41.
11. von Schoenberg M, Robinson P, Ryan R. Nasal packing after routine nasal surgery–is it justified? J Laryngol Otol 1993;107(10):902–5.
12. Weber R, Hochapfel F, Draf W. Packing and stents in endonasal surgery. Rhinology 2000;38(2):49–62.
13. Virgin FW, Bleier BS, Woodworth BA. Evolving materials and techniques for endoscopic sinus surgery. Otolaryngol Clin North Am 2010;43(3):653–72, xi.
14. Athanasiadis T, Beule AG, Wormald PJ. Effects of topical antifibrinolytics in endoscopic sinus surgery: a pilot randomized controlled trial. Am J Rhinol 2007;21(6):737–42.
15. Jameson M, Gross CW, Kountakis SE. FloSeal use in endoscopic sinus surgery: effect on postoperative bleeding and synechiae formation. Am J Otolaryngol 2006;27(2):86–90.
16. Chandra RK, Conley DB, Haines GK 3rd, et al. Long-term effects of FloSeal packing after endoscopic sinus surgery. Am J Rhinol 2005;19(3):240–3.
17. Chandra RK, Conley DB, Kern RC. The effect of FloSeal on mucosal healing after endoscopic sinus surgery: a comparison with thrombin-soaked gelatin foam. Am J Rhinol 2003;17(1):51–5.
18. Shrime MG, Tabaee A, Hsu AK, et al. Synechia formation after endoscopic sinus surgery and middle turbinate medialization with and without FloSeal. Am J Rhinol 2007;21(2):174–9.
19. Woodworth BA, Chandra RK, LeBenger JD, et al. A gelatin-thrombin matrix for hemostasis after endoscopic sinus surgery. Am J Otolaryngol 2009;30(1):49–53.
20. Kimmelman CP, Edelstein DR, Cheng HJ. Sepragel sinus (hylan B) as a postsurgical dressing for endoscopic sinus surgery. Otolaryngol Head Neck Surg 2001;125(6):603–8.
21. Wormald PJ, Boustred RN, Le T, et al. A prospective single-blind randomized controlled study of use of hyaluronic acid nasal packs in patients after endoscopic sinus surgery. Am J Rhinol 2006;20(1):7–10.
22. Woodworth BA, Chandra RK, Hoy MJ, et al. Randomized controlled trial of hyaluronic acid/carboxymethylcellulose dressing after endoscopic sinus surgery. ORL J Otorhinolaryngol Relat Spec 2010;72(2):101–5.
23. Antisdel JL, Janney CG, Long JP, et al. Hemostatic agent microporous polysaccharide hemospheres (MPH) does not affect healing or intact sinus mucosa. Laryngoscope 2008;118(7):1265–9.

SUGGESTED READINGS

Gunaratne DA, Barham HP, Christensen JM, et al. Topical concentrated epinephrine (1:1000) does not cause acute cardiovascular changes during endoscopic sinus surgery. Int Forum Allergy Rhinol 2016;6(2):135–9.

Kassam A, Snyderman CH, Carrau RL, et al. Endoneurosurgical hemostasis techniques: lessons learned from 400 cases. Neurosurg Focus 2005;19(1):E7.

Vaz-Guimaraes F, Su SY, Fernandez-Miranda JC, et al. Hemostasis in endoscopic endonasal skull base surgery. J Neurol Surg B Skull Base 2015;76(4):296–302.

Surgical Adhesives in Facial Plastic Surgery

Dean M. Toriumi, MD[a],*, Victor K. Chung, MD[b], Quintin M. Cappelle, MD[a]

KEYWORDS

- Hemostasis • Fibrin tissue adhesive • Fibrin glue • Facial plastic surgery
- Rhytidectomy • Skin grafts • Forehead lift

KEY LEARNING POINTS

At the end of this article, the reader will:

- Know when surgical adhesives are useful in facial plastic procedures.
- Be able to identify which step in the coagulation cascade fibrin tissue adhesives replicate.
- Know the potential risks of homologous fibrin tissue adhesives.
- Know which factors influence the efficacy of fibrin tissue adhesives.
- Be able to identify the indications for fibrin tissue adhesives in facial plastic surgery.
- Know the advantages and disadvantages of the different methods of application.
- Know the key steps for application of fibrin tissue adhesives in facial plastic procedures.

INTRODUCTION

Why is bleeding a problem in facial plastic surgery?
• Skin flap injury from cautery
• Extended operating time
• Delayed wound healing
• Poor aesthetic outcome
• Return to operating room

Surgical bleeding should be anticipated and controlled in facial plastic surgery. Excessive bleeding and accumulation of blood can inhibit optimal healing, resulting in poor outcomes. Aesthetic surgery patients are concerned with prolonged downtime secondary to postoperative edema and ecchymosis. Surgeons typically limit

[a] Division of Facial Plastic and Reconstructive Surgery, Department of Otolaryngology-Head and Neck Surgery, University of Illinois at Chicago, Chicago, IL, USA; [b] La Jolla Facial Plastic Surgery, San Diego, CA 92130, USA
* Corresponding author. 1855 West Taylor Street, 2nd Floor, Chicago, IL 60612.
E-mail address: dtoriumi@uic.edu

Otolaryngol Clin N Am 49 (2016) 585–599
http://dx.doi.org/10.1016/j.otc.2016.02.012
0030-6665/16/$ – see front matter © 2016 Elsevier Inc. All rights reserved.

electrocautery of superficial tissues, as it might injure the skin flap. Gaining hemostasis without electrocautery may extend operating time. Accumulation of postoperative bleeding may necessitate an emergent return to the operating room. In facial plastic surgery, surgical adhesives can be used to improve hemostasis and outcomes.

SURGICAL TISSUE ADHESIVES

Categories of surgical tissue adhesives

- Cyanoacrylates
- Fibrin tissue adhesives

When discussing surgical adhesives, both categories, cyanoacrylates and fibrin tissue adhesives, are frequently grouped together and considered the same product; however, the inherent properties of each provide important distinctions for their appropriate use. It should be clear that they have separate indications that do not overlap in application.

Cyanoacrylates

- Superficial wound closure
- No hemostatic property, only a tissue adhesive
- Elicit foreign body reaction when placed subdermally
- Longer-chain derivatives have decreased toxicity
- For example, Dermabond (Ethicon, Somerville, NJ)

During the development of cyanoacrylates, it was recognized that although they bonded and sealed tissue well, early cyanoacrylates generated a long-lasting inflammatory reaction within the body. By increasing the chain length of the molecule, the tissue reactivity decreased. These longer chain lengths can now be tolerated on the epidermis, but foreign body reactions still occur when cyanoacrylates are deposited below the dermis. Furthermore, this category of surgical adhesive has no hemostatic properties, limiting its application to superficial wound closure in facial plastic surgery (**Fig. 1**).[1]

Fibrin tissue adhesives

- Mechanism of action occurs on the coagulation cascade, replicating the body's natural hemostasis pathway
- Conversion of fibrinogen to fibrin initiates clot formation
- Fibrin tissue adhesives are composed of 2 components that activate when mixed together

---

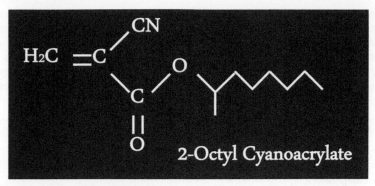

Fig. 1. Cyanoacrylate chemical formula.

Fibrin tissue adhesives, however, do have hemostatic properties. The body has an excellent mechanism to achieve blood clot formation. Blood clot formation occurs through the coagulation cascade of clotting factors within the blood plasma. The final result of that pathway is the conversion of the inactive fibrinogen to the active fibrin, which is one of the main components of clots. The 2 components of fibrin tissue adhesives take advantage of this physiology. To understand fibrin tissue adhesives' mechanisms of action, an understanding of the body's natural coagulation cascade must be reviewed.[1]

Coagulation pathway

- Extrinsic and intrinsic pathways give way to the common pathway
- The last step in the common pathway is the conversion of fibrinogen to fibrin
- Fibrinogen in the plasma is converted to fibrin in the presence of thrombin and calcium chloride
- Factor XIII catalyzes fibrin molecules to cross-link to form a clot

---

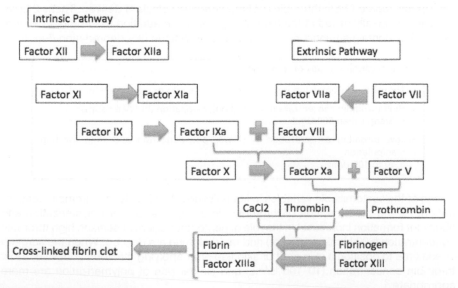

Fig. 2. Coagulation pathway.

As seen in **Fig. 2**, the extrinsic and intrinsic pathways converge into the common pathway. Fibrinogen is circulating within the plasma at baseline. When fibrinogen is in the presence of thrombin and calcium chloride, either endogenously or exogenously, it is converted to fibrin. Fibrin tissue adhesives take advantage of this natural pathway by supplying the coenzymes/factors necessary to complete the final steps of native coagulation. By activating a natural process, fibrin tissue adhesives artificially induce cross-linking and clot formation.[1]

Fibrin tissue adhesive components

- Component 1
  - Fibrinogen, calcium chloride, factor XIII
- Component 2
  - Thrombin and antifibrinolytic agent

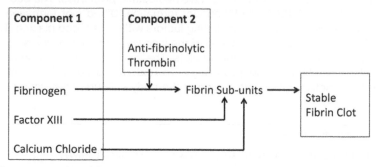

Fig. 3. Components 1 and 2.

Fibrin tissue adhesives contain exactly what is needed in clot formation. The catalysts (thrombin, calcium chloride, and factor XIII) convert the substrate (fibrinogen) into its stable product (cross-linked fibrin). In reactions, the substrate and catalysts are stored as separate components to prevent preemptive interaction. Fibrinogen must be kept segregated from thrombin until the time hemostasis is desired. These 2 components are ideally mixed at the time of application. In addition to thrombin, component 2 may contain an antifibrinolytic agent to slow fibrin clot degradation (**Fig. 3**).[1,2]

Optimal concentrations of thrombin

- Thrombin concentration is proportional to the rate of polymerization
- High thrombin concentration = rapid polymerization and hemostasis
  - Greater than 500 U/mL
- Low thrombin concentration = slower polymerization and time for flap manipulation
  - 10 to 100 U/mL

One of the customizable variables in fibrin tissue adhesives is the thrombin concentration. As the concentration of thrombin increases, the rate of polymerization and fibrin clot formation increases. In the role of hemostatic agent or sealant, high thrombin concentration (500 U/mL or greater) and rapid clotting are desired. When the surgeon needs time to position a skin graft or skin flap after applying the fibrin adhesive, a low thrombin concentration (10–100 U/mL) and slower rate of polymerization are more appropriate.[2]

Methods of application

• Single-barrel syringe
  ○ Less uniform mixing
  ○ Cumbersome
 	
• Double-barrel syringe
  ○ Clogging issues
 	
• Gas-pressurized spray
  ○ Requires pressurized air source
  ○ Increased expense

Another variable is how the product is applied to the tissues. Of the available fibrin tissue delivery systems, sequential delivery of components 1 and 2 from 2 single-barrel syringes is the simplest. Less uniform mixing of the components and clumsy handling of multiple syringes limit this technique. A double-barrel syringe, such as Duploject (Immuno AG, Vienna, Austria), improves uniform mixing; however, early mixing and stasis result in clogging of the applicator needle. The aerosol spray device in **Fig. 4** uses a pressurized gas stream at 5 to 10 L/min to maximally mix and evenly distribute the fibrin tissue adhesive. With a pressure-assisted system, the surgeon can achieve efficient mixing and, as a result, maximal strength of the glue with minimal volume (**Fig. 4**).[1,2]

Autologous fibrin tissue adhesives

• Patient's own blood, autologous
  ○ Collected preoperatively
  ○ No risk of disease transmission or immune reaction
 	
• Centrifugation isolates the platelet-rich plasma layer
  ○ Fibrinogen collected at a natural concentration
 	
• Combined with premade mixture of thrombin-calcium chloride
  ○ Low risk of factor V cross-reactivity with bovine thrombin
 	
• Selphyl device (Aesthetic Factors, LLC, Princeton, NJ)

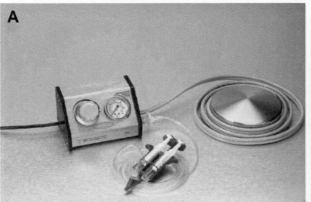
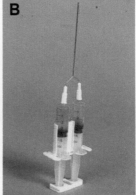

Fig. 4. (*A*) Aerosol spray device. (*B*) Double barrel syringe. (*From* Mobley SR, Hilinski J, Toriumi D. Surgical tissue adhesives. Facial Plast Surg Clin N Am 2002;10:147–54; with permission.)

Within fibrin tissue adhesives, there are 2 derivatives: autologous and homologous. The advantage of an autologous hemostatic agent is no risk of immune reaction or contraction of blood-borne pathogens from donors. Venipuncture is performed preoperatively, and the collected blood is centrifuged to isolate the fibrinogen containing platelet-rich plasma layer. Selphyl (Aesthetic Factors, LLC, Princeton, NJ) is an example of a device designed for this process. At the time of application, the autologous fibrinogen is combined with a prefabricated mixture of thrombin and calcium chloride. Disadvantages of autologous fibrin tissue adhesives include additional time needed to collect and prepare the product, low risk of factor V cross-reactivity with bovine thrombin, and functional limitations inherent to the patient's own clotting ability (**Fig. 5**).[2,3]

Homologous fibrin tissue adhesives

- Pooled donors, homologous
- Greater concentration of fibrinogen compared with platelet-rich plasma
- Identical substrates of fibrinogen, thrombin, calcium chloride, factor XIII
- Theoretic risks associated with homologous products (transmission of human immunodeficiency virus [HIV] and hepatitis)
- For example, Tisseel and Artiss (Baxter Healthcare Corp, Deerfield, IL); Evicel (formerly Crosseel; Omrix Biopharmaceuticals, Israel)

Homologous products are different from autologous in a few distinctions. Homologous fibrin tissue adhesives are produced by pooling multiple donors' blood. The substrates of homologous and autologous products are the same: fibrinogen, thrombin, calcium chloride, and factor XIII. However, with a larger blood source, the homologous fibrinogen can be condensed to achieve greater concentrations for a proposed more effective hemostasis. Because the blood is coming from other human beings, homologous products have the theoretic risk of transmitting blood-borne pathogens such as

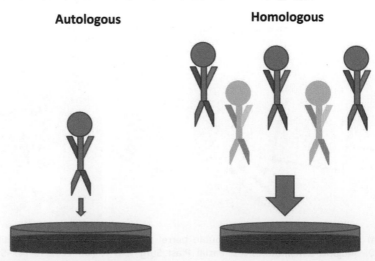

Autologous   **Homologous**

Fig. 5. Autologous versus homologous.

HIV, hepatitis B and C, and parvovirus B19. Conversely, autologous products are without that theoretic risk.[4]

Risk of viral transmission from homologous products

- One reported case of B19 parvovirus transmission
  - Risk estimated at 1:500,000
- No reported cases of HIV, hepatitis B, or hepatitis C
  - Risk estimated at less than 1×10^{15}

Despite the theoretic risk of viral transmission through the pooled products, the actual risk of transmission has been significantly decreased through screening protocols of blood donors and laboratory testing after donation. The components are processed by vapor heat treatment to eliminate potential pathogens. To date, after millions of applications in Europe, no transmission of chronic viral illnesses, such as HIV, hepatitis B or hepatitis C, has been documented. There has been 1 case of an active infection of B19 parvovirus. The estimated risk of B19 transmission is 1:500,000; whereas, the estimated risk of HIV and hepatitis B and C each is less than 1×10^{15}.[2,4]

What are the proposed benefits of fibrin tissue adhesives in facial plastic surgery?

- Improved hemostasis
- Expedited operating time
- Decreased edema
- Decreased ecchymosis
- Expedited postoperative recovery

Fibrin tissue adhesives promote the formation of stable clot, improving hemostasis. With less bleeding to address intraoperatively, the surgeon can limit the use of electrocautery. Overall operating time should decrease. Sealing both blood vessels and lymphatics reduces the potential space for fluid accumulation. Postoperatively, the potential decreased risk for hematoma, seroma, edema, and ecchymosis would improve patient outcomes in many facial plastic procedures.[2,3]

FDA off-label use

- Fibrin combined with thrombin since 1944
- FDA approval in 1998
- Artiss (Baxter Healthcare Corp, Deerfield, IL)
  - Adhere autologous skin grafts to surgically prepared wound beds resulting from burns in adult and pediatric populations
- Tisseel (Baxter Healthcare Corp)
  - Prevent leakage from colonic anastomoses, adjunct to hemostasis in adults and pediatric patients undergoing surgery
- Evicel (formerly Crosseel; Omrix Biopharmaceuticals)
  - Adjunct to hemostasis in patients undergoing liver surgery

---

Fibrin tissue adhesives have been used for many years. The current version, combining fibrinogen and thrombin for hemostasis, has existed since 1944. Before US Food and Drug Administration (FDA) approval in 1998, homologous fibrin products had millions of applications in Europe without disease transmission. Under the category of fractionated plasma products, there are 3 (Artiss, Tisseel, and Evicel) approved by the FDA for skin grafting burn patients, preventing leakage at colonic anastomosis sites, and as an adjunct to hemostasis refractory to traditional surgical techniques. The following applications are off-label indications. More importantly, a clear discussion and informed consent are obtained from the patient before the use of any homologous fibrin tissue adhesives.[1,2,5–7]

Applications in facial plastic and reconstructive surgery

- Historic use
  - 1944—first application
- Grafts and Flaps
  - Obliterate dead space
  - Promote hemostasis
  - Decrease seroma formation
  - Aid in neovascularization of graft or flap

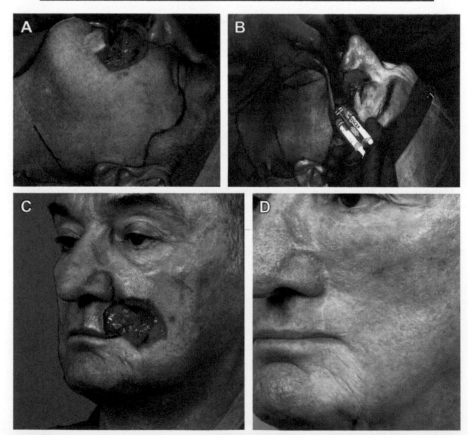

Fig. 6. Grafts and flaps. (*A*) Preoperative Mohs defect of the left cheek and upper lip. (*B*) Double-barrel syringe application of fibrin tissue adhesive. (*C*) Preoperative view of Mohs' defect site. (*D*) Postoperative view of reconstructed defect site. (*Courtesy of* [*A, B*] Baxter, Deerfield, IL; with permission.)

Historically, fibrin tissue adhesive was used as early as 1944 in the setting of skin grafts. Promoting hemostasis, obliterating dead space, and decreasing seromas, fibrin tissue adhesives optimize the conditions for graft or flap survival. Large facial skin flaps are a good opportunity to use a lower thrombin concentration (10–100 U/mL). With a lower thrombin concentration, the slower polymerization rate allows time for manipulation of a large flap or graft. First, the flap is trimmed to size. Tacking sutures are placed but not tied. A pressurized spray evenly distributes a thin layer of the fibrin tissue adhesive under the flap. The flap is positioned and the tacking sutures are now tied. Lastly, pressure is applied while polymerization process comes to completion (**Fig. 6**).[2,8]

Optimal application thickness

- Higher skin graft survival with thin application of fibrin sealant (vs thicker application)
- Similar survival between thin application group and the control
- Decreased survival with thicker application versus the control
- Fibrinogen concentration did not affect skin graft survival
- Critical for grafts but less important for well-vascularized flaps

---

- **Thinner layer FTA**   • **Thicker FTA**

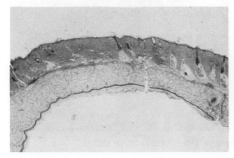 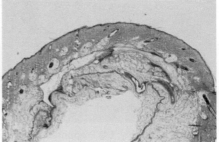

Fig. 7. Histology: thick versus thin application of Fibrin tissue adhesive (FTA).

Evenly spraying a thin layer under a flap is a classic example of "less is more." In a study evaluating the optimal thickness of fibrin tissue adhesive applied to a free skin graft, 3 mL of fibrin tissue adhesive was compared with 6 mL applied to the same surface area. The thin application and the control were similar in graft survival. Thicker applications of fibrin tissue adhesive decreased skin graft survival. This is seen histologically in **Fig. 7**. A second variable, fibrinogen concentration, was measured, and it was found to have no effect on graft survival. Well-vascularized flap survival was found to be independent of fibrin application thickness. It is postulated that the thick layer of adhesive may act as a nidus for infection or hinders neovascularization of the overlying graft.[9]

> **Fibrin tissue adhesive use in facial plastic surgery: rhytidectomy**
>
> - Randomized, prospective, blinded trials—trend toward reduced drainage from indwelling suction drains and no effect on hematoma
> - Retrospective (large) reduced hematoma rate in fibrin sealant group 3.4% versus 0.4%; $P = .01$
> - Sequential trials with unilaterally treated face: reduced both drainage and hematoma
> - Fibrin glue reduced drainage, but there was no difference in hematoma rates

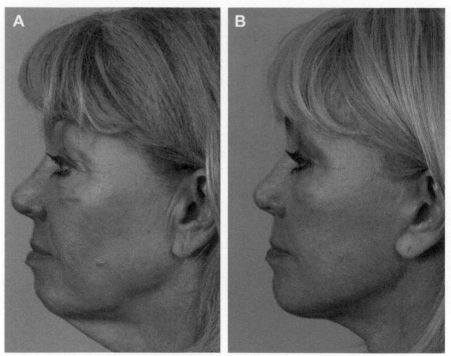

Fig. 8. Rhytidectomy: (*A*) Preoperative lateral view. (*B*) Postoperative lateral view.

Another application for fibrin tissue adhesives in facial plastic surgery is rhytidectomy (**Fig. 8**). Considering that hematoma is the most common major complication of rhytidectomy, any measure to decrease the possibility of emergently taking the patient back to the operating room may be beneficial. Looking closely at the data supporting fibrin tissue adhesives, the evidence does not show a statistically significant difference in hematoma/seroma rates. Fibrin tissue adhesives reduced drain output; therefore, drains could be avoided. With fibrin tissue adhesive, rates of postoperative morbidity—prolonged edema, induration, and ecchymosis—were decreased by a statistically significant difference. This reduction is meaningful to aesthetic surgery patients concerned with delays in recovery and prolonged downtime.[10]

Fibrin tissue adhesive use in facial plastic surgery: rhytidectomy

Technique

- Lower thrombin concentration
- Designed and tailored skin flaps
- Placed, but not tied fixation sutures
- Pressurized spray application
- Positioned skin flap
- Sutures tied
- Pressure applied
- No drain placement

Before the end of the procedure, thrombin is prepared at a lower concentration (10–100 U/mL). Polymerization at a slower rate provides time to manipulate the large cervico-facial flaps into the appropriate position. The skin flaps are designed and cut. Tacking sutures are placed but not tied. Using a pressurized spray applicator, a uniform and thin layer is applied under the flap (**Fig. 9**). The skin flap is positioned appropriately before tying the tacking sutures. Until polymerization is completed, pressure should be applied to the flap. No drains are necessary.[2]

Fibrin tissue adhesive use in facial plastic surgery: endoscopic forehead lift

- Seals blood vessels
- Around orbital rim
- Glabellar and corrugator musculature
- Decrease postoperative edema and ecchymosis

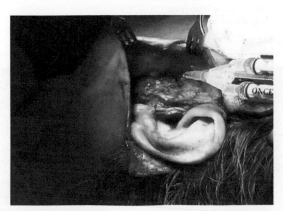

Fig. 9. Rhytidectomy intraoperative.

As the trend in surgery is moving toward minimally invasive and keyhole procedures, a technique such as endoscopic forehead surgery becomes another opportunity to use fibrin tissue adhesives for both hemostasis and fixation (**Fig. 10**). The elevation and release of periorbita and division of glabellar and corrugator musculature is prone to edema, hemorrhage, and ecchymosis. The fibrin tissue adhesive can seal vessels and lymphatics and cut muscle fibers around the orbital rim to decrease postoperative edema and ecchymosis.[1,2]

Fibrin tissue adhesive use in facial plastic surgery: endoscopic forehead lift

- Technique
  - Subperiosteal dissection
  - Release of arcus marginalis
  - Division of procerus and corrugator muscles
  - Temporal dissection and lateral suture fixation
  - Fixation with suture and fibrin tissue adhesive
  - Fixation sutures are placed but not tied
  - 2 mL of homologous fibrin tissue adhesive along orbital rim and on divided muscles
  - Normal thrombin concentration
  - 15 cm malleable double-barrel applicator tip
  - Fixation sutures are tied
  - Pressure to glabella 5 to 10 minutes

From 2 access points behind the hairline, a subperiosteal dissection is continued down to the arcus marginalis. After releasing that structure, the procerus and corrugator muscles are divided. A temporal dissection gives access to place a lateral fixation suture. Bone tunnels are made to allow passage of fixation sutures. Fixation sutures are placed but not tied. Using a normal thrombin concentration, 2 mL of homologous fibrin tissue adhesive is applied through a 15-cm malleable double-barrel applicator tip along the orbital rim and over the cut muscles under endoscopic guidance (**Fig. 11**). The fixation sutures are then tied and pressure is applied to the midline structures for 5 to 10 min while the fibrin tissue adhesive completes polymerization. Postoperatively, the patients have little bruising or edema. Some surgeons will use fibrin tissue adhesive as the sole method of fixation.[2]

Fibrin tissue adhesive use in facial plastic surgery: selecting cases

- Recommended for use in case by case basis
  - Excess intraoperative bleeding
  - Augmenting traditional fixation
- No supported role in rhinoplasty

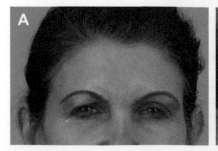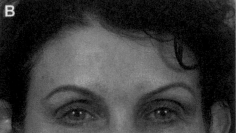

Fig. 10. Endoscopic forehead lift. (*A*) Preoperative photograph. (*B*) Postoperative photograph.

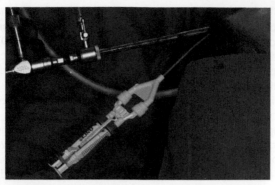

Fig. 11. Endoscopic forehead lift application.

Ultimately, it is up to the surgeon whether to integrate fibrin tissue adhesives into his or her armamentarium. Intraoperative bleeding or concern for the adherence of the soft tissue may prompt a surgeon to use a fibrin tissue adhesive. Concern for adequate tissue adherence may prompt the addition of fibrin tissue adhesives to a skin graft or flap procedure. Currently, there is no supported recommendation for blanket use of fibrin tissue adhesives in facial plastic surgery. In addition, no studies have been performed to identify patient or locoregional characteristics that would promote its use. Although hemostasis is important in rhinoplasty, fibrin tissue adhesives have no current application to improve outcomes in nasal surgery.

SUMMARY

Fibrin tissue adhesives are an adjunct to traditional surgical techniques for hemostasis. As a hemostatic and adhesive agent, fibrin tissue adhesives have a utility in skin grafts, flaps, rhytidectomy, and endoscopic forehead lift procedures.

When applied under elevated tissue, they help promote hemostasis, obliterate dead space, preclude the need for drains, decrease postoperative edema, and possibly aid in neovascularization of the flap. Hematoma and seroma rates in rhytidectomy are clinically but not statistically improved by fibrin tissue adhesives. By improving hemostasis and wound healing, fibrin tissue adhesives can benefit the facial plastic surgery patient.

Post-Test Questions (Correct answers are in italics)

1. What protein is obtained in higher concentrations from pooled homologous fibrin tissue adhesive products?
   A. fibrin
   B. *fibrinogen*
   C. thrombin
   D. Factor XIII
2. When applying fibrin tissue adhesive, what factor is known to decrease skin graft survival?
   A. thin layer of application
   B. *thick layer of application*
   C. low fibrinogen concentration
   D. high fibrinogen concentration

3. All of the following are potential applications of fibrin tissue adhesives, EXCEPT
   A. rhytidectomy
   B. *superficial skin closure*
   C. endoscopic forehead lift
   D. skin grafting
4. Which is an incorrect statement regarding issues with applicators?
   A. Single barrel: less uniform mixing of components I and II
   B. Double barrel: clogging of the application needle
   C. *Gas-Pressurized spray: requires multiple passes for adequate thickness*
   D. Applicators must keep thrombin-calcium chloride and fibrinogen separated because a stable cross-linked fibrin clot can form in seconds.

SUPPLEMENTARY DATA

Supplementary PDF slides related to this article can be found online at http://www. oto.theclinics.com/.

REFERENCES

1. Mobley SR, Hilinski J, Toriumi D. Surgical tissue adhesives. Facial Plast Surg Clin North Am 2002;10:147–54.

2. Saltz R, Toriumi DM, editors. Tissue glues in cosmetic Surgery. St Louis (MO): QMP; 2004. Chapter 5.

3. Farrior E, Ladner K. Platelet gels and hemostasis in facial plastic surgery. Facial Plast Surg 2011;27(4):308–14.

4. Horowitz B, Busch M. Estimating the pathogen safety of manufactured human plasma products: application to fibrin sealants and to thrombin. Transfusion 2008;48(8):1739–53.

5. Available at: http://www.fda.gov/BiologicsBloodVaccines/BloodBloodProducts/ApprovedProducts/LicensedProductsBLAs/FractionatedPlasmaProducts/ucm089262.htm. Accessed July 11, 2014.

6. Available at: http://www.fda.gov/BiologicsBloodVaccines/BloodBloodProducts/ApprovedProducts/LicensedProductsBLAs/FractionatedPlasmaProducts/ucm089269.htm. Accessed July 11, 2014.

7. Available at: http://www.fda.gov/BiologicsBloodVaccines/BloodBloodProducts/ApprovedProducts/LicensedProductsBLAs/FractionatedPlasmaProducts/ucm089267.htm. Accessed July 11, 2014.

8. Egan KK, Kim DW, Toriumi DM. Tissue adhesives. In: Papel I, Frodel JL, Holt GR, et al, editors. Facial plastic and reconstructive surgery. New York: Thieme; 2009. p. 91–7.

9. O'Grady KM, Agrawal A, Bhattacharyya TK, et al. An evaluation of fibrin tissue adhesive concentration and application thickness on skin graft survival. Laryngoscope 2000;110(11):1931–5.

10. Mustoe TA, Park E. Evidence-based medicine: face lift. Plast Reconstr Surg 2014; 133(5):1206–13.

SUGGESTED READINGS

Farrior E, Ladner K. Platelet gels and hemostasis in facial plastic surgery. Facial Plast Surg 2011;27(4):308–14.

Autologous fibrin tissue adhesive is isolated from the patient's body by centrifuging whole blood. The concentrated fibrinogen recombines with thrombin-calcium to stimulate clot formation. Homologous fibrin tissue adhesive uses many donors for increased concentrations of homologous fibrinogen and clotting factors. Small studies have suggested decreased ecchymosis and hematomas in rhytidectomies using fibrin sealants. Similarly decreased ecchymosis and edema is observed in rhinoplasty patients with osteotomies.

Kamer FM, Nguyen DB. Experience with fibrin glue in rhytidectomy. Plast Reconstr Surg 2007;120(4):1045–51.

This is one of the largest prospective, controlled trials investigating fibrin glue in the setting of rhytidectomy. The authors compared fibrin glue versus nonglue patients for expanding hematoma, seroma, prolonged induration, edema, and ecchymosis. They also surveyed patients with a pain score and satisfaction score. The authors report that there were some benefits associated with the use of fibrin glue in the setting of rhytidectomy. Fibrin glue eliminated the use of drains. Lower hematoma and seroma rates were clinically, but not statistically significant in the fibrin glue patients. Fibrin glue was most effective in eliminating prolonged induration, postoperative edema, and ecchymosis. Patient satisfaction and pain surveys showed no difference. As an adjunct to meticulous surgical technique, fibrin glue was found to decrease the postoperative morbidity of rhytidectomy patients in this large prospective trial.

Hemostasis in Pediatric Surgery

Soham Roy, MD*, Jo-Lawrence Bigcas, MD, Laura Vandelaar, MD

KEYWORDS

• Hemostasis • Pediatric • Epistaxis • Tonsillectomy • Von Willebrand

KEY LEARNING POINTS

At the end of this article, the reader will:

• Be able to make a thorough preoperative assessment of pediatric patients with respect to risk of surgical bleeding.
• Be familiar with common bleeding disorders affecting pediatric patients.
• Be able to discuss hemostatic strategies used in common pediatric surgeries such as adenotonsillectomy, posttonsillectomy hemorrhage, and middle ear surgery.

PREOPERATIVE EVALUATION

> **Clinical indicators of bleeding disorders**
>
> • Patient history: prolonged bleeding (spontaneous, epistaxis, dental extractions, surgeries), spontaneous bruising, excessive bruising after surgery, medications affecting platelet function (anticoagulants, nonsteroidal anti inflammatory drugs, aspirin), diseases (malignancies, hepatic, renal, hematologic).
>
> • Family history: bleeding tendencies, inheritable diseases (von Willebrand, hemophilia), easy bruising.
>
> • Physical examination: petechiae and ecchymoses (thrombocytopenia or functionally deficient platelets), telangiectasias (liver disease or hereditary hemorrhagic telangiectasia), hematomas, evidence of hemarthroses and joint deformities.

If there are any signs of family or personal history of bleeding issues, then preoperative laboratory evaluations are indicated. Preoperative investigations without positive findings in history and physical examination have not been found to be beneficial in either retrospective or prospective studies.[1,2]

Department of Otolaryngology, University of Texas at Houston McGovern Medical School, 6431 Fannin Street, MSB 5.036, Houston, TX 77030, USA
* Corresponding author.
E-mail address: soham.roy@uth.tmc.edu

Otolaryngol Clin N Am 49 (2016) 601–614
http://dx.doi.org/10.1016/j.otc.2016.03.007
0030-6665/16/$ – see front matter © 2016 Elsevier Inc. All rights reserved.

oto.theclinics.com

> **Preoperative laboratory evaluation**
>
> - Prothrombin time (PT): assesses the extrinsic pathway of clotting, and coagulation factors in the common pathway.
> - Partial thromboplastin time (PTT): assesses the intrinsic coagulation pathway and final common pathway.
> - Platelet count (**Table 1**).
> - Bleeding time: assess platelet function.
> - Hemoglobin: greater than 10 g/dL before surgery for pediatric patients.

PT assesses the extrinsic pathway of clotting, which consists of tissue factor and factor VII, and coagulation factors in the common pathway (factors II [prothrombin], V, and X, and fibrinogen). PTT assesses the intrinsic coagulation pathway (prekallikrein, high molecular weight kininogen, factors XII, XI, IX, and VIII) and final common pathway (factors II, V, and X, and fibrinogen). In general, a platelet count of greater than 80,000 is desirable to minimize bleeding risk during major surgical procedures (see **Table 1**). Bleeding time classically assesses platelet function but it is not a good predictor of intraoperative or postoperative bleeding. A retrospective study found a 5% positive predictive value of the bleeding time and a 95% negative predictive value.[2] **Table 2** provides common causes of abnormal PT and/or PTT.

It is generally suggested that the hemoglobin should be greater than 10 g/dL before surgery for pediatric patients. However, in infants younger than 6 months, the hematologic system is not fully matured and they have physiologic anemia owing to decreased erythropoietin; thus, they are more susceptible to adverse side effects of transfusion. In this age group, it is more important to take into account the severity of the surgery, likelihood of excessive bleeding, and the severity of the anemia before transfusing.

PEDIATRIC BLEEDING AND BLOOD DISORDERS IN SURGERY

von Willebrand disease (vWD) is a family of disorders caused by quantitative or qualitative defects of von Willebrand factor (VWF), a plasma protein that plays a role in both platelet adhesion and fibrin formation. Between 75% and 80% of patients have type 1 vWD.[3] This is a quantitative abnormality of the vWF molecule that results in decreased amounts of VWF protein. The clinical symptoms of type 1 VWD include mucosal bleeding, easy bruising, menorrhagia, and postoperative hemorrhage. Patients with type 1 vWD usually have mild to moderate platelet-type bleeding. Type 2 vWD is seen in 15% to 20% of patients with vWD. There are different subtypes, but all involve a qualitative defect in the VWF protein. Patients with type 2 vWD usually have moderate to severe bleeding that presents in childhood or adolescence (**Table 3**).

> **Perioperative considerations**
>
> - vWD type 1
>   - Desmopressin: increases release of vWF, overcoming quantitative defect in type 1 vWD
>   - vWF concentrate
> - vWD type 2
>   - vWF concentrate is effective
>   - Desmopressin: not effective owing to qualitative defect in vWF molecule

Table 1
Desired platelet count ranges for prevention of bleeding

Clinical Scenario	Platelet Count
Prevention of mucocutaneous bleeding	>10,000–20,000
Insertion of central venous catheter	>20,000–50,000
Minor surgical procedures	>50,000–80,000[a]
Major surgical procedures	>80,000–100,000

Adapted from Fogarty PF, Minichiello T. Chapter 14. Disorders of hemostasis, thrombosis, & antithrombotic Therapy. In: Papadakis MA, McPhee SJ, Rabow MW, editors. CURRENT Medical diagnosis & treatment 2014. New York: McGraw-Hill; 2014.

Table 2
Causes of a prolonged prothrombin time (PT) and/or activated partial thromboplastin time (aPTT)

Test Result		Causes of Test Result Pattern
PT	aPTT	

Prolonged	Normal	Inherited
		    Factor VII deficiency
		Acquired
		    Acquired factor VII deficiency
		    Mild vitamin K deficiency
		    Liver disease
		    Warfarin administration
		    Inhibitor of factor VII
		    Lupus anticoagulant (rare; may be associated with
		        bleeding rather than thrombosis)

Normal	Prolonged	Inherited
		    Deficiency of factors VIII, IX, or XI
		    Deficiency of factor XII, prekallikrein, or HMW kininogen[a]
		    von Willebrand disease (variable)
		Acquired
		    Heparin administration
		    Inhibitor of factors VIII, IX, XI, or XII
		    Acquired von Willebrand disease
		    Lupus anticoagulant[b]

Prolonged	Prolonged	Inherited
		    Deficiency of prothrombin, fibrinogen, or factors V or x
		    Combined factor deficiencies
		Acquired
		    Liver disease
		    Disseminated intravascular coagulation
		    Supratherapeutic doses of anticoagulants
		    Severe vitamin K deficiency
		    Combined heparin and warfarin administration
		    Angatroban with or without warfarin administration
		    Inhibitor of prothrombin, fibrinogen, or factors V or X
		    Primary amyloidosis-associated factor X deficiency

[a] Not associated with a bleeding diathesis.
[b] May be associated with thrombosis rather than bleeding.
From UpToDate. Causes of a prolonged prothrombin time (PT) and/or a prolonged activated partial thromboplastin time (aPTT). 2016. Available at: http://www.uptodate.com/contents/image?imageKey=HEME/79969. Accessed March 1, 2016; with permission.

Table 3
von Willebrand's Disease (vWD)

Type 1	Type 2
75%–85% of patients with vWD	15%–20% of patients with vWD
Quantitative defect of vWF	Qualitative defect of vWF
Mild-moderate platelet bleeding	Moderate-severe platelet bleeding
Can present in childhood or adulthood	Usually presents in childhood/adolescence
Treat with Desmopressin or vWF concentrate	Treat with only vWF concentrate

In vWD type 1, desmopressin (DDAVP) can be used effectively. It increases release of vWF, overcoming quantitative defect in type 1 vWD (see **Table 3**). The dose of DDAVP is 0.3 µg/kg intravenously in 50 mL saline over 20 minutes, or nasal spray 300 µg for weight greater than 50 kg or 150 µg for less than 50 kg every 12 to 24 hours, maximum of 3 doses in a 48-hour period. If more than 2 doses are used in a 12- to 24-hour period, free water restriction and/or monitoring for hyponatremia is essential.

vWF concentrate can be given at a dose is 60 to 80 recombinant factor units per kilogram intravenously every 12 hours initially followed by lesser doses at longer intervals once hemostasis has been established.

For vWD type 2, desmopressin is generally not effective owing to qualitative defect in vWF molecule and vWF concentrate is required (see **Table 3**).

Hemophilia

- Hemophilia A: 1 per 5000 live male births.
- Hemophilia B: 1 in 25,000 live male births.
- X-linked recessive inheritance.
- Testing is indicated for asymptomatic male infants with a hemophilic pedigree.
- Hemophilia diagnosis: isolated reproducibly low factor VIII or factor IX activity, in the absence of other conditions.

The frequency of hemophilia A is 1 per 5000 live male births, whereas hemophilia B occurs in approximately 1 in 25,000 live male births. It is an X-linked recessive inheritance, leading to affected males and carrier females. Severe hemophilia presents in infant males or in early childhood with spontaneous bleeding into joints, soft tissues, or other locations. Spontaneous bleeding is rare in patients with mild hemophilia, but bleeding may occur with a significant hemostatic challenge (eg, surgery, trauma) Testing is indicated for asymptomatic male infants with a hemophilic pedigree, for male infants with a family history of hemophilia who experience excessive bleeding, or for an otherwise asymptomatic adolescent or adult who experiences unexpected excessive bleeding with trauma. Hemophilia is diagnosed by demonstration of an isolated reproducibly low factor VIII or factor IX activity level, in the absence of other conditions. If the PTT is prolonged, it typically corrects upon mixing with normal plasma.

Perioperative Considerations

- Hemophilia A (mild).
  - Desmopressin: treat for 3 to 10 days for major bleeding or following surgery, keeping factor activity level at 50% to 80% initially. Adjunctive aminocaproic acid may be useful for mucosal bleeding or procedures.
- Hemophilia A (moderate to severe).
  - Factor VIII concentrate: dose is 50 U/kg intravenously initially followed by 25 U/kg every 8 hours, followed by lesser doses at longer intervals once hemostasis has been established.
- Hemophilia B (mild, moderate, or severe).
  - Factor IX concentrate: dose is 100 U/kg intravenously initially, followed by 50 U/kg every 8 hours, followed by lesser doses at longer intervals once hemostasis has been established.

SICKLE CELL DISEASE

- Patients are prone to anemia and often require transfusions preoperatively. This helps to avoid anesthetic complications, sickle cell complications, and severe anemia postoperatively.
- Preoperative transfusion may not be necessary in children and adults undergoing elective, minor, low-risk surgery such as myringotomy.
- Treatment.
  - A simple transfusion regimen in the perioperative period to increase the hemoglobin to 10 g/dL is suggested rather than an aggressive exchange transfusion regimen to reduce the Sickle-cell hemoglobin concentration to less than 30%.

Compared with an aggressive regimen, a conservative approach provides equivalent outcomes, similar rates of major complications, and fewer transfusion-related complications.

THROMBOCYTOPENIA

- Evident based on bleeding history or preoperative platelet counts, also congenital disorders or acquired syndromes may have additional symptoms.
- Can be caused by
  - Reduced platelet production in the bone marrow (eg, amegokaryocytic thrombocytopenia, Wiskott Aldrich syndrome, Fanconi anemia)
  - Excessive peripheral destruction of platelets (eg, immune thrombocytopenic purpura, disseminated intravascular coagulation, heparin-induced thrombocytopenia)
  - Hypersplenism (eg, myeloproliferative disorders, sickle cell disease).
- May require platelet transfusion preoperatively depending on preoperative platelet counts. For minor surgical procedures platelet count should be greater than 50,000, for major procedures platelet count should be greater than 80,000 (see **Table 1**).

Occasionally, undiagnosed bleeding disorders are discovered during the perioperative period. In addition to obtaining hemostasis, a multidisciplinary approach in further evaluation and management is necessary.

METHODS OF HEMOSTASIS DURING SURGERY

Mechanical[4]

Pressure

Sutures

Ligating clips

Bone wax

Chemical

Oxymetazoline

Epinephrine

Silver nitrate

Cocaine

Biomaterials

Gelatin-based (Floseal, GelFoam, Surgifoam)

Collagen based (Ativene, Helistat, Ultrafoam)

Cellulose based (Surgicel, Oxycel)

MECHANICAL HEMOSTASIS

Application of gentle pressure finger or gauze, sponges, or sponge sticks to a site of bleeding for 20 to 30 seconds or until bleeding decreases is often effective. The compression of capillaries allows for platelet aggregation and thrombus formation. It typically controls arterial bleeding better than venous bleeding. The use of surgical instruments can also be beneficial, especially with applying pressure with a needle driver or hemostat. Frequently, gauze packing can be used during adenoidectomy and tonsillectomy. When placed in the adenoid or tonsillar fossae, it applies pressure to the bleeding vessels and promotes clot formation. Tonsillar packs need to be removed before the end of the surgery, whereas adenoid packs can be removed the next morning if the patient is remaining in the hospital.

Sutures and ties can be used to ligate blood vessels and control bleeding, there are multiple characteristics to consider when suturing.

Suture characteristics to consider

- Physical characteristics: tensile strength, elasticity, single strand or multistrand, memory.
- Handling: slippage, knot tying capability, tissue drag, pliability.
- Tissue reaction: inflammatory effects, allergic reactions, infection potential, absorption qualities.

Blood vessels can be directly ligated using ligating to facilitate hemostasis and may be preferred owing to ease of application and less risk of a foreign body reaction compared with sutures.

Bone wax does not have chemical hemostatic properties and acts by physical occlusion of blood vessels. It is used most commonly for surgery on spongy bone, such as mastoid surgery. It functions by occluding the channels that contain the mastoid emissary veins. It should not be used in a contaminated field, and it can cause foreign body reaction and reactive granuloma formation.

CHEMICAL HEMOSTASIS

Oxymetazoline (Afrin) is an alpha-1 agonist and partial alpha-2 agonist that causes smooth muscle constriction of blood vessels. It is typically used for its nasal decongestant effects in otolaryngology. Intraoperatively it can be used for vasoconstriction and hemostasis. It is often used as Afrin-soaked pledgets along with pressure to better achieve hemostasis.

Epinephrine activates adrenoreceptor activation causing vasoconstriction and hemostasis and is highly effective at concentrations from 1:1000 to 1:1,000,000. It is often used in cutaneous surgeries, either injected in combination with an anesthetic agent to help potentiate the anesthetic effects, or directly applied to induce vasoconstriction.

Silver nitrate causes hemostasis by free silver ions binding to tissue proteins and causing precipitants that obstruct small bleeding vessels. This action causes a black eschar to form, which is eventually shed. Silver nitrate is often used to obtain hemostasis during intranasal surgeries and epistaxis. There is a risk of a tattoo effect at area of application; extreme caution is required for its use on visible skin surfaces. There is a risk of septal perforation, especially when used bilaterally for cautery.

Cocaine is a potent sympatheticomimetic agent that blocks the reuptake of norepinephrine. It has a quick onset of action and lasts up to 1 hour. The maximum dose is 1 mg/kg; however, reaction and metabolism are extremely variable in pediatric patients. Factors to be considered with dosage include tissue vascularity, site of administration, and route of administration. In some centers, cocaine is used commonly for surgeries in the oral and nasal cavity and larynx.

BIOMATERIALS

Gelatin-based (eg, Floseal, GelFoam, Surgifoam) biomaterials provide a matrix for clot formation and forms a mechanical barrier to bleeding.

- Generally used in minimal cases of bleeding
- Available in powder, paste, sponge, and viscous gel forms
- Commonly combined with saline, epinephrine, or procoagulant factors such as thrombin
- Conforms easily to wounds so it is useful in irregular wounds
- Widely used in intranasal bleeding and hemostasis

Collagen-based biomaterials (eg, Ativene, Helistat, Ultrafoam) are activated on contact with blood, forming a scaffold that platelets can adhere to. It also promotes platelet aggregation, degranulation and release of clotting factors.

- Used to control venous, capillary, and small arterial bleeding.
- Often combined with procoagulant factors such as thrombin.
- Ativene powder often used for tonsillectomy and intranasal procedures.

For cellulose-based biomaterials (eg, Surgicel, Oxycel), the exact mechanism of action is unknown; however, when placed on a bleeding surface it increases in size and forms a physical meshwork that aids in clot formation by activation of the extrinsic and intrinsic coagulation pathways.

- Used to control venous, capillary, and small arterial bleeding.
- Available in mesh, gauze, woven strips, or sponges, which can be cut to size needed intraoperatively.
- Surgicel comes in 2 forms, a woven knitted patch (Nu-Knit) and a fibrillar form (Fibrillar).
- Surgicel Nu-Knit is often used in intranasal surgery.
- Surgicel Fibrillar is often used in mastoid surgery.
- Maximal effect when applied dry, do not soak in saline, epinephrine, or thrombin.
- Major advantage is that it has bacteriostatic properties.

HEMOSTASIS IN PEDIATRIC TONSILLECTOMY AND ADENOTONSILLECTOMY

- One of the most common surgical procedures in pediatric population.
- Typically involves little intraoperative blood loss; management of posttonsillectomy hemorrhage is more concerning.
- Bleeding can occur from either the tonsillar beds or the adenoid pad.
- Posttonsillectomy hemorrhage is the most serious, most common, and life-threatening complication of surgery.

Intraoperative hemostasis[5]

- Cold dissection versus "hot" dissection.
  - Two common operative techniques.
  - Cold dissection involves ligation of bleeding vessels after dissection with scalpel.
  - Hot dissection encompasses the use of diathermy, both bipolar and monopolar, which can be single-tip or forceps, and coblation, argon.
  - Hot dissection is associated with lower intraoperative bleeding, although it has no effect on decreasing postoperative hemorrhage.
- Gauze packing and/or oxymetazoline-soaked packing can be placed tonsillar and adenoid fossae intraoperatively works to apply pressure, whereas oxymetazoline also vasoconstricts bleeding vessels.
- Ligation of vessels can be used, typically with a cold dissection technique.
- Electrocautery can be used to cauterize bleeding vessels.
- For adenoidectomy, direct visualization using mirrors and rubber catheter placement to elevate soft palate can help identify vessels or retained tissue causing bleeding.
- Hemostatic biomaterial (FloSeal, Surgicel) can be used to achieve intraoperative hemostasis with no adverse effects in the pediatric population.

POSTOPERATIVE HEMORRHAGE

- Surgical technique (cold dissection, diathermy, ultrasonic scalpel, coblation, etc) has not been shown to affect postoperative hemorrhage.[1,5]
- Primary postoperative hemorrhage (<24 hours postoperatively).
  - Incidence between 0% and 1.4%.[6]
  - Associated with surgical technique.
  - Usually owing to reopening of small vessels in the wound.
  - More serious complication than delayed (secondary) hemorrhage.
  - Dangerous owing to lack of responsiveness and protective airway reflexes are blunted because of effects of anesthesia and narcotics. This puts the patient at risk for aspiration and laryngospasm.
  - Typically requires surgical intervention for hemostasis.
- Secondary postoperative hemorrhage (>24 hours postoperatively).[6]
  - Incidence between 2% and 7%.
  - Some studies report that secondary hemorrhage is lower in children compared with adults.
  - Generally occurs between 5 and 10 days postoperatively.
  - Thought to be owing to loss of eschar, local infection, or trauma from food.
  - Rarely, it could be owing to a hereditary or acquired hemostatic deficiency.

Management of postoperative hemorrhage[7]

- Patient Assessment
  - Ensure stability of airway, if needed cuffed endotracheal tube works best to secure airway with bleeding from the tonsillar bed.
  - Obtain intravenous (IV) access.
  - Obtain laboratory tests (hemoglobin/hematocrit, PT/PTT, blood type and screen).
  - Start administering crystalloid fluids.

- Assess severity of bleeding.
  - Formed clot, no active bleeding.
    - Remove clot, assess wound for further interventions.
  - Mild to moderate bleeding (based on clinical assessment).
    - Oxymetazoline-soaked packing.
    - Local injection of epinephrine.
    - Local anesthesia with ligation or electrocautery of bleeding vessel if available.
  - Severe bleeding (based on clinical assessment).
    - Return to the operating room.
    - Clot removal, evaluation of eschar.
    - Use of vasoconstricting agents: oxymetazoline and epinephrine.
    - Use of pressure and packings.
    - Identification and ligation or electrocauterization of vessel.
    - If bleeding unable to be controlled, can perform external carotid artery ligation. This is rare.
    - Evaluate hemodynamic stability and hemoglobin/hematocrit and need for blood transfusion.

The management of secondary hemorrhage is complex and does not have precise guidelines for management. Pediatric patients typically have a lower rate of secondary hemorrhage, and if they present to the emergency department or the clinic with bleeding, they tend achieve spontaneous hemostasis more commonly than adult patients. However, it is important to understand how to manage these patients. When a patient presents, first evaluate the severity of the bleeding and the stability of the airway. With severe hemorrhage, it may be necessary to intubate the patient with a cuffed endotracheal tube to prevent aspiration. Then, gain intravenous line access; obtain a hemoglobin and hematocrit, coagulation profile, and blood type and screen. Next, fully assess the tonsillar bed, looking for clot, eschar, and active bleeding. The severity of bleeding is based on clinical assessment.

If the patient is not actively bleeding and there is a small clot in the tonsillar bed, it can be removed in the emergency department or clinic and the wound can be further evaluated. Conservative management with observation and cold water rinses can also be considered. Other methods, such as oxymetazoline-soaked packing, injection of epinephrine, can be considered.

Severe bleeding necessitates administration of general anesthesia and evaluation in the operating room. Here, the wound needs to be evaluated for large clots and removal of these in a controlled setting. Also, the presence or absence of an eschar should be noted and if there is any bleeding through the eschar it should be cauterized. The operating room allows the surgeon to fully use the electrocautery and ligation to control hemorrhage as well as vasoconstrictors, pressure packings and biomaterials (Surgicel, Gelfoam). If bleeding is unable to be controlled, external carotid artery ligation can be performed.

HEMOSTASIS IN PEDIATRIC MIDDLE EAR SURGERY

- Myringotomy with tympanostomy tube insertion.[8]
- Other middle ear surgeries,[9] including but not limited to myringoplasty, tympanomastoidectomy, and stapedectomy.

Surgical hemostasis is crucial in middle ear surgery owing to the small operating field and is necessary for visualization. Myringotomy with tympanostomy tube insertion, also referred to as middle ear ventilating tubes or grommets, is a common pediatric surgery. Usually does not require hemostatic measures in routine surgeries, because blood loss is minimal and patients achieve spontaneous hemostasis. Care must be taken to avoid ear canal injury, because blood loss from here can impede visualization of the tympanic membrane owing to confined surgical space. In this situation, mild bleeding from the incision can be controlled with administration of a cottonoid soaked with oxymetazoline.

Significant bleeding during myringotomy procedures can be encountered in patients with high jugular bulbs, dehiscent jugular bulbs, or, less commonly, aberrant carotid arteries in the middle ear. The only finding on examination, if any, that will warn a surgeon of a high or dehiscent jugular bulb is a bulging blue tympanic membrane, although this is not always present. Usually jugular bulb does not mature until 2 years of age, although cases have been reported of dehiscent and high jugular bulbs in children under the age of 2. If severe bleeding is encountered, hemostasis can be achieved by packing the external auditory canal with gauze or absorbable packing. Oxidized cellulose (Surgicel) can be applied to the gauze packing if additional hemostasis is needed. Blood loss can be extensive with jugular bulb bleeding or carotid artery, monitor hemoglobin/hematocrit and transfuse if needed.

Other Middle Ear Surgeries[9]
- Preoperative local injection
- Skin and soft tissue hemostasis
  - Apply pressure with speculum or other instruments
  - Electrocauterization with monopolar or bipolar electrocautery
  - Apply cellulose-based biomaterial (Surgicel) if bleeding or oozing continues
- Mucosa in tympanic cavity and tympanomeatal flap
  - Avoid using electrocautery to prevent thermal damage to the structures of the middle ear cavity
  - Cottonoids soaked in saline with lidocaine and epinephrine can be applied
- Bone
  - Diamond burrs are frequently used first to achieve hemostasis
  - Bone wax can be used and pressure can be applied with cottonoids if additional hemostasis is needed
- Jugular bulb
  - Bipolar electrocautery can be used at a very low setting because the structure is very fragile to avoid unwanted damage
  - If hemostasis is not achieved with bipolar electrocautery, oxidized cellulose (Surgicel) can be applied to the structure to achieve hemostasis
- Dura
  - Bipolar electrocautery can be used
  - Never use monopolar electrocautery because it can cause a perforation

INDICATIONS FOR BLOOD VOLUME REPLACEMENT

- Rapid blood loss[10]
- Impaired oxygenation
- General medical condition
- When amount of blood loss is the maximum allowable blood loss

In the presence of rapid blood loss, impaired oxygenation, and poor general medical condition of the child, transfusion may be required. Children are more susceptible to these metabolic complications and they occur more frequently in children. It is an option to replace blood loss with 3:1 of lactated ringers until approximate blood loss reaches maximum allowable blood loss, after which blood transfusion should be initiated: maximum allowable blood loss = [(starting hematocrit – target hematocrit) ÷ starting hematocrit] × estimated blood volume (**Table 4**). Transfuse approximately 0.5 mL

Table 4 Estimated pediatric blood volume	
Age	**Estimated Blood Volume (mL/kg)**
Premature Infant	90–100
Term infant – 3 mo	80–90
Children >3 mo old	70
Very obese children	65

Data from Arya VK. Basics of fluid and blood transfusion therapy in pediatric surgical patients. Indian J Anaesth 2012;56(5):454–62.

packed red blood cell for each milliliter of blood loss beyond the maximum allowable blood loss.

Possible Complications of Packed Red Blood Cell Transfusion

- Hypocalcemia
- Hypokalemia
- hypothermia

Post-Test Questions (Correct answers are in italics)

1. How should you manage operative patients preoperatively?
   A. Obtain hemoglobin/hematocrit, PT/PTT on all patients
   B. *Obtain laboratory tests based on patient and family history of bleeding tendencies*
   C. Never obtain preoperative laboratory tests on pediatric patients
2. The hemoglobin level in pediatric patients preoperatively should ideally be
   A. 8 g/dL
   B. *10 g/dL*
   C. 12 g/dL
3. What should the preoperative platelet count be for a pediatric patient undergoing a major surgical procedure?
   A. Greater than 10,000 to 20,000
   B. Greater than 20,000 to 50,000
   C. Greater than 50,000 to 80,000
   D. *Greater than 80,000 to 100,000*
4. Oxymetazoline is a useful hemostatic agent in which of the following procedures?
   A. Nasal surgeries
   B. Tonsillectomy
   C. Myringotomy with tympanostomy tube insertion
   D. *All of the above*
5. Airway stabilization, if needed, in patients with posttonsillectomy bleeding should ideally be established by which method?
   A. *Cuffed endotracheal tube*
   B. Uncuffed endotracheal tube
   C. Tracheostomy
   D. Laryngeal mask airway (LMA)
6. All of these hemostatic methods can routinely be used on visible skin except:
   A. Epinephrine
   B. Oxymetazoline
   C. *Silver nitrate*
   D. Sutures
7. When should you initiate pediatric blood transfusion?
   A. Blood loss or greater than 1 L
   B. Loss of one-quarter of the EBV (estimated blood volume)
   C. *Blood loss above the maximum allowable blood loss*
   D. Loss of one-half of the EBV (estimated blood volume)

8. What procedure can be done to ultimately control tonsillar bed bleeding if other methods have failed?
   A. *External carotid artery ligation*
   B. Internal carotid artery ligation
   C. Internal jugular vein ligation

9. Which of these is best to control bleeding from bone?
   A. Surgicel
   B. Cocaine
   C. *Bone wax*
   D. GelFoam

10. When performing middle ear surgery on a pediatric patient, if hemorrhage is encountered in the dura, which hemostatic method should *never* be used?
    A. *Monopolar electrocautery*
    B. Bipolar electrocautery
    C. Epinephrine
    D. Surgicel

SUPPLEMENTARY DATA

Supplementary PDF slides related to this article can be found online at http://www.oto.theclinics.com/.

REFERENCES

1. Howells RC 2nd, Wax MK, Ramadan HH. Value of preoperative prothrombin time/partial thromboplastin time as a predictor of postoperative hemorrhage in pediatric patients undergoing tonsillectomy. Otolaryngol Head Neck Surg 1997; 117(6):628–32.
2. Coture S. Preoperative assessment of hemostasis. UpToDate. 2014.
3. Fogarty PF, Minichiello T. Chapter 14. Disorders of hemostasis, thrombosis, & antithrombotic therapy. In: Papadakis MA, McPhee SJ, Rabow MW, editors. CURRENT Medical diagnosis & treatment 2014. New York: McGraw-Hill; 2014. Available at: http://accessmedicine.mhmedical.com/content.aspx?bookId=330&Sectionid=44291016.
4. Acar B, Babademez MA, Karabulut H. Topical hemostatic agents in otolaryngologic surgery. Kulak Burun Bogaz Ihtis Derg 2010;20(2):100–9.
5. Steketee KG, Reisdorff EJ. Emergency care for posttonsillectomy and postadenoidectomy hemorrhage. Am J Emerg Med 1995;13(5):518–23.
6. Kim DW, Koo JW, Ahn SH, et al. Difference of delayed post-tonsillectomy bleeding between children and adults. Auris Nasus Larynx 2010;37:456–60.
7. Sasi S, Larrier D. Common postoperative complications in otolaryngology presenting to the pediatric emergency department. Clinical Pediatric Emergency Medicine 2010;11(2):131–6.
8. Atmaca S, Elmali M, Kucuk H. High and dehiscent jugular bulb: clear and present danger during middle ear surgery. Surg Radiol Anat 2014;36:369–74.
9. Sanna, M, Sunose, H. Chapter 4: general technical considerations. middle ear and mastoid microsurgery.
10. Arya VK. Basics of fluid and blood transfusion therapy in paediatric surgical patients. Indian J Anaesth 2012;56(5):454–62.

SUGGESTED READINGS

Acar B, Babademez MA, Karabulut H. Topical hemostatic agents in otolaryngologic surgery. Kulak Burun Bogaz Ihtis Derg 2010;20(2):100–9.

This article goes into further detail about the coagulation cascade and management of pediatric bleeding disorders for the pediatric otolaryngology patient.

Bluestone CD, Stool SE, Kenna MA. Pediatric hematology: the coagulation system and associated disorders. Pediatric Otolaryngology. Philadelphia: Saunders; 1996.

This article details the different uses of chemical hemostatic agents in otolaryngologic surgery.

Hemostasis in Tonsillectomy

Ryan M. Mitchell, MD, PhD[a], Sanjay R. Parikh, MD[a,b,*]

KEYWORDS

- Tonsillectomy • Hemorrhage • Transfusion • Complication • Hemostasis
- Tonsillotomy

KEY LEARNING POINTS

At the end of this article, the reader will:

- Appreciate the incidence of bleeding complications associated with tonsillectomy.
- Be able to review the relevant surgical vascular anatomy.
- Gain familiarity with methods of obtaining hemostasis during tonsillectomy and managing posttonsillectomy hemorrhage.

WHAT IS THE INCIDENCE OF POSTTONSILLECTOMY HEMORRHAGE?

Incidence of posttonsillectomy hemorrhage

- Overall hemorrhage rate of 3% to 5% is generally accepted[1]
- Primary posttonsillectomy hemorrhage: ~2%
- Secondary posttonsillectomy hemorrhage: most commonly between 5 and 10 days after surgery: ~3.7%
- Reported rates of posttonsillectomy mortality resulting from hemorrhage reported 1 per 7000 to 1 per 170,000[2,3]

---

[a] Department of Otolaryngology-Head and Neck Surgery, University of Washington, 1959 NE Pacific St, Box 256515, Seattle, WA 98195, USA; [b] Division of Pediatric Otolaryngology-Head and Neck Surgery, Seattle Children's Hospital, 4800 Sand Point Way Northeast, OA.9.329, Seattle, WA 98105, USA
* Corresponding author. Division of Pediatric Otolaryngology-Head and Neck Surgery, Seattle Children's Hospital, 4800 Sand Point Way Northeast, OA.9.329, Seattle, WA 98105.
E-mail address: sanjay.parikh@seattlechildrens.org

Otolaryngol Clin N Am 49 (2016) 615–626
http://dx.doi.org/10.1016/j.otc.2016.03.008
0030-6665/16/$ – see front matter © 2016 Elsevier Inc. All rights reserved.

oto.theclinics.com

Tonsillectomy and/or adenoidectomy is performed over several hundred thousand times per year in adults and children in the United States.[4] There are significant variations in the reported incidence of posttonsillectomy hemorrhage (PTH) among studies, which may be caused by various definitions of hemorrhage, technique of tonsillectomy, postoperative care, and the study populations. Hemorrhage after tonsillectomy is not a rare event, but mortality caused by hemorrhage is rare. Primary PTH occurs within 24 hours of surgery and is considered to usually result from blood vessels not effectively controlled during surgery. Secondary PTH occurs after 24 hours of surgery and is thought to occur from exposed blood vessels after sloughing of the eschar.

What is the source of hemorrhage following tonsillectomy?

- Blood supply to the palatine tonsils arises from the
  - Tonsillar branch of the facial artery
  - Dorsal lingual artery
  - Ascending pharyngeal artery
  - Lesser palatine artery
  - Ascending palatine artery

The lateral surface of the palatine tonsils is covered by a condensation of pharyngobasilar fascia, which has septae extending into the tonsils that transmits arteries, veins, and nerves. On removal of the tonsils, transected blood vessels may spasm and reduce blood loss or stop bleeding altogether.

Primary PTH may result from a blood vessel that initially spasms and later resumes bleeding if a method is not used to promote coagulation. Some surgeons elect to treat only sites observed to bleed during the tonsillectomy to reduce surrounding tissue damage. Other surgeons elect to treat all potential bleeding sites with the goal of potentially reducing the risk of PTH,[5] although this may slow tissue healing and increase postoperative pain and need for analgesics.

Vascular anomalies and anatomic variations may cause some concern for potential injury or increased risk of PTH. In particular, the course of the cervical internal carotid artery has a high reported rate of variable anatomy, particularly in association with velocardiofacial syndrome.[6] However, there are no data to support an increased risk of PTH because of variable vascular anatomy.

What factors have been proposed to affect hemorrhage during tonsillectomy?

- Surgical technique
  - Cold dissection (sharp, blunt, snares) and hemostasis with ties or diathermy
  - "Hot" dissection
    - Diathermy or electrocautery
      - Direct contact with tissue (monopolar, bipolar)
      - Indirect (argon)
    - Laser
  - Bipolar radiofrequency ablation (coblation)
  - Harmonic scalpel
  - Argon
  - Intracapsular tonsillectomy/tonsillotomy

- Patient factors
  - Age
  - Indication for tonsillectomy
  - Coagulopathy
  - Vascular anatomy, aberrant blood vessels

Numerous studies have sought to identify which tonsillectomy method is associated with the lowest risk of PTH, although no technique has definitively been shown to have a clinically significant benefit. A possible explanation is that secondary PTH is generally thought to occur from sloughing of fibrinous exudate approximately 7 days after tonsillectomy. By this point in time, the method of dissection may be less relevant. Suturing of the faucial pillars, which is also performed with many uvulopalatopharyngoplasty techniques, has been proposed to reduce bleeding that occurs from exposed blood vessels after fibrinous sloughing. One study showed that this technique was associated with a lower risk of needing operative management of PTH, and may reduce the overall risk of PTH, although this study was underpowered.[7]

Cold dissection tonsillectomy

- Fischer knife, snare, microdebrider, other methods
- Hemostasis must be achieved as a second step
- May have higher intraoperative blood loss compared with "hot" techniques
- May have lower PTH rates because of reduced thermal injury to adjacent muscle compared with "hot" techniques

---

Cold dissection depends on operator skill for dissection and hemostasis. A variety of methods have been reported for achieving hemostasis following cold dissection, and allow the operator to target sources of bleeding and reduce tissue damage in nonbleeding regions. The risk of PTH with cold dissection may be lower because of reduced collateral tissue injury, therefore a reduced thickness of fibrinous slough; however, larger studies are required to substantiate this. Cold dissection technique for tonsillectomy is currently standard of practice against which outcomes and complications of newer techniques are compared.

Electrocautery

- Monopolar cautery: high-frequency electrical current passing through tissue as either continuous ("cut" mode), interrupted ("coag" mode), or a mixture of current flow
- Tissue temperatures near the active electrode frequently exceed 200°C
- Continuous current flow creates higher tissue temperatures and results in explosive vaporization
- Bipolar cautery also uses high-frequency electrical current, but the current is limited to the tissue between the two electrodes

---

Electrocautery is frequently used in tonsillectomy, either for dissection and hemostasis, or for hemostasis following other dissection techniques. A variety of active electrode shapes are used with the monopolar cautery, including a needle tip; a funnel-shaped tip; or a broad, flat electrode. A suction cautery device with a round, hollow electrode through which the surgeon may also suction is frequently used for hemostasis alone (**Fig. 1**).

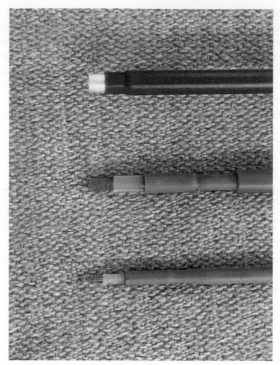

Fig. 1. An example of monopolar electrocautery tips used for tonsillectomy hemostasis. (*Top*) Suction monopolar tip. (*Middle*) Insulated blade monopolar tip. (*Bottom*) Insulated needle monopolar tip.

Radiofrequency ablation
• First approved by the US Food and Drug Administration for tonsillectomy in 2001 (Coblation device, Smith & Nephew, London, UK)
• Capable of tissue dissection and achieving hemostasis
• Potentially less surrounding thermal tissue injury than monopolar cautery
• Reduced thermal injury has been proposed to reduce postoperative pain and possibly the risk of hemorrhage
• Similar hemorrhage rates compared with electrocautery

Radiofrequency is a relatively new technique compared with electrocautery methods of tonsillectomy. This technique uses radiofrequency signals to produce an electrodissociation effect to generate a plasma of excited ions or an ionized field. Two electrodes immersed in electrolyte solution are used to create a plasma field of high energy charged particles that break molecular bonds between 40°C and 70°C. Monopolar cautery is frequently compared with coblation because of similar applications and technique, although the disposable Coblator handpieces are significantly more expensive than typical monopolar cautery handpieces. Monopolar cautery may still be used with radiofrequency for brisk bleeding control. One large study with 1918 children (<20 years old) showed overall 4.5% incidence of PTH.[8] There was no association between surgeon experience and rate of PTH, and 1% required electrocautery for intraoperative hemostasis. The English National Tonsillectomy Audit showed that coblation was associated with a 1.6 to 2.7 times greater hemorrhage rate than cold dissection techniques.[9] However, there were some confounding factors and a larger study is required to examine this further.

Harmonic scalpel

- Vibration of a blade at 55.5 kHz over a distance of 50 to 100 μm transmits ultrasonic energy to tissue and heats it to 55°C to 100°C, and causes denaturation and coagulation of proteins

- Capable of tissue dissection and achieving hemostasis

- Causes surrounding tissue thermal injury

- Most studies reported no primary hemorrhages; however, most also report a secondary method was frequently used to achieve hemostasis

---

Harmonic scalpel is capable of performing dissection and hemostasis; however, other methods are frequently needed to achieve hemostasis.[10] This obscures the data regarding the true amount of intraoperative hemorrhage and incidence of PTH related to the harmonic scalpel. A systematic review failed to show overall difference in hemorrhage rate compared with any other method; however, this review was limited by poor reporting within studies and small sample sizes.[11]

ARGON PLASMA COAGULATION

- Ability to dissect and achieve hemostasis
- Used for the theoretical benefit of improved homogenous coagulation of bleeding vessels with a more limited depth of coagulation compared with electrocautery
- Studies using argon plasma coagulation in pediatric and adult populations have failed to show any improvement in the rate of PTH in both groups

---

Intracapsular tonsillectomy, also known as tonsillotomy

- Removal of tonsil tissue medial to capsule

- Mostly used in pediatric patients with obstructive sleep-disordered breathing

- Less postoperative pain and low risk of hemorrhage as a result of leaving capsule in vivo[12,13]

- Multiple studies suggest reduced risk of PTH (<1%)[14,15]

During tonsillotomy, the intracapsular portion of tonsil tissue is shaved or thermally reduced by multiple reported methods (eg, microdebrider, electrocautery, radiofrequency ablation, laser). Hemostasis of residual tonsil bed is usually achieved by electrocautery. With this method, there is a potential for tonsil regrowth (1% rate) and thus has tempered enthusiasm for this approach. However, because of its potential to reduce the risk of PTH, there is renewed interest in some centers to introduce this technique as the favored technique for management of tonsils for sleep-disordered breathing. Larger studies are needed, particularly to examine the incidence of tonsillar regrowth and the effects of this on airway obstruction. Ultimately, tonsillotomy may be offered as an option depending on a patient's or caregiver's preference for reduced risk of hemorrhage and pain with the caveat that tonsillar regrowth may be more common with this technique.

Data from the English and Northern Ireland National prospective tonsillectomy audit (2003–2004) collected data from 15,000 tonsillectomies.[9] The results for five common tonsillectomy techniques are summarised below:

Tonsillectomy technique and risk of post tonsillectomy hemorrhage and return to theatre.

1. Cold steel tonsillectomy using ties and/or packs: postoperative hemorrhage (1.3%), return to theatre (1.0%).
2. Cold steel dissection with bipolar or monopolar diathermy hemostasis: hemorrhage 2.7% and 2.9%, respectively; 0.7% and 0.8% of the patients, respectively, returned to theatre.
3. Bipolar (forceps) diathermy for dissection and hemostasis: hemorrhage rate of 4.6%; 1.0% of the patients returned to theatre.
4. Monopolar diathermy for dissection and hemostasis: hemorrhage rate of 6.6%; 1.6% of the patients returned to theatre.
5. Coblation for dissection and hemostasis: hemorrhage rate of 4.6%; 1.8% of the patients returned to theatre.

Tissue dissection techniques that do not achieve hemostasis require a second step to address bleeding sources. This is particularly necessary after cold dissection.

How is primary hemostasis achieved during tonsillectomy or secondary hemostasis after postoperative hemorrhage?

- Pressure
- Suture ligation: absorbable suture material placed around obvious sites of significant bleeding
- Injection of epinephrine ± local anesthetic near bleeding vessels to cause constriction and coagulation
- Electrocautery
  - Monopolar
  - Bipolar
- Procoagulants
  - Floseal (Baxter Healthcare Corp, Deerfield, IL)
  - Surgicel (Ethicon Inc, Bridgewater, NJ): absorbable woven sheet of cellulose thought to act as a scaffold for platelet aggregation
    - May be used for primary or secondary hemostasis when no obvious bleeding source is identified[11]
  - Fibrin glue

Floseal

- Matrix of human thrombin and gelatin granules
- Associated with less intraoperative blood loss and quicker hemostasis when used for primary hemostasis following adenoidectomy or adenotonsillectomy in children[16]
- Seems effective for primary hemostasis after cold dissection, and does not seem to increase the rate of primary PTH[17]
- No data suggest improved rates of secondary PTH in adults or children

Although multiple authors have shown that Floseal may improve primary hemostasis following adenoidectomy or tonsillectomy, no data suggest that it improves PTH rates, although studies have had very small sample sizes. This may reflect the idea that secondary PTH results after sloughing of the healing eschar, and it is expected that any remaining Floseal would be removed (**Fig. 2**).

FIBRIN GLUE

- Available as component system of separated solutions of fibrinogen with factor XIII and thrombin with calcium. Some preparations also may include an antifibrinolytic agent.
- All commercially available products derived from human donors.
- Has been used for primary hemostasis after cold dissection and as prophylactic after hemostasis achieved with electrocautery in small pilot studies.

Fibrin glue has been used for primary hemostasis and as a prophylactic agent to prevent postoperative hemorrhage, but sufficiently powered studies are lacking to assess the true impact of glue on PTH.[18]

Does postoperative care affect rate of PTH?

- Medications
  - Nonsteroidal anti-inflammatory drugs (NSAIDS)
  - Corticosteroids
  - Tranexamic acid
  - Aminocaproic acid (Amicar)

- Diet: no evidence of effect

- Activity: increased physical exertion possibly associated with increased risk of hemorrhage

---

There are limited data examining the effect of activity level on the rate of PTH. In one study in which 413 adenoidectomies and 387 adenotonsillotomies were performed in children between the ages of 3 and 13, those patients with no restrictions had more episodes of postoperative hemorrhage.[19] However, caregivers reported difficulty

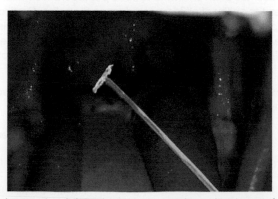

Fig. 2. A simulated example of thrombin/gelatin matrix application to the tonsillar fossa.

restricting physical activity levels of the patients. In this same study, eliminating hot and hard foods and liquids from the patients' postoperative diets had no impact on the rate of PTH. A smaller study in 150 patients older than age 16 also showed no effect of diet on PTH.[20–22]

Does the use of NSAIDs affect PTH?

- NSAIDs reduce platelet aggregation by inhibiting platelet cyclooxygenase and preventing formation of thromboxane A_2
- NSAIDs are commonly used in pediatric patients for postoperative analgesia after tonsillectomy
- Ketorolac, ibuprofen, and celecoxib are all frequently used
- A Cochrane review showed that use of NSAIDs does not significantly increase risk of postoperative hemorrhage or need for surgical control of hemorrhage in children[18]
- Meta-analysis for ketorolac showed increased rate of postoperative hemorrhage in adults (relative risk = 5.64) but not in children[19]

Postoperative analgesia following tonsillectomy typically consists of a combination of acetaminophen, NSAIDs, and narcotics. Because of a concern about the sedating effects of narcotics and the potential for suppression of respiratory drive, some clinicians prefer to avoid narcotics, particularly in pediatric patients. This may increase reliance on NSAIDs combined with acetaminophen for postoperative analgesia. The reasons for increased risk of PTH in adults treated with ketorolac are unclear, but are consistent with reports that adults have an elevated overall risk of PTH.

Does the use of postoperative steroids affect PTH?

- Reduces postoperative nausea, vomiting, and pain
- Improves the ability of children to advance their diet
- No conclusive data to recommend against using corticosteroids with respect to risk of increased postoperative hemorrhage[23]

Corticosteroid use has been shown to reduce postoperative nausea, vomiting, and pain and improves the ability of children to advance their diet. Corticosteroids are hypothesized to impair wound healing, possibly leading to increased risk of postoperative hemorrhage. A large multicenter observational study recently showed a statistically significant, but not clinically significant increased risk of revisit for PTH (0.40% increase in standardized risk, $P = .003$).[23]

- Included 139,715 patients aged 1 to 18 who were discharged on the day of tonsillectomy ± adenoidectomy
  - Excluded children with coagulopathies
  - Assumed a conservative clinically significant increase in bleeding was 1.5%

TRANEXAMIC ACID

Tranexamic acid is a synthetic lysine analogue that inhibits the activation of plasminogen to plasmin. It is used for patients at increased risk of intraoperative hemorrhage or PTH. A systematic review of tranexamic acid in patients without bleeding disorders showed nonsignificant reduction in PTH in 1670 patients.[24] Rare adverse reactions have been reported.

AMINOCAPROIC ACID (AMICAR)

This is a lysine analogue that competitively binds plasminogen and prevents conversion to plasmin. It has been studied for prophylactic and therapeutic use in patients with von Willebrand disease (VWD). A study with 41 pediatric patients with VWD receiving three perioperative doses of DDAVP (desmopressin) and 5 days of perioperative aminocaproic acid reported secondary PTH in seven patients (17%), five of whom required cautery for hemostasis.[25]

One study reported PTH in 8 of 99 pediatric patients, an average of 8.6 days after surgery[26]: 93 of 99 received perioperative DDAVP, and 46 of 99 received perioperative aminocaproic acid. Use of aminocaproic acid did not decrease risk of hemorrhage, but this study was underpowered.

What patient factors affect PTH?

- Age
  - Multiple studies show increasing rates of PTH with increasing age[14,27]
  - Younger children who experience PTH may have greater chance of spontaneous hemostasis compared with older children or adults[28]

- Coagulopathies
  - von Willebrand disease
  - Hemophilia
    - Small studies with few patients suggest high rate of PTH even after factor replacement[29]
  - Preoperative screening of all tonsillectomy patients for coagulopathies generally is not performed and is not cost-effective[30]

- Indication for tonsillectomy
  - Peritonsillar abscess, recurrent tonsillitis, chronic tonsillitis, obstructive sleep apnea
    - Overall, data are inconclusive for an association between indication for tonsillectomy and the incidence of PTH[9,31–33]

Most patients who experience significant intraoperative blood loss or PTH have no identified coagulopathy. Patients with coagulopathies have higher rates of PTH,[34] but preoperative screening is only recommended for patients with a significant personal or family history of abnormal bleeding.

VON WILLEBRAND DISEASE

VWD is the most common inherited coagulopathy and results in quantitative or qualitative deficiencies of von Willebrand factor (VWF). It is classified into six different forms (1, 2A, 2B, 2M, 2N, and 3), most of which are inherited in an autosomal-dominant pattern. Many centers test patients for responsiveness to DDAVP, and infusion of DDAVP perioperatively is recommended for responders.[35] DDAVP increases circulating VWF in some patients with type 1 or type 2 VWD. Plasma-derived VWF concentrates may be used for patients with qualitative VWF deficiencies or nonresponders to DDAVP. Although prophylactic medications are typically used for patients with VWD undergoing surgery, patients are still at increased risk of PTH. One large study reported 1.6% incidence of primary hemorrhage and 15% incidence of secondary hemorrhage.[36]

Post-Test Questions (Correct answers are in italics)

1. Which hemostatic agent consists of human thrombin and gelatin granules?
   a. Surgicel
   b. *Floseal*
   c. Arista
   d. TISSEEL
2. Secondary PTH occurs during which timeframe?
   a. Between 0 and 24 hours
   b. *After 24 hours*
   c. Between 7 and 14 days
   d. After 14 days
3. Use of a microdebrider is an example of what tonsillectomy technique?
   a. "Hot" dissection
   b. Bipolar radiofrequency ablation
   c. *"Cold" dissection*
   d. Hemostasis
4. Data suggest which is NOT associated with intracapsular tonsillectomy/tonsillotomy compared with tonsillectomy?
   a. Less pain
   b. Reduced risk of PTH
   c. Regrowth of tonsils
   d. *Improved airway obstruction*
5. Which surgical instrument results in the highest tissue temperatures?
   a. *Monopolar cautery*
   b. Coblator
   c. Harmonic scalpel
   d. Microdebrider

SUPPLEMENTARY DATA

Supplementary PDF slides related to this article can be found online at http://www.oto.theclinics.com/.

REFERENCES

1. Blakley BW. Post-tonsillectomy bleeding: how much is too much? Otolaryngol Head Neck Surg 2009;140(3):288–90.

2. Goldman JL, Baugh RF, Davies L, et al. Mortality and major morbidity after tonsillectomy: etiologic factors and strategies for prevention. Laryngoscope 2013; 123(10):2544–53.

3. Windfuhr JP. Serious complications following tonsillectomy: how frequent are they really? ORL J Otorhinolaryngol Relat Spec 2013;75(3):166–73.

4. Cullen KA, Hall MJ, Golosinskiy A. Ambulatory surgery in the United States, 2006. Natl Health Stat Rep 2009;(11):1–25.
5. Ulualp SO. Rate of post-tonsillectomy hemorrhage after elective bipolar micro-cauterization of nonbleeding vessels. Eur Arch Otorhinolaryngol 2012;269(4): 1269–75.
6. Paulsen F, Tilmann B, Christofides C, et al. Curving and looping of the internal carotid artery in relation to the pharynx: frequency, embryology and clinical implications. J Anat 2000;197(Pt 3):373–81.
7. Senska G, Schroder H, Putter C, et al. Significantly reducing post-tonsillectomy haemorrhage requiring surgery by suturing the faucial pillars: a retrospective analysis. PLoS One 2012;7(10):e47874.
8. Walner DL, Miller SP, Villines D, et al. Coblation tonsillectomy in children: incidence of bleeding. Laryngoscope 2012;122(10):2330–6.
9. National prospective tonsillectomy audit. The Royal College of Surgeons of England; 2005.
10. Kamal SA, Basu S, Kapoor L, et al. Harmonic scalpel tonsillectomy: a prospective study. Eur Arch Otorhinolaryngol 2006;263(5):449–54.
11. Neumann C, Street I, Lowe D, et al. Harmonic scalpel tonsillectomy: a systematic review of evidence for postoperative hemorrhage. Otolaryngol Head Neck Surg 2007;137(3):378–84.
12. Wang H, Fu Y, Feng Y, et al. Tonsillectomy versus tonsillotomy for sleep-disordered breathing in children: a meta analysis. PLoS One 2015;10(3): e0121500.
13. Goodman RS. Surgicel in the control of post-tonsillectomy bleeding. Laryngoscope 1996;106(8):1044–6.
14. Gallagher TQ, Wilcox L, McGuire E, et al. Analyzing factors associated with major complications after adenotonsillectomy in 4776 patients: comparing three tonsillectomy techniques. Otolaryngol Head Neck Surg 2010;142(6):886–92.
15. Walton J, Ebner Y, Stewart MG, et al. Systematic review of randomized controlled trials comparing intracapsular tonsillectomy with total tonsillectomy in a pediatric population. Arch Otolaryngol Head Neck Surg 2012;138(3):243–9.
16. Mathiasen RA, Cruz RM. Prospective, randomized, controlled clinical trial of a novel matrix hemostatic sealant in children undergoing adenoidectomy. Otolaryngol Head Neck Surg 2004;131(5):601–5.
17. Mozet C, Prettin C, Dietze M, et al. Use of Floseal and effects on wound healing and pain in adults undergoing tonsillectomy: randomised comparison versus electrocautery. Eur Arch Otorhinolaryngol 2012;269(10):2247–54.
18. Stoeckli SJ, Moe KS, Huber A, et al. A prospective randomized double-blind trial of fibrin glue for pain and bleeding after tonsillectomy. Laryngoscope 1999; 109(4):652–5.
19. Zagolski O. Do diet and activity restrictions influence recovery after adenoidectomy and partial tonsillectomy? Int J Pediatr Otorhinolaryngol 2010;74(4):407–11.
20. Cook JA, Murrant NJ, Evans KL, et al. A randomized comparison of three post-tonsillectomy diets. Clin Otolaryngol Allied Sci 1992;17(1):28–31.
21. Lewis SR, Nicholson A, Cardwell ME, et al. Nonsteroidal anti-inflammatory drugs and perioperative bleeding in paediatric tonsillectomy. Cochrane Database Syst Rev 2013;(7):CD003591.
22. Chan DK, Parikh SR. Perioperative ketorolac increases post-tonsillectomy hemorrhage in adults but not children. Laryngoscope 2014;124(8):1789–93.
23. Mahant S, Keren R, Localio R, et al. Dexamethasone and risk of bleeding in children undergoing tonsillectomy. Otolaryngol Head Neck Surg 2014;150(5):872–9.

24. Chan CC, Chan YY, Tanweer F. Systematic review and meta-analysis of the use of tranexamic acid in tonsillectomy. Eur Arch Otorhinolaryngol 2013;270(2):735–48.
25. Witmer CM, Elden L, Butler RB, et al. Incidence of bleeding complications in pediatric patients with type 1 von Willebrand disease undergoing adenotonsillar procedures. J Pediatr 2009;155(1):68–72.
26. Rodriguez KD, Sun GH, Pike F, et al. Post-tonsillectomy bleeding in children with von Willebrand disease: a single-institution experience. Otolaryngol Head Neck Surg 2010;142(5):715–21.
27. Walker P, Gillies D. Post-tonsillectomy hemorrhage rates: are they technique-dependent? Otolaryngol Head Neck Surg 2007;136(Suppl 4):S27–31.
28. Kim DW, Koo JW, Ahn SH, et al. Difference of delayed post-tonsillectomy bleeding between children and adults. Auris Nasus Larynx 2010;37(4):456–60.
29. Watts RG, Cook RP. Operative management and outcomes in children with congenital bleeding disorders: a retrospective review at a single haemophilia treatment centre. Haemophilia 2012;18(3):421–5.
30. Cooper JD, Smith KJ, Ritchey AK. A cost-effectiveness analysis of coagulation testing prior to tonsillectomy and adenoidectomy in children. Pediatr Blood Cancer 2010;55(6):1153–9.
31. Perkins JN, Liang C, Gao D, et al. Risk of post-tonsillectomy hemorrhage by clinical diagnosis. Laryngoscope 2012;122(10):2311–5.
32. Achar P, Sharma RK, De S, et al. Does primary indication for tonsillectomy influence post-tonsillectomy haemorrhage rates in children? Int J Pediatr Otorhinolaryngol 2015;79(2):246–50.
33. Hessén Söderman AC, Ericsson E, Hemlin C, et al. Reduced risk of primary postoperative hemorrhage after tonsil surgery in Sweden: results from the National Tonsil Surgery Register in Sweden covering more than 10 years and 54,696 operations. Laryngoscope 2011;121(11):2322–6.
34. Werner EJ. Preoperative hemostatic screening for pediatric adenotonsillar surgery: worthwhile effort or waste of resources? Pediatr Blood Cancer 2010; 55(6):1045–6.
35. Federici AB, Mannucci PM. Management of inherited von Willebrand disease in 2007. Ann Med 2007;39(5):346–58.
36. Sun GH, Auger KA, Aliu O, et al. Posttonsillectomy hemorrhage in children with von Willebrand disease or hemophilia. JAMA Otolaryngol Head Neck Surg 2013;139(3):245–9.

SUGGESTED READINGS

Chan DK, Parikh SR. Perioperative ketorolac increases post-tonsillectomy hemorrhage in adults but not children. Laryngoscope 2014;124(8):1789–93.

Cooper JD, Smith KJ, Ritchey AK. A cost-effectiveness analysis of coagulation testing prior to tonsillectomy and adenoidectomy in children. Pediatr Blood Cancer 2010; 55(6):1153–9.

Lewis SR, Nicholson A, Cardwell ME, et al. Nonsteroidal anti-inflammatory drugs and perioperative bleeding in paediatric tonsillectomy. Cochrane Database Syst Rev 2013;(7):CD003591.

Mahant S, Keren R, Localio R, et al. Dexamethasone and risk of bleeding in children undergoing tonsillectomy. Otolaryngol Head Neck Surg 2014;150(5):872–9.

Walner DL, Miller SP, Villines D, et al. Coblation tonsillectomy in children: incidence of bleeding. Laryngoscope 2012;122(10):2330–6.

Surgical Management of Severe Epistaxis

Giant Lin, MD[a], Benjamin Bleier, MD[b],*

KEYWORDS

- Epistaxis • Sphenopalatine artery ligation • Anterior ethmoid artery ligation
- Hemostasis • Endoscopic sinus surgery

KEY LEARNING POINTS

At the end of this article, the reader will:

- Be familiar with passive methods of bleeding management to optimize endoscopic visualization.
- Understand the anatomy of the anterior ethmoid artery and surgical approaches to ligate this artery.
- Understand the anatomy of the sphenopalatine artery (SPA) and the surgical steps in endoscopic SPA ligation.
- Know the results of SPA ligation for control of primary epistaxis.

INTRODUCTION

The true incidence of spontaneous epistaxis is unknown, but it is estimated that 60% of individuals experience epistaxis in their lifetime. Of these, 6% seek medical treatment.[1] No standard definition of severe epistaxis exists, but a reasonable definition is any epistaxis that requires surgical intervention, extensive nasal packing, or blood products. In one study,[2] 45% of patients hospitalized for epistaxis had systemic conditions that can contribute to severe epistaxis. Although high-dose aspirin increases bleeding risk and leads to higher chance of rebleeding after intervention for epistaxis, low-dose aspirin (81 mg daily) increases epistaxis risk only slightly (19.1 vs 16.7% in one study).[3] Hypertension as a primary cause of severe epistaxis is controversial. If possible, systemic conditions should be addressed along with surgical intervention in severe cases of epistaxis.

PATIENT OPTIMIZATION

Many patients with severe epistaxis benefit from endoscopic intervention for control of bleeding. However, active bleeding worsens endoscopic visualization. A few initial

[a] Advocare Aroesty Ear, Nose, and Throat Associates, 400 Valley Road, Suite 105, Mount Arlington, NJ 07856, USA; [b] Department of Otolaryngology, Harvard Medical School, Massachusetts Eye and Ear Infirmary, 243 Charles Street, Boston, MA 02114, USA
* Corresponding author.
E-mail address: bleierb@gmail.com

Otolaryngol Clin N Am 49 (2016) 627–637
http://dx.doi.org/10.1016/j.otc.2016.01.003
0030-6665/16/$ – see front matter © 2016 Elsevier Inc. All rights reserved.
oto.theclinics.com

Systemic causes of bleeding
• Alcohol
• Connective tissue disease
• Medications: aspirin, nonsteroidal anti-inflammatory drugs, clopidogrel, warfarin, other antiplatelet or anticoagulant therapy
• Renal disease
• Liver failure
• Hematologic malignancies
• Vitamin C deficiency
• Vitamin K deficiency
• Idiopathic thrombocytopenic purpura
• Disseminated intravascular coagulation
• Genetic bleeding tendency (eg, von Willebrand disease, hemophilia, Bernard-Soulier syndrome)
• Hereditary hemorrhagic telangiectasia
• Alternative medicinals (garlic, ginkgo, ginseng)

maneuvers help the surgeon decrease the blood loss encountered at surgery to more accurately visualize, locate, and control the hemorrhage.

What are some nonsurgical methods of bleeding management?
• Head of bed elevation as part of endoscopic surgical setup
• Topical epinephrine and other decongestants
• Intranasal injections
• Greater palatine injection
• Warm saline irrigation
Anesthetic strategies
• Blood pressure control to decrease bleeding
• Consider use of clonidine as a premedication

Elevation of the head of bed increases venous return and thus decreases overall bleeding in the surgical field. The optimal angle of head elevation is 15° to 20°.[4] One study[4] compared blood loss of sinus surgery performed at 5°, 10°, and 20° of head elevation. Blood loss was 231 mL, 230 mL, and 135 mL, respectively.

Topical decongestants include epinephrine, cocaine, oxymetazoline, phenylephrine, and Moffett solution (2 mL of 10% cocaine, 1 mL of 1:1000 epinephrine, and 2 mL of sodium bicarbonate). No randomized trials exist comparing one decongestant with another in endoscopic sinus surgery. One study[5] showed no difference in blood loss between surgery performed using 1:100,000 and 1:200,000 epinephrine. The 1:1000 epinephrine causes particularly robust vasoconstriction and has been proven to be safe assuming the use of proper safeguards to prevent inadvertent injection.[6] Regardless of surgeon preference, topical decongestants are all effective in producing vasoconstriction and improving surgical visualization.

Selective injection of local anesthetic/decongestant in areas of bleeding is effective in managing epistaxis. Injections can decrease local hydrostatic pressure and also produce vasoconstriction. Greater palatine injection effectively decreases posterior nasal blood supply. It can be performed before endoscopic evaluation of epistaxis by bending a 25-gauge needle 45°, 25 mm from the needle tip.[7] The needle is inserted transorally into the greater palatine canal and the pterygopalatine fossa infiltrated with 1:100,000 epinephrine.

Warm saline irrigation at 49°C has been shown to decrease the rate of bleeding, but endoscopic visualization improves only in longer surgical cases.[8] However, warm saline irrigation can be used to help identify the primary source of bleeding, which can then be treated effectively.

Controlled, hypotensive anesthesia can decrease intraoperative blood loss and improve visualization during surgery. One benefit may be decreased heart rate in addition to decreased blood pressure. Regardless of theoretic advantages, trials regarding the true efficacy of total intravenous anesthesia have not been entirely conclusive or convincing.[9,10] This anesthetic technique remains controversial but can certainly be added to the surgeon and anesthesiologist armamentarium.

A more recent development in efforts to decrease blood loss during endoscopic sinus surgery is the use of clonidine as a premedication. Clonidine activates α_2 receptors within the central nervous system to decrease peripheral sympathetic tone. There is also α_1 agonist activity to a lesser extent, resulting in some peripheral vasoconstriction within the mucosal bed.[11,12] More studies are required to demonstrate the benefit of this medication in endoscopic sinus surgery.

Surgical techniques

- Major vascular targets and techniques to control epistaxis
- Sphenopalatine artery (SPA)
- Anterior ethmoid artery (AEA)
- Posterior ethmoid artery (PEA)
- Vidian and pharyngeal artery
- Carotid artery
- Venous bleeding

Sphenopalatine artery ligation

- Sphenopalatine foramen (SPF) most commonly in the transition zone between middle and superior meatus
- Accessory foramen in 10%
- SPA may exit in multiple branches through the foramen in 35% to 40%
- SPA is generally identified emerging from posterior to the endoscopic landmark, crista ethmoidalis of the palatine bone
- Surgical clipping or diathermy or both?

ANATOMY

The SPA is a branch of the internal maxillary artery and is the major blood supply of the posterior nasal cavity. Epistaxis from this arterial source is generally more severe than anterior epistaxis. The artery enters the nasal cavity from the pterygopalatine fossa via the SPF. Knowledge of the anatomic variations of the SPA and SPF improves surgical results. This article focuses on anatomy pertinent to endoscopic SPA ligation. Transantral ligation of internal maxillary artery branches is of historical interest and is not discussed.

The SPF is located most frequently (87%) at the transitional zone between the superior and middle meatus.[13] It is less frequently found in the superior meatus. The crista ethmoidalis is a bony crest of the palatine bone that points to the SPF. The SPF lies behind this crest and may rest above or straddle this bony crest.[14] A single foramen is usually encountered, but an accessory foramen exists in 10% of patients.[14,15] Terminal branches of the SPA include the posterior septal artery and the posterior lateral nasal artery branches. The SPA exits the SPF as a single branch in 60% to 75%, as two branches in 20% to 30%, and three or more branches in less than 10%.[13,15,16]

SURGICAL APPROACH FOR ENDOSCOPIC SPHENOPALATINE ARTERY LIGATION

The entry zone of the SPA within the nasal cavity is located approximately at the tail of the middle turbinate. The mucosa just anterior to the middle turbinate tail is infiltrated with local anesthetic (usually 1% lidocaine with 1:100,000 epinephrine). Next, the posterior fontanelle of the maxillary sinus and the perpendicular plate of the palatine bone are palpated. A standard maxillary antrostomy is optional for this procedure, but is often valuable in defining the area of mucosal incision at the palatine bone behind the antrostomy and back wall of the maxillary sinus. A vertical mucosal incision at the orbital process of the palatine bone is made, and submucosal dissection proceeds posteriorly to identify the crista ethmoidalis. The crista can be removed with Kerrison rongeurs but this is not always necessary. SPA branches are identified by wide exposure of soft tissue behind the crista ethmoidalis (**Fig. 1**). A ball-probed seeker is helpful in this dissection because it can help define arterial branches with minimal trauma. Awareness of the considerable variation in the number of arterial branches and thorough dissection via wide exposure are critical. Arterial occlusion can be performed by Ligaclips or bipolar electrocoagulation on all isolated arterial branches. The mucosa previously elevated for this dissection is returned to original position.

EFFICACY OF SPHENOPALATINE ARTERY LIGATION

Success rate of SPA ligation for severe epistaxis ranges from 88% to 98%.[17,18] One report showed statistically better control of bleeding with a combination of surgical clips and diathermy.[18] Because of anatomic variations, it is possible to miss arterial

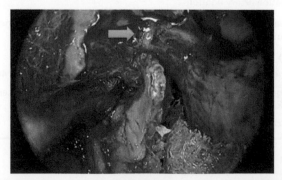

Fig. 1. Example of right SPA dissection before ligation. The *arrow* points to the SPA as it exits the sphenopalatine foramen. SPA branches are identified by wide exposure of soft tissue behind the crista ethmoidalis before ligation.

branches during surgical dissection. One report suggests extending the dissection medially and posteriorly toward the lower sphenoid rostrum to locate the posterior septal branch because this artery may enter the nose through a separate foramen posterior to the SPA. Another option to ensure that all pertinent vessels are addressed is to follow the SPA laterally into the pterygopalatine fossa to ligate the vessel more proximally before any branching occurs. Complications of SPA ligation are uncommon but include rebleeding, sinusitis, and palatal/nasal numbness. Inferior turbinate necrosis was reported in one case.[19] Postoperative care for the procedure involves regular saline rinse as per standard endoscopic sinus surgery.

ANTERIOR ETHMOID ARTERY LIGATION
Surgical Anatomy

The AEA is a branch of the ophthalmic artery that supplies mucosa of the anterior nasal cavity before entering intracranially to form meningeal branches. The artery traverses the ethmoid roof via a bony mesentery in 36% in one cadaveric study (**Fig. 2**).[20] Otherwise, the AEA is protected by the fovea ethmoidalis along the skull base. From an endoscopic approach, the AEA is identified on average 17.5 mm from the axilla of the middle turbinate.[21] From an external, transorbital approach, the artery averages 24 mm from the anterior lacrimal crest.

Severe epistaxis from the AEA is less common than from the SPA. Possible causes include spontaneous, postsinus surgery, and traumatic bleeding. When endoscopic examination suggests an anterior source of intractable bleeding, AEA ligation can be considered.

Approaches

> **Surgical approaches for AEA ligation**
>
> - Open approach
>   - Lynch incision
>   - Transcaruncular incision
>
> - Endoscopic approach
>   - Transethmoid (direct)
>   - Transorbital

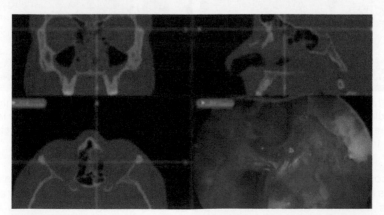

Fig. 2. Anatomy of the left AEA. The AEA in this example traverses the left ethmoid roof via bony mesentery below the skull base. The image-guided frontal probe (*bottom right image*) confirms the location of the artery.

External approach: the Lynch incision

The Lynch incision is performed by making a curvilinear incision at a midpoint between the medial canthus and the middle of the anterior nasal bone. A subperiosteal dissection is performed, identifying the lacrimal crests without injuring the lacrimal apparatus. The AEA is identified in the frontoethmoidal suture line, approximately 24 mm behind the anterior lacrimal crest. Surgical clips or bipolar electrocautery can be used for ligation.

Transcaruncular approach

A transcaruncular approach provides access to the AEA while avoiding a transfacial incision. This medial conjunctival incision along the semilunar fold avoids the lacrimal drainage pathways by staying deep to the posterior fibers of the pretarsal orbicularis muscle (Horner muscle). Dissection in a natural plane between Horner muscle and the medial orbital septum exposes the posterior lacrimal crest, which is the attachment of Horner muscle. Next, the periorbita along the posterior lacrimal crest is incised to expose the medial orbital wall. Subperiosteal dissection then allows access to the medial wall (**Fig. 3**A). The AEA is then ligated (**Fig. 3**B). The periorbita does not require closure, whereas the caruncle and conjunctiva are closed using 6–0 resorbable sutures.

Endoscopic anterior ethmoid artery ligation

> **Endoscopic landmarks of AEA**
>
> - AEA runs posterior to the bulla lamella (posterior to frontal recess)
> - AEA runs in posterolateral to anteromedial direction
> - Can be found approximately 17.5 mm from the axilla of middle turbinate.

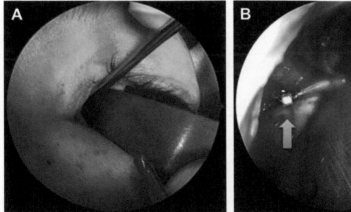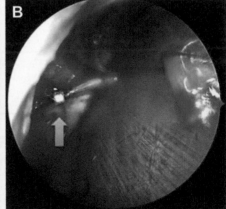

Fig. 3. Trancaruncular approach in a left orbit for control anterior ethmoid artery ligation. The medial orbital wall is exposed (*A*) after incising periorbital along the posterior lacrimal crest. The anterior ethmoid is identified and ligated (*B*). The *arrow* points to the surgical clip applied to the artery.

Endoscopic ligation of the AEA begins with injections of local anesthetic and vasoconstrictors into the middle turbinate axilla and maxillary line. A standard maxillary antrostomy is performed and anterior ethmoid air cells cleared to identify the lamina papyracea and fovea ethmoidalis. An angled telescope aids in identification of the AEA, which crosses the ethmoidal skull base in an anteromedial direction from orbit to cribiform plate. In cases where the AEA is easily identifiable in a bony mesentery, direct clipping or bipolar cautery of the artery may be possible (**Fig. 4**).

A more reliable technique for AEA ligation involves partial removal of the medial orbital wall. A small opening is made through the lamina papyracea just below the area of the AEA. Care is taken to avoid penetrating the periorbita because prolapse of orbital fat narrows the endoscopic corridor and makes positive identification of the AEA difficult. After removal of a small piece of lamina papyracea, gentle retraction of the orbit contents laterally helps identify the AEA. Elevation anterior and posterior to the artery exposes the artery for endoscopic clip placement. No closure is necessary for the endoscopic approach.

Efficacy of Anterior Ethmoid Artery Ligation

Objective data addressing the efficacy of AEA ligation alone in the treatment of severe epistaxis are limited. Most reports on this topic are cadaveric feasibility studies, and AEA ligation is often performed in conjunction with SPA ligation. One cadaveric study showed that endoscopic clipping was successful in only 50% in cases with bony mesentery based on intraoperative computed tomography scan results.[22] Another study showed successful endoscopic AEA ligation in three patients with severe epistaxis.[23] Possible complications include rebleeding, orbital injury, and skull base disruption.

POSTERIOR ETHMOID ARTERY LIGATION

PEA is also a branch of the ophthalmic artery. In an endoscopic study, the PEA is 14.9 mm behind the AEA and 8.1 mm in front of the anterior wall of the sphenoid sinus.[21] The artery is in front of the sphenoid rostrum in 98% of cases when present but may be congenitally absent in up to 50% of patients.[24] Ligation of the PEA is rarely necessary or indicated in severe epistaxis.

VIDIAN AND PHARYNGEAL ARTERY CAUTERY

Bleeding from the vidian and pharyngeal arteries is exceptionally rare except in cases of endonasal tumor resection and other transpterygoid skull base approaches. The pharyngeal artery is a branch of the internal maxillary artery that enters the palatovaginal canal at the sphenoid floor. The vidian artery runs with the vidian nerve in the vidian canal, which is located 3.78 mm lateral to the palatovaginal canal.[25] This artery can be controlled definitively with electrocautery (**Fig. 5**).

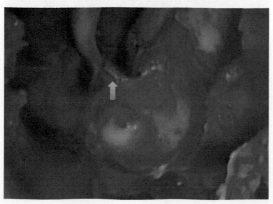

Fig. 4. The bipolar cautery is applied to the left anterior ethmoid artery (*arrow*).

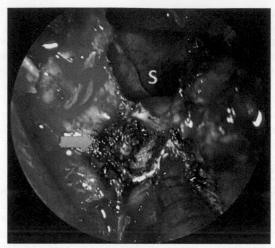

Fig. 5. This right vidian canal (*arrow*) is cauterized as part of a juvenile angiofibroma resection, in this case to decrease blood supply to the tumor from the internal carotid artery system. S, sphenoid sinus.

CAROTID ARTERY BLEEDING

Carotid injury during endoscopic endosnasal skull base surgery is a feared complication, with an incidence of 0.3%.[26] Detailed management protocols are discussed elsewhere in this issue (see Gardner PA, Snyderman CH, Fernandez-Miranda JC, et al: Management of Major Vascular Injury During Endoscopic Endonasal Skull Base Surgery, in this issue).

MANAGEMENT OF VENOUS BLEEDING

Venous bleeding is typically encountered at the pterygopalatine venous plexus, cavernous sinus, and basilar venous plexus during endoscopic skull base surgery. These can be controlled via tamponade. In addition, application of gelatin-based

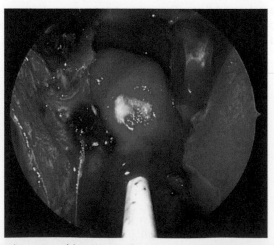

Fig. 6. In this example, venous bleeding in the pterytopalatine venous plexus is controlled with a gelatin-based hemostatic agent.

hemostatic agents provides excellent and rapid control of high-flow venous bleeding (**Fig. 6**). A review of hemostatic agents available for this application is detailed elsewhere in this issue (see Barham HP, Sacks R, Harvey RJ: Hemostatic Materials and Devices, in this issue).

SUMMARY

Advances in endoscopic technique and instrumentation have improved the care of the patient with severe epistaxis. Many patients with severe epistaxis benefit from endoscopic intervention for control of bleeding. The high success rate of SPA ligation should decrease the need for long-term nasal packing for posterior epistaxis. Although less common, intractable bleeding from the anterior nasal cavity may call for anterior ethmoid ligation. Endoscopic approaches for AEA ligation are now possible, but further studies are needed to assess outcomes.

Post-Test Questions (Correct answers are in italics)

1. Which of the listed medications below are both an α_2 agonist and a weak α_1 agonist?
   a. Sevoflurane
   b. Propofol
   c. *Clonidine*
   d. Sufentanil
2. In the transcaruncular approach, what is the immediate plane of dissection after initial conjunctival incision?
   a. *Dissection just deep to Horner muscle*
   b. Dissection just superficial to Horner muscle
   c. Subperiosteal dissection
   d. Just medial to the medial rectus muscle in a posterior direction
3. Which bony structure is located immediately anterior to the SPF and is a critical landmark for endoscopic SPA ligation?
   a. Superior turbinate
   b. Middle turbinate
   c. Uncinate process
   d. *Crista ethmoidalis*
4. An accessory SPF is found in what percentage of patients?
   a. 5%
   b. *10%*
   c. 20%
   d. 30%
5. Which of the following reasons could explain intractable ipsilateral spontaneous posterior epistaxis following SPA clipping (select one or more that apply)
   a. *Incomplete clipping of bleeding vessel, need for clipping and diathermy*
   b. *Wrong vessel clipped because of multiple branches, need for further exploration, and control of bleeding vessel*
   c. *Bleeding from posterior nasal artery emerging from a separate accessory foramen*
   d. Bleeding from vidian artery, need for further exploration and ligation of vidian artery

SUPPLEMENTARY DATA

Supplementary PDF slides related to this article can be found online at http://www.oto.theclinics.com/.

REFERENCES

1. Viehweg TL, Roberson JB, Hudson JW. Epistaxis: diagnosis and treatment. J Oral Maxillofac Surg 2006;64:511–8.
2. Awan MS, Iqbal M, Imam SZ. Epistaxis: when are coagulation studies justified? Emerg Med J 2008;25:156–7.
3. Ridker PM, Manson JE, Gaziano JM, et al. Low-dose aspirin therapy for chronic stable angina. A randomized, placebo-controlled clinical trial. Ann Intern Med 1991;114:835–9.
4. Gan EC, Habib AR, Rajwani A, et al. Five-degree, 10-degree, and 20-degree reverse Trendelenburg position during functional endoscopic sinus surgery: a double-blind randomized controlled trial. Int Forum Allergy Rhinol 2014;4:61–8.
5. Moshaver A, Lin D, Pinto R, et al. The hemostatic and hemodynamic effects of epinephrine during endoscopic sinus surgery: a randomized clinical trial. Arch Otolaryngol Head Neck Surg 2009;135:1005–9.
6. Orlandi RR, Warrier S, Sato S, et al. Concentrated topical epinephrine is safe in endoscopic sinus surgery. Am J Rhinol Allergy 2010;24:140–2.
7. Douglas R, Wormald PJ. Pterygopalatine fossa infiltration through the greater palatine foramen: where to bend the needle. Laryngoscope 2006;116:1255–7.
8. Gan EC, Alsaleh S, Manji J, et al. Hemostatic effect of hot saline irrigation during functional endoscopic sinus surgery: a randomized controlled trial. Int Forum Allergy Rhinol 2014;4(11):877–84.
9. DeConde AS, Thompson CF, Wu EC, et al. Systematic review and meta-analysis of total intravenous anesthesia and endoscopic sinus surgery. Int Forum Allergy Rhinol 2013;3:848–54.
10. Beule AG, Wilhelmi F, Kuhnel TS, et al. Propofol versus sevoflurane: bleeding in endoscopic sinus surgery. Otolaryngol Head Neck Surg 2007;136:45–50.
11. Wawrzyniak K, Burduk PK, Cywinski JB, et al. Improved quality of surgical field during endoscopic sinus surgery after clonidine premedication: a pilot study. Int Forum Allergy Rhinol 2014;4:542–7.
12. Mohseni M, Ebneshahidi A. The effect of oral clonidine premedication on blood loss and the quality of the surgical field during endoscopic sinus surgery: a placebo-controlled clinical trial. J Anesth 2011;25:614–7.
13. Padua FG, Voegels RL. Severe posterior epistaxis-endoscopic surgical anatomy. Laryngoscope 2008;118:156–61.
14. Wareing MJ, Padgham ND. Osteologic classification of the sphenopalatine foramen. Laryngoscope 1998;108:125–7.
15. Midilli R, Orhan M, Saylam CY, et al. Anatomic variations of sphenopalatine artery and minimally invasive surgical cauterization procedure. Am J Rhinol Allergy 2009;23:e38–41.
16. Gras-Cabrerizo JR, Adema-Alcover JM, Gras-Albert JR, et al. Anatomical and surgical study of the sphenopalatine artery branches. Eur Arch Otorhinolaryngol 2014;271:1947–51.
17. Kumar S, Shetty A, Rockey J, et al. Contemporary surgical treatment of epistaxis. What is the evidence for sphenopalatine artery ligation? Clin Otolaryngol Allied Sci 2003;28:360–3.

18. Nouraei SA, Maani T, Hajioff D, et al. Outcome of endoscopic sphenopalatine artery occlusion for intractable epistaxis: a 10-year experience. Laryngoscope 2007;117:1452–6.
19. Moorthy R, Anand R, Prior M, et al. Inferior turbinate necrosis following endoscopic sphenopalatine artery ligation. Otolaryngol Head Neck Surg 2003;129: 159–60.
20. Floreani SR, Nair SB, Switajewski MC, et al. Endoscopic anterior ethmoidal artery ligation: a cadaver study. Laryngoscope 2006;116:1263–7.
21. Han JK, Becker SS, Bomeli SR, et al. Endoscopic localization of the anterior and posterior ethmoid arteries. Ann Otol Rhinol Laryngol 2008;117:931–5.
22. Solares CA, Luong A, Batra PS. Technical feasibility of transnasal endoscopic anterior ethmoid artery ligation: assessment with intraoperative CT imaging. Am J Rhinol Allergy 2009;23:619–21.
23. Pletcher SD, Metson R. Endoscopic ligation of the anterior ethmoid artery. Laryngoscope 2007;117:378–81.
24. Bleier BS, Healy DY Jr, Chhabra N, et al. Compartmental endoscopic surgical anatomy of the medial intraconal orbital space. Int Forum Allergy Rhinol 2014; 4:587–91.
25. Herzallah IR, Amin S, El-Hariri MA, et al. Endoscopic identification of the pharyngeal (palatovaginal) canal: an overlooked area. J Neurol Surg B Skull Base 2012; 73:352–7.
26. Gardner PA, Tormenti MJ, Pant H, et al. Carotid artery injury during endoscopic endonasal skull base surgery: incidence and outcomes. Neurosurgery 2013; 73:261–9 [discussion: 269–70].

SUGGESTED READINGS

Kumar S, Shetty A, Rockey J, et al. Contemporary surgical treatment of epistaxis. What is the evidence for sphenopalatine artery ligation? Clinical otolaryngology and allied sciences 2003;28:360–3.

Nouraei SA, Maani T, Hajioff D, et al. Outcome of endoscopic sphenopalatine artery occlusion for intractable epistaxis: a 10-year experience. The Laryngoscope 2007;117:1452–6.

Treatment of Hereditary Hemorrhagic Telangiectasia–Related Epistaxis

Nathan B. Sautter, MD*, Timothy L. Smith, MD, MPH

KEYWORDS

- Hereditary hemorrhagic telangiectasia (HHT) • Osler-Weber-Rendu • Epistaxis
- Septodermoplasty • Laser photocoagulation • Young's procedure • Bevacizumab

KEY LEARNING POINTS

At the end of this article, the reader will:

- Know how to diagnose a patient with HHT and discover the key examination findings.
- Know what additional workup is required in a patient with HHT.
- Understand the Epistaxis Severity Score and how it is used.
- Know the nonsurgical options for treatment of mild or moderate epistaxis related to HHT.
- Know the surgical options available for treatment of HHT.
- Understand the role of Avastin (bevacizumab) in treatment of HHT.

 Video content accompanies this article at http://www.oto.theclinics.com

INTRODUCTION

HHT is a rare, autosomal dominant disease with prevalence of 1:5000 characterized by formation of multiple mucocutaneous telangiectasias as well as formation of AVMs within the pulmonary, cerebral, and gastrointestinal vasculature. Patients are particularly prone to formation of telangiectasias within the sinonasal mucosa, and recurrent, spontaneous epistaxis is the most common symptom at time of presentation. More than half of patients with HHT will develop troublesome epistaxis by the third decade of life, and severity of epistaxis increases with age. More than 90% of

Conflicts of Interest: There is no relevant conflict of interest or financial disclosure for Dr N.B. Sautter. Dr T.L. Smith is a consultant for IntersectENT (Palo Alto, CA) which provided no financial support for this publication.
Department of Otolaryngology - Head and Neck Surgery, Oregon Sinus Center, Oregon Health and Science University, 3181 Southwest Sam Jackson Park Road, Portland, OR 97239, USA
* Corresponding author. Department of Otolaryngology, Head and Neck Surgery, Providence St. Vincent Medical Center, 9135 Southwest Barnes Road, Suite 963, Portland, OR 97225.
E-mail address: nsautter@gmail.com

Otolaryngol Clin N Am 49 (2016) 639–654
http://dx.doi.org/10.1016/j.otc.2016.02.010
0030-6665/16/$ – see front matter © 2016 Elsevier Inc. All rights reserved.

> **What is HHT?**
>
> - HHT is hereditary hemorrhagic telangiectasia, also known as Osler-Weber-Rendu disease
> - Autosomal dominant inheritance, approximately 1:5000 prevalence
> - Recurrent, spontaneous epistaxis is most common presenting symptom
> - Spontaneous formation of multiple mucocutaneous telangiectasias
> - Patients are also at risk for multiorgan vascular dysplasia with formation of arteriovenous malformations (AVMs) in the brain, lungs, and gastrointestinal (GI) tract

patients with HHT experience recurrent epistaxis at some point in life. Severity and frequency of epistaxis varies widely between patients, from mild, occasional epistaxis to severe, life-threatening nosebleeds. In general, severity of epistaxis increases with age.[1]

ETIOLOGY

> **What causes formation of telangiectasias and AVMs?**
>
> - Mutations in genes associated with transforming growth factor-beta (TGF-β) superfamily signaling pathway
> - Dysregulation of vascular endothelial tissue remodeling results in weakened integrity of vessel wall leading to formation of telangiectasias and AVMs
> - Three gene mutations have been identified: endoglin (ENG), activin receptor-like kinase (ACVRL1 or ALK1), and MADH4

Various members of the transforming growth factor (TGF)-β superfamily have been implicated in the pathogenesis of HHT. Remodeling of the vascular endothelium within mucosal vessels occurs in a dysregulated fashion, leading to loss of elasticity and dilation of arteriole-venule communications. As a result, fragile and thin-walled telangiectasias form within the nasal cavity in regions with high airflow prone to dryness or repeated mechanical trauma. Telangiectasias tend to congregate along the anterior septum, head of inferior turbinates, anterior lateral nasal wall, and anterior nasal floor. Recurrent and spontaneous epistaxis results from traumatic rupture of the ectatic vessel wall lacking contractile and elastic elements. Elevated plasma levels of vascular endothelial growth factor (VEGF) are present in patients with HHT, which has provided rationale for treatment with VEGF inhibitors in certain cases.[2]

Two distinct mutations account for 90% of cases of HHT: ENG mutation is known at HHT1, and ACVRL1 mutation is known as HHT2.[3] Another gene, MADH4 (mothers against decapentaplegic homolog 4) has been implicated in both juvenile polyposis and a small proportion of cases of HHT.[4] Recently, mutation in bone morphogenetic protein-9 (BMP9) has been described as resulting in a vascular anomaly syndrome with phenotypic similarity to HHT.[5]

Distinct phenotypic variations have been described in HHT1 and HHT2. Patients with HHT1 are more likely to present with epistaxis earlier in life as well as pulmonary AVMs. Patients with HHT2 are more likely to develop hepatic AVMs.[6]

DIAGNOSIS

> ### What are the diagnostic criteria for HHT?
>
> - The Curaçao criteria include 4 different clinical criteria: a definite diagnosis is made if 3 criteria are present (Table 1)
> - Positive genetic testing may also provide a definite diagnosis, although testing is expensive and indicated in only a minority of cases

The diagnosis of HHT is based on various clinical and physical examination criteria known as the Curaçao criteria. The Curaçao criteria (see Table 1) were established in 2000 by an expert consensus panel, consisting of 4 different clinical criteria: recurrent and spontaneous epistaxis, mucocutaneous telangiectasias, visceral AVMs, and family history. Three positive criteria are necessary for a "definite" diagnosis, whereas 2 criteria allow for "possible/suspected" diagnosis. Diagnosis is "unlikely" with only 1 criterion present.[7]

Genetic testing may also provide a definite diagnosis of HHT, and standard testing for ENG and ACVRL1 mutation is available. Current genetic testing may not be positive in all patients with HHT due to presence of an unrecognized genetic mutation. Routine genetic testing, therefore, is not recommended in patients with suspected HHT. Expert guidelines have established indications for testing in specific situations, such as prenatal screening, index cases within a family, and establishing or excluding a definite diagnosis in members with few symptoms in a family with known HHT.[7]

EVALUATION

> ### What are characteristic examination findings in patients with HHT?
>
> - Multiple mucocutaneous telangiectasias involving skin (face, fingertips), lips, oral cavity (hard palate), tongue, and sinonasal cavity
> - Differential diagnosis includes CREST syndrome (calcinosis, Raynaud disease, esophageal dysmotility, sclerodactyly, and telangiectasia), essential telangiectasia, ataxia-telangiectasia
> - Telangiectasias vary in morphology from small, flattened, and stellate lesions to large, raised conglomerate lesions
> - Crusting and dryness of nasal mucosa as well as septal perforation are common findings in patients with history of multiple nasal procedures for treatment of epistaxis
> - Iron deficiency in conjunction with low ferritin and elevated transferrin is characteristic in patients with moderate to severe epistaxis

Table 1
Curaçao criteria for diagnosis of hereditary hemorrhagic telangiectasia

Criteria	Description
Epistaxis	Spontaneous and recurrent
Telangiectases	Multiple, at characteristic sites: lips, oral cavity, fingers, nose
Visceral lesions	Gastrointestinal telangiectasia, pulmonary, hepatic, cerebral, or spinal arteriovenous malformations
Family history	A first-degree relative with HHT according to these criteria

Patients with HHT will present to the otolaryngologist with a history of recurrent, spontaneous epistaxis. Some patients will identify particular triggers, such as dietary factors, emotional state, and seasonal variations.[8] Other complaints include sequelae of recurrent epistaxis or prior treatments, such as crusting, foul odor, nasal obstruction, and septal perforation. In addition to the nasal cavity, mucosal telangiectasias involving the lips, hard palate, and tongue are characteristic, and patients may request treatment for these lesions as well. Multiple cutaneous telangiectasias are commonly seen on the skin of the face, ears, and fingertips, and referral to the dermatologist or facial plastic surgeon may be helpful in patients seeking treatment for these lesions. In a patient presenting with intranasal telangiectasias without a prior diagnosis of HHT, other conditions such as CREST syndrome, essential telangiectasia, and ataxia-telangiectasia syndrome should be considered in the differential diagnosis.

A complete examination of the upper aerodigestive tract should be performed during the initial evaluation of the patient with HHT. Anterior rhinoscopy and nasal endoscopy may detect presence of telangiectasias. Nasal endoscopy is performed in a careful, atraumatic manner to prevent bleeding. Patients with a history of severe, high-volume epistaxis may wish to defer nasal endoscopy in the office. Intranasal crusting and blood clots are typically present overlying larger telangiectasias, and debridement, if indicated, should be performed carefully to prevent bleeding. Nasal crusting is particularly prevalent in patients with a history of septodermoplasty. Cotton balls soaked with oxymetazoline or equivalent topical decongestant are a useful adjunct during the examination. Nasal endoscopy is useful to evaluate for septal perforation, scarring, and more posterior telangiectasias that may not be evident on anterior rhinoscopy.

Intranasal telangiectasias vary widely with regard to morphology and number of lesions present. Mahoney and Shapshay[9] described 3 distinct vessel patterns associated with nasal telangiectasias in HHT: small, punctate isolated telangiectasias (type I) (**Fig. 1**), diffuse interconnecting lesions with "feeder" vessels (type II) (**Fig. 2**), and large, solitary AVM (type III). Type I lesions are more likely associated with mild

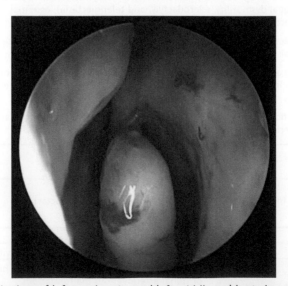

Fig. 1. Endoscopic view of left nasal cavity and left middle turbinate in patient with Shapshay type I (small, stellate) telangiectasias.

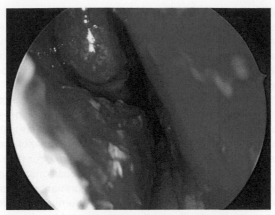

Fig. 2. Endoscopic view of right nasal cavity and middle turbinate in a patient exhibiting Shapshay type II (large, diffuse, interconnecting) telangiectasias.

epistaxis, whereas type II and type III lesions are often associated with moderate or severe epistaxis. Morphologic characterization and quantifying number of lesions may be useful for treatment planning. For example, smaller punctate type I lesions tend to respond well to laser treatment, whereas larger, raised type II and III lesions are better addressed with coblation or electrocautery.[10] Additionally, patients with fewer, predominantly anterior lesions are better candidates for in-office treatment as compared with patients with more numerous, more posterior telangiectasias.

What should be included in the initial evaluation in patients with HHT?

- Nasal endoscopy performed atraumatically, with careful debridement of crusts so as to characterize number and size of telangiectasias

- The Epistaxis Severity Score is a normalized, validated scoring tool used to quantify severity of epistaxis

- Patients with HHT should undergo pulmonary AVM screening with bubble echocardiogram at time of diagnosis and every 5 to 10 years thereafter. Brain MRI is indicated at time of diagnosis. Gastrointestinal (GI) endoscopy is indicated in patients with anemia disproportionate to degree of epistaxis

- Complete blood count and type and cross are recommended before any surgical intervention. Patients with unknown pulmonary AVM status undergoing surgery should undergo bubble echocardiogram screening before surgery

---

A careful history with attention to family history as well as symptoms of visceral AVMs should be performed. A history of stroke, heart failure, and GI bleeding warrant further investigation. The Curaçao criteria expert guidelines recommend screening for pulmonary AVMs and cerebrovascular malformations in all patients with HHT at time of diagnosis.[7] Bubble echocardiogram is a screening test recommended every 5 to 10 years following initial screening to rule out formation of new AVMs. If positive, bubble echocardiogram is followed by chest computed tomography (CT) scan to fully characterize size and number of AVMs. Patients with pulmonary AVMs should be referred to a pulmonologist, interventional radiologist, or thoracic surgeon for treatment. Brain MRI is recommended at time of diagnosis, and presence of cerebrovascular malformations warrants referral to neurosurgery. Routine GI endoscopy is not indicated; however, patients with a history of GI bleeding and/or anemia disproportionate to epistaxis severity should undergo GI endoscopy for diagnosis and treatment of GI AVMs. The wide range of organ systems potentially affected in patients with HHT underlines the need for a multidisciplinary approach.

The Epistaxis Severity Score (ESS) is a validated, normalized scoring tool composed of questions related to nosebleed frequency, severity, presence of anemia, need for medical treatment, and need for blood transfusion.[11] This is the only validated patient questionnaire for HHT-related epistaxis, and is a useful tool for evaluating treatment success as well as following nosebleed severity over time.

Severity of HHT-related epistaxis ranges from mild, occasional nasal bleeding to severe, life-threatening epistaxis. Mild nosebleeds are primarily a quality-of-life issue, whereas moderate bleeding may be associated with anemia or iron deficiency. Microcytic iron deficiency anemia with elevated transferrin and low ferritin is characteristic of moderate or severe HHT-related epistaxis. Expert guidelines recommend annual hemoglobin and hematocrit screening in patients older than 35 years.[7]

Laboratory testing before surgical intervention should include a complete blood count with type and screen or type and crossmatch. Patients should be questioned regarding need for recent blood transfusions, and prepared for possible transfusion during surgery. Patients with unknown pulmonary AVM status should be screened with bubble echocardiogram before surgery. Patients with a positive or unknown history of pulmonary AVM should receive antibiotic prophylaxis before any procedure. Additionally, intravenous filters should be considered in patients with a positive or unknown history of pulmonary AVMs to prevent air embolism.[7]

MANAGEMENT

What nonsurgical treatments are available for patients with HHT-related epistaxis?

- Nosebleed prevention is the mainstay of therapy for any patient with HHT-related epistaxis

- Nonmedicinal prevention measures include avoidance of triggers, use of nasal emollients, proper nasal hygiene, and avoidance of blood thinning medications if possible

- Pressure tamponade and use of topical spray decongestants are useful for nosebleed treatment

- Nondissolvable nasal packing should be avoided in most cases

- Topical medical treatments include bevacizumab (Avastin), estriol, tranexamic acid, thalidomide, and timolol

---

Treatment of HHT-related epistaxis includes nasal hygiene and avoidance of triggers.[8] Regardless of treatment modality (with exception of nasal closure), nosebleeds will continue. In most patients, treatment goals include decreasing the frequency, volume, and severity of epistaxis and to improve quality of life. Less commonly, treatment is pursued to relieve severe anemia or prevent life-threatening epistaxis. There are few randomized, prospective studies of treatment modalities for HHT-related epistaxis. Most reports are retrospective case series or based on expert opinion. No standard treatment algorithm is available; however, a graduated treatment strategy beginning with conservative topical therapies progressing to more invasive surgical treatments is recommended. **Table 2** summarizes the treatment options with associated level of evidence.

Prevention of nasal dryness and crusting is essential in all patients with HHT. Various topical nasal emollients are available to maintain nasal humidification. Many commercial products with a strong safety profile are available for frequent, daily use. In general, saline gels formulated with hyaluronic acid are more effective than saline mist sprays at maintaining a high level of nasal hydration. Several other emollient products have been proposed for daily use in patients with HHT, including mupirocin ointment, petroleum jelly, and tranexamic acid gel.[12–14] A recent cohort study demonstrated a significant improvement in ESS using compounded topical sesame/rose geranium oil in patients with HHT.[15] Nasal saline irrigations may be effective at preventing crusting and dryness, but should be administered carefully in an atraumatic manner as they may be a trigger for nosebleeds in some patients.

Bevacizumab (Avastin, Roche/Genentech, San Francisco, CA) is a monoclonal antibody inhibitor of the VEGF-A receptor that has been proposed as a preventive treatment modality for HHT-related epistaxis. Several case series have demonstrated efficacy with this treatment modality. Limitations include cost and lack of insurance coverage due to off-label use. When used topically, benefits of treatment generally extend for 2 weeks following cessation of use. The largest published case series to date evaluated treatment of 52 patients with HHT with topical and/or injected bevacizumab in conjunction with potassium-titanyl phosphate (KTP) laser photocoagulation. Significant improvement in ESS was noted up to 46 months after treatment. Submucosal injection of bevacizumab in the region of the cartilaginous septum was associated with a high risk of septal perforation in this series.[16,17]

Studies evaluating treatment for HHT-related epistaxis using estrogen and selective estrogen receptor modifiers such as raloxifene have demonstrated some efficacy.[18–20] Two prospective, randomized studies evaluating raloxifene treatment in patients with HHT demonstrated improvement in severity and frequency of nosebleeds, in addition to improvement in hemoglobin levels in a subset of patients. Topical estriol therapy has also proven effective in reducing HHT-related epistaxis.[21,22] Patients will often report worse epistaxis following menopause, and hormonal replacement should be considered in those patients not at increased risk of breast or endometrial cancer.

Recently, topical timolol therapy (0.5% ophthalmic solution, 1 drop each nostril 3 times a day) has been described as a successful treatment for HHT-related epistaxis, although evidence is limited to a single case report.[23]

What surgical interventions are available for HHT-related epistaxis?

- Surgical treatment should be tailored to the individual patient and severity of epistaxis
- In-office treatments useful for mild to moderate epistaxis include injection sclerotherapy or bipolar electrocautery
- Use of silver nitrate cautery should be avoided in patients with HHT
- Cauterization treatment options in the operating room (OR) for moderate to severe epistaxis include laser photocoagulation, electrocautery, and electrosurgical plasma coagulation (coblation)
- More aggressive surgical options include septodermoplasty and nasal closure (Young procedure) for cases of moderately severe or severe epistaxis

Table 2
Summary of treatments for hereditary hemorrhagic telangiectasia–related epistaxis with level of evidence

Therapy	Indications	Advantages	Disadvantages	Level of Evidence	References
Estrogen/antiestrogen therapy	Mild, moderate or severe epistaxis	Prevention of osteoporosis	May only be used in female patients	Prospective, randomized, placebo-controlled trials (Level I)	Albinana et al,[18] 2010; Jameson & Cave,[19] 2004; Yaniv et al,[20] 2009
Topical estrogen	Mild epistaxis	No systemic effects as compared with oral administration	Long-term use results in squamous metaplasia of nasal mucosa; efficacy is not well established	Single randomized placebo-controlled trial (Level II)	Vase,[21] 1981
Bevacizumab (topical application)	Mild to moderate epistaxis	Ease of application	Need for daily, ongoing use; safety profile has not been well studied for topical application; currently not approved by the Food and Drug Administration for topical intranasal use	Prospective, randomized placebo-controlled multi-institutional trial is ongoing, Level I (pending)	—
Bevacizumab (injection)	Moderate to severe epistaxis	May provide additional benefit when combined with surgical treatment	Septal perforation if injected into cartilaginous septum	Single case series, Level IV	Karnezis & Davidson,[17] 2010
Injection sclerotherapy (sodium tetradecyl sulfate or polydocanol)	Mild or moderate epistaxis	In-office procedure	Safety profile not well defined	Retrospective case series, Level IV	Boyer et al,[24] 2011; Hanks et al,[26] 2014; Morais et al,[25] 2012
Bipolar cautery	Mild to moderate epistaxis	Readily available, may be combined with laser photocoagulation	Deeper degree of thermal injury compared with laser photocoagulation	Single case series, Level IV	Ghaheri et al,[34] 2006

Treatment	Indication	Advantages	Disadvantages	Level of Evidence	References
KTP laser	Moderate to severe epistaxis	Useful for smaller, punctate lesions, very precise	Risk of injury to patient, OR personnel, airway fire; bleeding during procedure can limit visualization	Few case series, Level IV	Harvey et al,[30] 2008; Karnezis & Davidson,[17] 2010
Nd:YAG laser	Moderate to severe epistaxis	Useful for smaller, punctate lesions, very precise	Risk of injury to patient, OR personnel, airway fire; deeper thermal injury can result in septal perforation	Several case series, Level IV	Kuhnel et al,[31] 2005; Mahoney & Shapshay,[9] 2006; Kluger et al,[28] 1987
Coblation	Moderate to severe epistaxis	Ease of use, higher degree of OR safety compared with laser treatments; useful for larger, conglomerate lesions; may be combined with laser therapy	Not well studied, deeper degree of thermal injury and less precise than laser treatments	Prospective, randomized trial (Level II)	Luk et al,[10] 2014
Septodermoplasty	Severe epistaxis, or moderate epistaxis not responsive to more conservative treatment	Effective for near-cessation of bleeding for up to 2 y	Destructive, loss of native nasal mucosa resulting in increased crusting; donor site morbidity for skin graft	Several case series, Level IV	Lesnik et al,[37] 2007; Harvey et al,[30] 2008; Ross & Nguyen,[35] 2004
Young procedure	Life-threatening or severely recalcitrant epistaxis	Complete cessation of bleeding in most reports	Loss of nasal function, obligatory mouth breathing	Several case series, Level IV	Ross & Nguyen,[35] 2004; Gluckman & Portugal,[38] 1994; Hosni & Innes,[39] 1994; Lund & Howard,[40] 1997

In-office treatment has gained in popularity in recent years following initial descriptions of intranasal injection sclerotherapy. Intranasal sclerotherapy is useful for mild or mild to moderate cases of HHT-related epistaxis. One of the primary advantages of in-office treatment includes avoidance of general anesthesia, which is a significant benefit in patients suffering from pulmonary or cardiac sequelae of HHT. Disadvantages of in-office treatment include diminished access to more posterior lesions and decreased ability to control higher volume bleeding in an awake patient. Boyer and colleagues[24] provided the first description of in-office injection sclerotherapy using sodium tetradecyl sulfate (Sotradecol, AngioDynamics, Latham, NY). A large European case series describes use of polidocanol injection sclerotherapy with equal efficacy.[25] The sclerosant is diluted in a 4:1 fashion with air and foamed by vigorously passing the solution between 2 Luer lock syringes. Following application of local anesthetic, up to 3 mL foamed sclerosant is injected peripherally into telangiectasias in a submucosal fashion. Generally, benefits of injection sclerotherapy will last up to 4 months.[24–26]

Monopolar electrocautery and silver nitrate cautery have been associated with increased risk of septal perforation. Monopolar suction electrocautery may be used prudently in the OR when other modalities fail to achieve hemostasis (Video 1). In general, silver nitrate cautery should be avoided in patients with HHT as it is relatively imprecise and has a tendency to worsen epistaxis severity.[27]

Endoscopic intranasal laser photocoagulation has been a mainstay of operative treatment for HHT-related epistaxis since it was first described nearly 30 years ago.[28] Both the KTP and neodymium-doped yttrium aluminum garnet (Nd:YAG) lasers have been described for this use. The advantages of this method include precise coagulation of vessels with relatively minimal depth of thermal injury. Disadvantages of laser treatment include cost and lack of availability at some centers. Additionally, eye protection is required by all OR personnel, and special precautions, such as moist eye pads and wet towel drapes, are necessary during use.[29] Several retrospective series have described success with this treatment modality, with decrease in nosebleed frequency and severity for approximately 1 to 2 years following treatment.[28,30–33] In general, patients with smaller, punctate telangiectasias fare well with laser photocoagulation, whereas those with larger, conglomerate lesions are better treated with other modalities, such as coblation or septodermoplasty. Lesions are treated in a "rosette" fashion, starting at the periphery of the lesion so as to address feeding vessels, then proceeding inward. Laser photocoagulation is relatively ineffective in situations with active bleeding (Video 2).

Bipolar electrocautery and electrosurgical plasma coagulation (coblation) are both effective surgical treatments for HHT-related epistaxis. Bipolar is generally preferred over monopolar electrocautery due to improved precision and decreased depth of thermal injury.[34] Several bipolar forceps designed for endoscopic nasal surgery are available commercially, such as the Landolt, Wormald, and Stammberger instrument designs. The coblation wand (PROcise EZ and EXcise PDX wands; ArthroCare ENT, Austin, TX) combines irrigating bipolar function along with coblation function, which is useful for ablation of large, conglomerate telangiectasias. The coblation wand is particularly effective during active bleeding (**Fig. 3**, Video 3). A recent randomized, prospective trial demonstrated similar efficacy comparing coblation treatment with KTP laser photocoagulation.[10]

Septodermoplasty is an effective treatment for patients with HHT with moderate to severe epistaxis, or in those patients who prefer to avoid repeat surgical cautery treatments. This technique involves removal of the superficial layer of septal mucosa while carefully preserving the underlying perichondrium. This may be accomplished using curettage or with the microdebrider. A split-thickness skin graft is positioned over the denuded septal mucosa, and nasal packing is left in place for several days to prevent disruption of the graft (**Fig. 4**). Some investigators describe staged unilateral

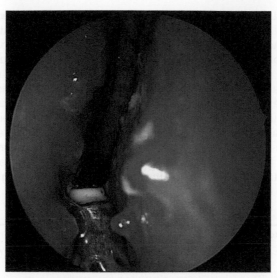

Fig. 3. The coblation wand positioned between the inferior turbinate and septum as the surgeon prepares to coblate a bulky, raised telangiectasia on the nasal septum.

procedures; bilateral procedure may be performed safely in one session. In patients with prominent telangiectasias along the nasal floor, inferior turbinates, and lateral nasal wall, the graft may be extended to cover the nasal floor and lateral nasal wall after removal of the inferior turbinates.[35] A handful of case series have described success with this technique as measured by improved quality of life and decreased need for blood transfusion in previously transfusion-dependent patients with HHT. Patients should expect a significant reduction in epistaxis for at least 2 years, at which point neovascularization with formation of new telangiectasias within and around the graft starts to occur. Invariably, patients experience loss of normal mucociliary function in the region of the graft with resulting crusting and foul odor, and a daily nasal hygiene regimen may be necessary in these patients.[30,35–37]

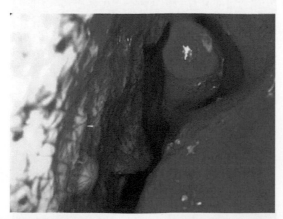

Fig. 4. Endoscopic view of the left nasal cavity in a patient undergoing septodermoplasty procedure for HHT-related epistaxis. The split-thickness skin graft has been positioned in place over the left septum using a quilting Vicryl Rapide suture. The skin graft is distinguished by its relatively pale color.

Complete closure of the nasal vestibule, also known as the Young procedure, is used in patients with severe, transfusion-dependent or life-threatening epistaxis. This technique achieves complete nasal closure by raising mucocutaneous flaps through an endonasal or alotomy approach. This procedure results in obligatory mouth breathing and loss of olfaction. Although patients are often reluctant to lose the ability to breathe through their nose, this can be an effective and potentially life-saving procedure in cases in which prior treatment with cautery and/or septodermo-plasty has been unsuccessful. This technique also may be performed in a unilateral fashion, and closure can be reversed at any time if the patient desires. Several small case series have described success with this technique when other less aggressive treatments have failed.[38–40] Ting and colleagues[41] described a case of severe life-threatening epistaxis in a patient with HHT following the Young procedure that required reversal of nasal closure and endovascular treatment.

> **What are potential complications of treatment?**
>
> - Surgical treatment: septal perforation, scarring, chronic nasal crusting, bleeding, and infection
> - Septodermoplasty: Crusting and foul odor are expected
> - Recurrent epistaxis is not a complication, but epistaxis may increase in severity after treatment
> - Life-threatening epistaxis has been reported following the Young procedure

Septal perforation is one of the most common complications of surgical treatment for HHT-related epistaxis, and should be avoided if possible (**Fig. 5**). Injury to opposing sides of the cartilaginous septum deep to the perichondrium can result in a perforation. Septal perforation causes a disruption of laminar nasal airflow with subsequent dryness and crusting. This results in large telangiectasias at the posterior aspect of the

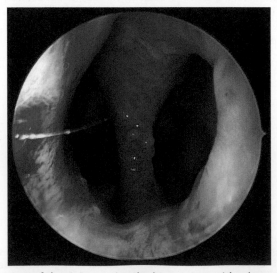

Fig. 5. Endoscopic view of the right nasal cavity in a patient with a large septal perforation resulting from multiple prior surgical treatments for HHT-related epistaxis.

perforation, and treatment of these lesions can enlarge the perforation. Collapse of the nasal dorsum with saddle nose deformity may occur from large septal perforations. Careful surgical technique while avoiding injury to opposing sides of the septum, and avoidance of excessive use of monopolar cautery or silver nitrate cautery will help prevent this complication. Submucosal injection of bevacizumab following surgical cautery increases risk of perforation.[16] A staged procedure should be considered when large, prominent telangiectasias are present on opposing areas of the anterior nasal septum.

Scarring is an expected outcome of most surgical cautery procedures. Scarring results in loss of mucociliary clearance and function, leading to crusting and mucostasis. Postoperative nasal hygiene and nasal debridement may help prevent adverse scarring. Scarring with formation of synechiae may result in obstruction of nasal airflow or outflow of sinonasal secretions, and this may be corrected in the office or during subsequent procedures.

Some patients may experience a worsening in epistaxis severity following treatment. In these cases, alternative treatment modalities should be considered. It is not uncommon for patients to experience increased epistaxis during the initial 2 weeks after surgery, and a regimen of aggressive nasal humidification along with a course of oral antibiotics may help speed healing in these cases. Use of bevacizumab in conjunction with surgical cautery may increase success rates in patients in whom standard treatments have failed to garner benefit.

SUMMARY

Several medical and surgical treatments are available for HHT-related epistaxis. Severity of epistaxis varies widely among patients with HHT, from mild, annoying nosebleeds to severe, transfusion-dependent and potentially life-threatening epistaxis. Treatment should be tailored to the individual patient, and careful presurgical counseling is helpful to establish realistic expectations of surgical treatments. Generally, a graduated treatment approach is successful, starting with topical therapies and progressing to more invasive surgical procedures.

The HHT Foundation, now known as Cure HHT, is a valuable online resource for patients and their families (curehht.org).

Post-Test Questions (Correct answers are in italics)

1. Mutations in these 2 genes are responsible for most cases of HHT
   a. *ACVRL1 and Endoglin (ENG)*
   b. Endoglin (ENG) and MADH4
   c. TGF-beta and VEGF
   d. HHT1 and HHT2
2. The ____ criteria are used to make a clinical diagnosis of HHT
   a. HHT Foundation
   b. ESS
   c. *Curaçao*
   d. Faughnan
3. In addition to intranasal telangiectasias, patients with HHT are also at risk for AVMs involving these organ systems
   a. Pulmonary
   b. Gastrointestinal
   c. CNS
   d. *All of the above*

---

4. Which of the following methods of cautery are not generally recommended for treatment of HHT-related epistaxis?
   a. KTP laser
   b. *Silver nitrate*
   c. Bipolar
   d. Coblation

SUPPLEMENTARY DATA

Supplementary data related to this article can be found at http://dx.doi.org/10.1016/j.otc.2016.02.010.

Supplementary PDF slides related to this article can be found online at http://www.oto.theclinics.com/.

REFERENCES

1. Plauchu H, de Chadarevian JP, Bideau A, et al. Age-related clinical profile of hereditary hemorrhagic telangiectasia in an epidemiologically recruited population. Am J Med Genet 1989;32:291–7.
2. Sadick H, Riedel F, Naim R, et al. Patients with hereditary hemorrhagic telangiectasia have increased plasma levels of vascular endothelial growth factor and transforming growth factor-beta 1 as well as high ALK1 tissue expression. Haematologica 2005;90:818–28.
3. Lesca G, Burnichon N, Raux G, et al. Distribution of ENG and ACVRL1 (ALK1) mutations in French HHT patients. Hum Mutat 2006;27:598.
4. Gallione CJ, Repetto GM, Legius E, et al. A combined syndrome of juvenile polyposis and hereditary haemorrhagic telangiectasia associated with mutations in MADH4 (SMAD4). Lancet 2004;363:852–9.
5. Wooderchak-Donahue WL, McDonald J, O'Fallon B, et al. BMP9 mutations cause a vascular-anomaly syndrome with phenotypic overlap with hereditary hemorrhagic telangiectasia. Am J Hum Genet 2013;93:530–7.
6. Dupuis-Girod S, Bailly S, Plauchu H. Hereditary hemorrhagic telangiectasia: from molecular biology to patient care. J Thromb Haemost 2010;8:1447–56.
7. Faughnan ME, Palda VA, Garcia-Tsao G, et al. International guidelines for the diagnosis and management of hereditary haemorrhagic telangiectasia. J Med Genet 2011;48:73–87.
8. Silva BM, Hosman AE, Devlin HL, et al. Lifestyle and dietary influences on nosebleed severity in hereditary hemorrhagic telangiectasia. Laryngoscope 2013;123:1092–9.
9. Mahoney EJ, Shapshay SM. New classification of nasal vasculature patterns in hereditary hemorrhagic telangiectasia. Am J Rhinol 2006;20:87–90.
10. Luk L, Mace JC, Bhandarkar ND, et al. Comparison of electrosurgical plasma coagulation and potassium-titanyl-phosphate laser photocoagulation for treatment of hereditary hemorrhagic telangiectasia-related epistaxis. Int Forum Allergy Rhinol 2014;4(8):640–5.
11. Hoag JB, Terry P, Mitchell S, et al. An epistaxis severity score for hereditary hemorrhagic telangiectasia. Laryngoscope 2010;120(4):838–43.
12. Messick D, Hurtuk A. Effectiveness of a nasal saline gel in the treatment of recurrent anterior epistaxis in anticoagulated patients. Ear Nose Throat J 2011;90:E4–6.

13. Tibbelin A, Aust R, Holgersson M, et al. Effect of local tranexamic acid gel in the treatment of epistaxis. ORL J Otorhinolaryngol Relat Spec 1995;57:207–9.

14. Kubba H, MacAndie C, Botma M, et al. A prospective, single-blind, randomized controlled trial of antiseptic cream for recurrent epistaxis in childhood. Clin Otolaryngol 2001;26:465–8.

15. Reh DD, Hur K, Merlo CA. Efficacy of a topical sesame/rose geranium oil compound in patients with hereditary hemorrhagic telangiectasia associated epistaxis. Laryngoscope 2013;123:820–2.

16. Chen S, Karnezis T, Davidson TM. Safety of intranasal bevacizumab (Avastin) treatment in patients with hereditary hemorrhagic telangiectasia-associated epistaxis. Laryngoscope 2010;121:644–6.

17. Karnezis TT, Davidson TM. Efficacy of intranasal bevacizumab (Avastin) treatment in patients with hereditary hemorrhagic telangiectasia-associated epistaxis. Laryngoscope 2010;121:636–8.

18. Albinana V, Bernabeu-Herrero ME, Zarrabeitia R, et al. Estrogen therapy for hereditary haemorrhagic telangiectasia (HHT): effects of raloxifene on endoglin and ALK1 expression in endothelial cells. Thromb Haemost 2010;103:525–34.

19. Jameson JJ, Cave DR. Hormonal and antihormonal therapy for epistaxis in hereditary hemorrhagic telangiectasia. Laryngoscope 2004;114:705–9.

20. Yaniv E, Preis M, Hadar T, et al. Antiestrogen therapy for hereditary hemorrhagic telangiectasia: a doubleblind placebo-controlled clinical trial. Laryngoscope 2009;119:284–8.

21. Vase P. Estrogen treatment of hereditary hemorrhagic telangiectasia. A double-blind controlled clinical trial. Acta Med Scand 1981;209:393–6.

22. Sadick H, Ramin N, Oulmi J, et al. Plasma surgery and topical estriol: effects on the nasal mucosa and long-term results in patients with Osler's disease. Otolaryngol Head Neck Surg 2003;128:233–8.

23. Olitsky SE. Topical timolol for the treatment of epistaxis in hereditary hemorrhagic telangiectasia. Am J Rhinol 2012;33(3):375–6.

24. Boyer H, Fernandes P, Duran O. Office-based sclerotherapy for recurrent epistaxis due to hereditary hemorrhagic telangiectasia: a pilot study. Int Forum Allergy Rhinol 2011;1(4):319–23.

25. Morais D, Millas T, Zarrabeitia R, et al. Local sclerotherapy with polydocanol (Aethoxysklerol) for the treatment of epistaxis in Rendu-Osler-Weber or hereditary hemorrhagic telangiectasia (HHT): 15 years of experience. Rhinology 2012;50(1):80–6.

26. Hanks JE, Hunter D, Goding GS. Complications from office sclerotherapy for epistaxis due to hereditary hemorrhagic telangiectasia (HHT or Osler-Webe-Rendu). Int Forum Allergy Rhinol 2014;4(5):422–7.

27. McCaffrey TV, Kern EB, Lake CF. Management of epistaxis in hereditary hemorrhagic telangiectasia: review of 80 cases. Arch Otolaryngol 1977;103:627–30.

28. Kluger PB, Shapshay SM, Hybels RL, et al. Neodyminum-YAG laser intranasal photocoagulation for hereditary hemorrhagic telangiectasia: an update report. Laryngoscope 1987;97:1397–401.

29. Sliney DH. Laser safety. Lasers Surg Med 1995;16:215–25.

30. Harvey RJ, Kanagalingam J, Lund VJ. The impact of septodermoplasty and potassium-titanyl-phosphate (KTP) laser therapy in the treatment of hereditary hemorrhagic telangiectasia-related epistaxis. Am J Rhinol 2008;22:182–7.

31. Kuhnel TS, Wagner BH, Schurr CP, et al. Clinical strategy in hereditary hemorrhagic telangiectasia. Am J Rhinol 2005;19:508–13.

32. Shah RK, Dhingra JK, Shapshay SM. Hereditary hemorrhagic telangiectasia: a review of 76 cases. Laryngoscope 2002;112:767–73.

33. Lennox PA, Harries M, Lund VJ, et al. A retrospective study of the role of the argon laser in the management of epistaxis secondary to hereditary haemorrhagic telangiectasia. J Laryngol Otol 1997;111:34–7.
34. Ghaheri BA, Fong KJ, Hwang PH. The utility of bipolar electrocautery in hereditary hemorrhagic telangiectasia. Otolaryngol Head Neck Surg 2006;134:1006–9.
35. Ross DA, Nguyen DB. Inferior turbinectomy in conjunction with septodermoplasty for patients with hereditary hemorrhagic telangiectasia. Laryngoscope 2004;114: 779–81.
36. McCabe WP, Kelly AP Jr. Management of epistaxis in Osler-Weber-Rendu disease: recurrence of telangiectases within a nasal skin graft. Plast Reconstr Surg 1972;50:114–8.
37. Lesnik GT, Ross DA, Henderson KJ, et al. Septectomy and septal dermoplasty for the treatment of severe transfusion-dependent epistaxis in patients with hereditary hemorrhagic telangiectasia and septal perforation. Am J Rhinol 2007;21:312–5.
38. Gluckman JL, Portugal LG. Modified Young's procedure for refractory epistaxis due to hereditary hemorrhagic telangiectasia. Laryngoscope 1994;104:1174–7.
39. Hosni AA, Innes AJ. Hereditary hemorrhagic telangiectasia: Young's procedure. J Laryngol Otol 1994;108:754–7.
40. Lund VJ, Howard DJ. Closure of the nasal cavities in the treatment of refractory hereditary haemorrhagic telangiectasia. J Laryngol Otol 1997;111:30–3.
41. Ting JY, Remenschneider A, Holbrook EH. Management of severe epistaxis after Young's procedure: a case report. Int Forum Allergy Rhinol 2013;3:334–7.

SUGGESTED READINGS

Boyer H, Fernandes P, Duran O. Office-based sclerotherapy for recurrent epistaxis due to hereditary hemorrhagic telangiectasia: a pilot study. Int Forum Allergy Rhinol 2011;1(4):319–23.

This article provides the first description of in-office Sotradecol sclerotherapy treatment for HHT-related epistaxis, which has become a popular in-office treatment option for HHT patients over the past 5 years.

Faughnan ME, Palda VA, Garcia-Tsao G, et al. International guidelines for the diagnosis and management of hereditary haemorrhagic telangiectasia. J Med Genet 2011;48:73–87.

This article summarizes the expert consensus guidelines for diagnosis and HHT and provides recommendations for screening and other diagnostic studies.

Harvey RJ, Kanagalingam J, Lund VJ. The impact of septodermoplasty and potassium-titanyl-phosphate (KTP) laser therapy in the treatment of hereditary hemorrhagic telangiectasia-related epistaxis. Am J Rhinol 2008;22:182–7.

This article provides a good summary of both septodermoplasty and KTP laser treatment for HHT, and also provides some outcomes data.

Hoag JB, Terry P, Mitchell S, et al. An epistaxis severity score for hereditary hemorrhagic telangiectasia. Laryngoscope 2010;120(4):838–43.

This article summarizes the Epistaxis Severity Score, which is a validated questionnaire that is, useful for quantifying severity of nosebleeds in patients with HHT.

Silva BM, Hosman AE, Devlin HL, et al. Lifestyle and dietary influences on nosebleed severity in hereditary hemorrhagic telangiectasia. Laryngoscope 2013;123:1092–9.

This article provides the results of a large survey sent to patients with HHT inquiring about various dietary and lifestyle triggers for epistaxis.

Hemostasis in Endoscopic Sinus Surgery

Harshita Pant, BMBS, PhD

KEYWORDS

- Sinus • Skull base • Bleeding • Hemostasis • Surgical field • Endoscopic
- Hypotensive anesthesia • Total intravenous anesthesia

KEY LEARNING POINTS

At the end of this article, the reader will:

- Apply key perioperative preventive strategies to minimize bleeding during sinus surgery.
- Critically assess named vessels that may be at risk of injury during sinonasal surgery.
- Understand the rational application of local vasoconstrictors.
- Understand the effects of relevant hemodynamic parameters during general anesthesia on the surgical field.
- Apply a logical approach in the management of intraoperative bleeding.
- Apply a rational approach in the management of suspected orbital compartment syndrome caused by anterior ethmoid artery bleed.

INTRODUCTION

Broad classification of hemostasis during endoscopic sinus surgery

- Management of expected bleeding
  - Microvascular circulation: mucosa, bone, vascular tumors
- Management of inadvertent vascular injury
  - Macrovascular circulation: named vessels

Endoscopic sinus surgery (ESS) is considered to be a moderate bleeding risk surgery. Bleeding is anticipated during sinonasal surgery when treating inflammatory and vascular disorders, and is due in part to the inherently rich blood supply derived from the external and internal carotid arteries in this region. Expected surgical bleeding is encountered from mucosa, bone and vascular tumors, such as juvenile angiofibroma and metastatic renal cell carcinoma.

Department of Otolaryngology, Head and Neck Surgery, University of Adelaide School of Medicine, Frome Road, Adelaide, SA 5005, Australia
E-mail address: harshita.pant@adelaide.edu.au

Otolaryngol Clin N Am 49 (2016) 655–676
http://dx.doi.org/10.1016/j.otc.2016.03.011
0030-6665/16/$ – see front matter © 2016 Elsevier Inc. All rights reserved.

oto.theclinics.com

Why is hemostasis important in sinonasal surgery?

- To improve intraoperative surgical field and visualization
  - Avoid injury (vascular, cerebrospinal fluid leak, orbital)
  - Allow completion of the surgical procedure

- Minimize bleeding associated comorbidities
  - Nausea, emesis and aspiration
  - Significant blood loss, hypoxia and blood transfusion

- Prevent the need for nasal packing and related complications

- Prevent postoperative complications and improve healing
  - Hematoma and bleeding
  - Adhesions and scarring

Adequate hemostasis of the microvascular and macrovascular circulation is needed during endoscopic or open sinus surgery, performed under local or general anesthesia, to accomplish the surgical goals and avoid complications. A thorough risk assessment is required to prevent excessive bleeding. Correct assessment of the source of the bleeding, and a detailed knowledge of surgical vascular anatomy and of hemostatic techniques, is necessary to successfully manage intraoperative bleeding.

Risk of mucosal bleeding

- Disorders
  - Chronic rhinosinusitis with nasal polyps, eosinophilic mucus chronic rhinosinusitis (EMCRS), allergic fungal rhinosinusitis (AFRS)
  - Rhinitis medicamentosa
  - Infection, subperiosteal abscess
  - Thyroid eye disease for example, Graves ophthalmopathy
  - Immunopathology; for example, Sarcoidosis, Wegener granulomatosis, Churg-Strauss disease
  - Vascular tumors (juvenile angiofibroma, metastatic renal cell carcinoma)

- Prior surgery, radiotherapy

- Patient
  - Morbid obesity, hypertension
  - Chronic alcohol, liver, kidney disease
  - Smoking
  - Coagulopathies (congenital or acquired)

Risk of inadvertent vascular injury

- Incorrect diagnosis
  - Internal carotid artery aneurysm, vascular tumor

- Unfavorable vascular and sinonasal anatomy
  - Ethmoidal arteries (anterior, posterior, and sometimes middle)
  - Internal carotid artery
  - Onodi cell
  - Sphenoid sinus septations

- Previous sinonasal surgery
  - Bone dehiscence, scarring, altered or absent anatomic landmarks

- Surgical mistakes

APPROACH TO HEMOSTASIS IN SINUS SURGERY

- Prevention of excessive bleeding
  - Preoperative strategies
  - Intraoperative strategies
- Management of intraoperative bleeding
- Management of postoperative bleeding

Significant intraoperative bleeding can be minimized by preventive measures preoperatively, intraoperatively, and postoperatively. When bleeding is encountered, either intraoperatively or postoperatively, the surgeon has to be prepared to be able to manage this effectively.

BLEEDING PREVENTION: PREOPERATIVE

Some preventive preoperative hemostasis strategies

- Assessment and treatment of comorbid patient factors (see Tassler A, Kaye R: Preoperative assessment of risk factors, in this issue)

- Timely cessation of medications that increase the risk of bleeding (see McKean E: Quality control approach to anticoagulants and transfusion, in this issue)

- Minimize sinonasal inflammatory and vascular burden
  - Role of preoperative glucocorticosteroids (GCs)
  - Vascular tumors and preoperative embolization

- Thoroughly examine clinically relevant vascular anatomy on patient's sinus computed tomography (CT) scans

For a comprehensive review on the assessment and management of patient comorbid risk factors and medications, please see articles elsewhere in this issue (see Tassler A, Kaye R: Preoperative assessment of risk factors, in this issue; and McKean E: Quality control approach to anticoagulants and transfusion, in this issue). It should be noted that herbal supplements, in particular the 4 Gs (ginseng, garlic, ginger, and gingko biloba), also affect platelet function and should be stopped 10 days (based on the half-life of platelets) before surgery. Saw palmetto and high doses of vitamin E and omega-3 can increase bleeding risk as well.

Rhinitis medicamentosa should be recognized preoperatively and the offending topical decongestant discontinued as soon as possible. To minimize rebound congestion patients should be started on topical saline and corticosteroids. Chronic topical exposure to sympathomimetics (eg, phenylephrine) or imidazolines (eg, oxymetazoline, xylometazoline) causes dysregulation of vascular tone, thus intraoperative topical vasoconstrictors are ineffective in controlling the microvascular circulation. In such situations, tranexamic acid (TXA) (1 mg during induction), which acts to reduce clot breakdown, can be used.

Adequate perioperative management of hypertension is imperative to achieve optimum intraoperative conditions. The risk of surgical bleeding is estimated to increase 1.5-fold with aspirin but for most procedures the severity of bleeding is not increased.[1]

In this study, the mean estimated blood loss during ESS in patients on aspirin was slightly higher than in controls, especially when more sinuses were opened.[2] It is generally possible to safely perform ESS in patients on aspirin by using other strategies to manage the surgical field.

Because of the risks associated with a bloody field during ESS and no known reversible agents for aspirin, it is advisable to cease aspirin 10 days earlier. Before stopping aspirin, the risk of doing so needs to be discussed with the patient's cardiologist or primary care physician because 10% of acute cardiovascular events are preceded by aspirin withdrawal. In at-risk patients, the average time intervals from aspirin cessation to acute stroke and acute coronary syndrome are 14·3 and 8·5 days respectively.[3]

For emergency reversal of the effect of aspirin, donor platelet infusion is effective. In otherwise healthy aspirin-treated individuals, desmopressin (desamino-D-arginine vasopressin [DDAVP]) has been shown to reduce bleeding time,[4] and may be considered intraoperatively in selected situations. However, it is contraindicated in patients at cardiovascular risk and there are no data to support the efficacy of DDAVP in this group.

Do preoperative GCs improve the surgical field in ESS?

- Hypothesis
  - GCs minimize sinonasal inflammatory and vascular burden, thereby improving the surgical field
- Options
  - Topical intranasal GC[5]
  - From 5 to 10 days of prednisolone or other oral GC[6–8]
  - Single preoperative dose of oral GC[9]
- In nasal polyps, there is a trend toward reduced blood loss
- Some evidence that a single preoperative dose may be sufficient to improve surgical field

---

At present there are insufficient data to make strong recommendations on routine GC use in ESS to improve the surgical field. Despite the limitations of study design and control groups (patient selection, disorder, type of anesthesia, or vasoconstrictor use), there seems to be a trend toward a beneficial effect of preoperative GC in reducing the amount of blood loss during ESS for nasal polyps.

In patients with nasal polyps, a single preoperative dose of 1 mg/kg prednisolone compared with 5 days of therapy may be just as effective in reducing blood loss during ESS.[9] However, a control group without any treatment was not used for comparison. In contrast, a recent randomized controlled study showed no significant hemostatic benefit of preoperative GC.[8] It remains to be seen whether the addition of preoperative GC has a significant benefit in the presence of other hemostatic preventive strategies (eg, adequate patient positioning and general anesthesia conditions). Note also that many anesthetists administer a single dose of dexamethasone during induction for its beneficial effects on perioperative nausea and vomiting, but it may also have an independent positive effect on the surgical field.

Preoperative devascularization

- Not used for routine sinus surgery or inflammatory disorders
- Reserved for vascular tumors such as angiofibroma
- Internal maxillary artery: endoscopic transpterygoid, infratemporal fossa approaches
- Persistent bleeding postembolization: likely caused by internal carotid artery contribution to a vascular tumor, inherent tumor vascularity (eg, metastatic renal cell carcinoma)

What steps can be taken for a thorough preoperative assessment of a patient's sinonasal CT scans?

- Ensure the images belong to the correct patient
- Examine the most recent, high-resolution, fine-cut sinus CT scans
- Examine different planes: coronal, axial, and sagittal
- Systematic assessment
  - Cribriform plate: depth, symmetry, slope, dehiscence
  - Lamina papyracea: dehiscence
  - Onodi cell: if present, relationship to optic nerve, internal carotid artery, dehiscence
  - Sphenoid sinus: pneumatization, septations, dehiscence
  - Skull base: dehiscence, slope (examine sagittal plane)
  - Ethmoidal arteries: position (skull base or pedicle), symmetry
  - Diagnosis: confirm clinical with radiological characteristics

---

Potential vascular hazards can be identified preoperatively by examining high-resolution sinus CT scans systematically. Note that the right and left sides may be asymmetrical. Breaching its boundaries during ESS not only risks serious complications and vascular injury but causes bleeding from surrounding tissues, orbital fat, and dura.

A suggested approach is described, starting off with coronal sections to examine the relationship of the cribriform plate to the frontal recess and ethmoid sinuses, including lateral lamella.

The lamina papyracea can be followed posteriorly into the sphenoid sinus and from the skull base to the level of the roof of the maxillary sinus to look for bone dehiscence in both axial and coronal planes.

Next, determine whether the ethmoid arteries are against the skull base or running within a pedicle suspended below the skull base. This anatomy is best identified on a coronal scan and confirmed with sagittal images. The anterior ethmoid artery (AEA) is more likely to be on a pedicle than the posterior ethmoid arteries. In some patients there is a middle ethmoid artery.

Follow the posterior ethmoid cells and examine their relationship with the sphenoid sinuses. If the posterior ethmoid pneumatization extends beyond the sphenoid sinus (demarcated inferiorly by the choanal roof), it is most likely an Onodi cell, hence closely related to the optic nerve, and in some cases the internal carotid artery (ICA).

The sphenoid sinus should be assessed for the extent of pneumatization, dehiscence, and configuration of the intersinus septum. If the septum is lateralized, it often attaches to bone overlying the ICA. Care needs to be taken when taking down the septum and avoid through-biting instruments and twisting maneuvers closer to its posterior attachment. Here also, the relationship of the pituitary gland and ICA within the sphenoid sinuses can be examined. Determine whether the course of the ICA is predictable or aberrant, and look for vascular malformations, aneurysms, bone dehiscence, and relationship to the posterior ethmoid sinus.

The shape or slope of the skull base can be appreciated on sagittal images. The skull base may be high within the sphenoid sinus, low toward ethmoid sinuses, and high again at the frontal recess and anterior ethmoid sinuses. The extent of low ethmoid skull base can be evaluated in comparison with the adjacent orbital roof height on coronal scans.

In addition, reconfirm that the radiological characteristics are in keeping with the clinical diagnosis. Presence of skull base dehiscence should prompt further assessment with MRI and or CT/MR angiogram to exclude the possibility of disorders such as a vascular tumor (angiofibroma), ICA aneurysm, or meningoencephalocele.

BLEEDING PREVENTION: INTRAOPERATIVE

What are some preventive intraoperative hemostasis strategies?

- Patient position
- Local vasoconstriction
- General anesthetic technique
- TXA
- Surgical technique

Patient Position

How high to raise the head of the bed relative to chest (heart) position?

- Reverse Trendelenburg position
- Minimum of 10° head elevation to show a benefit in the surgical field
- Achieve a balance between improved surgical field and cerebral perfusion pressure
- Aim for 10° to 20° head elevation

Studies addressing this issue consistently show a reduced blood loss and better surgical field with an elevated head position. A reverse Trendelenburg position can achieve this by reducing venous pressure and mucosal blood flow. The surgical field improves during ESS with a 10° tilt, and the blood flow at the head of the inferior turbinate reduces by 38% with a 20° tilt.[10,11] Cerebral perfusion and blood flow are preserved with up to 20° to 30° of head elevation.[12] The level of tilt is often underestimated without objective measure. It is advisable to check with a clinometer (available on most handheld mobile devices) while the patient is positioned to appreciate the extent of tilt required to achieve 10° to 20°.

Local Vasoconstrictors

Local agents are widely used in ESS for mucosal vasoconstriction, reduced bleeding, and decongestion. Most surgeons use a combination of local injection and topical application of vasoconstrictors on pledgets within the nose. Although, for injection, usually varying concentrations of adrenaline mixed with a local anesthetic is most commonly used, the choice of topical vasoconstrictor varies considerably between surgeons worldwide.

What are some technical aspects of local vasoconstrictor application during ESS?

- Allow time to exert its effects

- Atraumatic manner

- Topical application sites (with pledgets (cottonoids, neuropatties or pieces of gauze))
  - Root of middle turbinate/middle meatus (sphenopalatine artery)
  - Sphenoid rostrum (posterior septal artery)
  - Anterior nasal cavity (working area, mucosal decongestion)
  - Anterior floor of nose (greater palatine artery at incisive foramen)

- Injection/infiltration site options include:
  - Septum
  - Inferior turbinate
  - Anterior buttress (axilla) of middle turbinate
  - Above axilla of middle turbinate (anterior ethmoid branches)
  - Root of middle turbinate (sphenopalatine artery)
  - Sphenoid rostrum (posterior septal artery)
  - Greater palatine canal via the oral cavity (greater palatine artery, internal maxillary artery within the pterygopalatine fossa)

Key factors in the efficacy of local vasoconstrictors are to allow time for its action, usually 15 minutes, with peak effect ~30 minutes, and an atraumatic technique. If applied soon after induction, it can work while the ESS setup is performed. In addition to the agent used, the sites of vasoconstrictor application should be considered, bearing in mind the hemostatic goals. It is reasonable to suggest that, where possible, vasoconstrictor application should target the major vascular supply to the sinonasal cavities.

Does the addition of local vasoconstrictor injection provide a better surgical field in ESS?

- Middle turbinate anterior buttress injection[13]
  - Bupivacaine 0.25%, 1:200,000 adrenaline
  - No significant benefit in surgical field or blood loss

- Middle turbinate, lateral nasal wall, agger nasi region, sphenopalatine foramen[14]
  - Adrenaline 1:100,000
  - No significant benefit in surgical field or blood loss

- Greater palatine canal injection (via oral cavity)
  - Bupivacaine solution (2 mL of 0.5%) injection for compressive effects[10]
    - Reduction of 4.7% in inferior turbinate blood flow
  - Xylocaine 1%, 1:100,000 adrenaline[15]
    - No significant benefit in surgical field or blood loss
  - Not recommended for routine ESS for this purpose
  - May have a role in the surgical management of unilateral epistaxis from the sphenopalatine region (posterior epistaxis)

Based on available data, if already using topical vasoconstrictors, additional injection of a vasoconstrictor may not provide further hemostatic benefit during routine ESS. However, injection of a long-acting local anesthetic may be considered for postoperative local pain control if not already diluting topical vasoconstrictors in a local anesthetic solution, such as ropivacaine. The septum and inferior turbinate may be injected if performing a septoplasty and turbinate reduction together with ESS.

Which topical vasoconstrictors achieve the best surgical field in ESS?

- Vasoconstrictor options for topical (not injectable) application
  - Adrenaline: nonselective α1, α2, and βreceptor agonist
  - Oxymetazoline: predominantly α1 receptor agonist
  - Phenylephrine: predominantly α1 receptor agonist
  - Cocaine: potentiates α1, α2, and βactivity of endogenous catecholamines
  - Variations of Moffett's solution (mix of cocaine, adrenaline and sodium bicarbonate solution)

- Recommend rational use based on knowledge of pharmacologic vascular anatomy and side-effect profile (discussed later)
  - Single agent
  - Judicious use

- Amount delivered to mucosa may vary on the surgical pledget (cottonoid, neuropatties or gauze) used. The more absorbent the material, the less available to mucosa

---

Except for cocaine, these vasoconstrictors act directly on endogenous neural mediator adrenergic receptors to regulate the sinonasal vasculature. Cocaine acts indirectly, by preventing the reuptake of noradrenaline, thereby potentiating its vasoconstrictor effects. Cocaine is also a naturally occurring local anesthetic and acts by blocking sodium channels and preventing the propagation of nerve action potentials.

The arterial system is largely innervated by alpha1-adrenoceptors and the venous system by alpha2-adrenoceptors. Stimulation of alpha1 reduces flow into the capillary network, and of postsynaptic alpha2 constricts venous sinusoids and promotes decongestion. In the sinonasal vasculature, postsynaptic alpha2 receptors (mediate vasoconstriction) predominate over presynaptic alpha2 receptors (mediates vasodilation), hence a generalized constriction and decongestion is achieved.

When used as a single agent, adrenaline or cocaine theoretically also reduce mucosal blood flow and congestion, and have recently been suggested to achieve similar surgical field scores and blood loss to each other during ESS.[16]

What are some relevant vasoactive pharmacokinetic and safety parameters of adrenaline?

- These data are based on the pharmacokinetics of adrenaline administered via the subcutaneous (injected) route in mediating local vasoconstriction
  - Dosage for effective vasoconstriction: 1:50,000 to 1:200,000
  - Onset of action: 5 to 15 minutes
  - Peak effect: 30 minutes
  - Duration: 1 to 4 hours
  - Metabolized in liver, intravenous half-life 2 to 5 minutes, but prolonged when administered subcutaneously

- Adrenaline is deactivated by oxidizing agents, alkalis (including sodium bicarbonate), and halogens

- Beta2 (vasodilatory) effects may predominate on blood vessels after 6 hours of adrenaline stimulation

- For skull base surgery anticipated to extend beyond this time, an alpha1 agonist such as oxymetazoline may be preferred

Adrenaline may be favored rather than cocaine because of the toxic profile of the latter. No significant adverse cardiovascular effects have been described with topical adrenaline of up to 1:1000 in ESS.[17–19] However, based on the principle of using the lowest concentration to achieve the desired effect, a more dilute formulation of 1:10,000, 1:50,000, 1:100,000, or 1:200,000 may also be effective.[20,21] However, these studies examined surgical site blood flow[20] and surgical field[21] following adrenaline injection in head and neck and dermatologic surgery.

The reported toxicities for cocaine during sinonasal surgery are confounded by concomitant adrenaline use,[22] thus advocating against mixing adrenaline with cocaine (variations of Moffett solution). Note that sodium bicarbonate, which is helpful for the pharmacologic activity of cocaine, renders adrenaline ineffective. Furthermore, adding adrenaline to cocaine solution makes absorption of cocaine highly unpredictable, without added pharmacologic benefit because cocaine in itself is a potent vasoconstrictor. Ultimately these agents are absorbed, resulting in systemic vasopressor responses, manifested by fluctuating heart rate (HR) and blood pressure, which adversely affect the surgical field (discussed later).

Phenylephrine and oxymetazoline are predominantly alpha1 agonists, with oxymetazoline also exerting partial alpha2 activity. Theoretically, oxymetazoline may provide better vasoconstriction and decongestion, but there is no substantive evidence. It is noteworthy that a systematic review of topical vasoconstrictors in nasal sinus surgery strongly discouraged the use of topical phenylephrine.[23] This advice was based largely on phenylephrine-associated morbidity and mortality, which led the New York State Department of Health to issue guidelines for intraoperative phenylephrine use. In these cases, phenylephrine dosage was excessive; it was frequently not measured and was confounded by a long-acting β-blocker used to treat hypertension resulting in pulmonary edema.[24] Oxymetazoline-associated toxicity is also reported,[25–27] likely caused by its inadvertent excessive use attributed in part to squeezing the bottle in an inverted position while patient was supine which dispensed a much higher volume.[25] The anesthetist should be made aware of the topical and injectable agents used. The key to avoiding morbidity and mortality due to phenylephrine or oxymetazoline induced hypertension is its diagnosis, because its treatment differs in that, non-specific -blockers should be avoided.[27] Serious complications with topical application of these two vasoconstrictors have been reported, predominantly in pediatric patients in nonsinus surgeries.

Taking into account the available evidence regarding their efficacy or toxicity profile, there are no solid grounds to advocate the use of one rather than another.

The available evidence lends support to the following suggestions with regard to either oxymetazoline or phenylephrine use:

- Only topical application (not for local injection/infiltration)

- Not to combine its use with other vasoconstrictors, hence single-agent use

- Phenylephrine dosage (assumes 100% bioavailability): Groudine et al.
  - In adults, initial dose should not exceed 0.5 mg
  - In children < 25 kg, should not exceed 20 μg/kg

- Oxymetazoline dosage:
  - No specific guidelines exist, use manufacturer's instructions

- Exercise caution by using:
  - A measured amount
  - The least amount required to achieve hemostasis

General Anesthesia

It is generally accepted that hemodynamic parameters during general anesthesia have a significant effect on the surgical field during ESS. There are several studies in the area, with inherent confounding factors that preclude a meta-analysis and firm recommendations regarding specific anesthetic agents and techniques for obtaining the best surgical field. Hence, it is important to define the key questions relevant to sinonasal hemostasis. First, some current questions are addressed here.

Does Hypotensive Anesthesia Achieve the Best Surgical Field in Endoscopic Sinus Surgery?

Hypotensive anesthesia, also known as controlled hypotension, is defined as a reduction of the systolic blood pressure to 80 to 90 mm Hg, a reduction of mean arterial pressure (MAP) to 50 to 65 mm Hg, or a 30% reduction of baseline MAP. Hypotensive anesthesia is hypothesized to reduce organ blood flow and consequently improve surgical field and blood loss. To answer this question, and to rationally interpret the available data for ESS, an understanding of the fundamental physiologic parameters that affect end-organ blood flow is helpful.

   Cardiac output = HR × Stroke volume

   In addition, the volume of blood delivered to the sinonasal surgical field is influenced by locoregional vascular autoregulation, effect of topical vasoconstrictors, inflammatory disorders, and extent of upper airway resistance.

   In most published ESS studies, a common factor associated with a good surgical field is hypotension without reflex tachycardia. This physiologic response can be appreciated by the following:

   MAP = Heart rate × Stroke volume × Systemic vascular resistance

   If vasodilators are used to reduce the MAP by primarily decreasing systemic vascular resistance (SVR), the surgical field does not improve significantly, owing to reflex tachycardia that maintains cardiac output. However, if HR and/or cardiac contractility (affects stroke volume) are reduced by centrally acting presynaptic alpha2 agonists (clonidine, dexmedetomidine), β-blockers (eg, esmolol), or magnesium sulfate, cardiac output is reduced and consequently results in good surgical field scores. This result is also evident from studies showing independent correlation between HR and surgical field.[28,29]

Is Total Intravenous Anesthesia Necessary to Achieve the Best Surgical Field?

The term total intravenous anesthesia (TIVA) refers to maintenance anesthesia delivered solely intravenously, without inhalational agents such as sevoflurane. TIVA, using propofol alone or in combination with an opioid such as remifentanil, is generally advocated to achieve the desired conditions of hypotension without reflex tachycardia. Compared with inhalational maintenance anesthesia, TIVA causes less variability in MAP and HR, and thus reduces the need for additional antihypertensive or β-blocker medication during surgery.

   However, these stable hemodynamic parameters can also be achieved with a combination of inhalational anesthesia and remifentanil infusion.[30] Remifentanil is a short-acting synthetic opioid that acts specifically as a mu-receptor agonist. Among other physiologic effects, it independently reduces HR and MAP. It therefore follows that, if ideal physiologic parameters were obtained with means other than propofol TIVA, the impact on surgical field would not be significantly different.[28,31] Thus if a remifentanil infusion with inhalational sevoflurane maintenance anesthesia achieves a stable MAP and HR, then this would be ideal from both anesthetic and surgical viewpoints, because one of the challenges with TIVA (using propofol) is of monitoring adequate depth of anesthesia and its longer duration of action (see Cordoba Amorocho M, Fat I: Anesthetic techniques in endoscopic sinus and skull base surgery, in this issue).

It cannot be emphasized enough that good communication with the anesthetist throughout surgery is invaluable for achieving hemodynamic conditions that are ideal for ESS. Ultimately it rests with the anesthetist to use an effective technique that achieves a balance between the physiologic parameters ideal for the surgical field and the level of hypotension and bradycardia that can be safely tolerated by an individual patient.

Tranexamic Acid

> **What is the current evidence for the hemostatic effect of TXA in ESS?**
>
> - TXA prevents clot breakdown (antifibrinolytic)
> - Systemic use preoperatively[32,33]
>   - Significantly improved visualization, reduced bleeding
> - Some concern regarding systemic TXA use and risk of deep vein thrombosis
> - Topical TXA (5%) in sinus surgery compared with no TXA[34]
>   - Significantly improved surgical field (in the first 30 minutes)
>   - Overall less bleeding in the TXA group

TXA has been used during surgery to reduce blood loss and is the standard treatment used to reduce the rate of perioperative transfusion in cardiac surgery.[35] Its efficacy has also been suggested in orthopedic and liver surgery.[36,37] In ESS, a single systemic preoperative dose has shown significant benefit in surgical field and reduced blood loss. Because of some concern with the risk of deep vein thrombosis, topical TXA may be used with the desired hemostatic effect. TXA use in ESS may be considered, especially in diseases with high risk of bleeding (eg, nasal polyps) and where topical vasoconstrictors may not be effective (eg, rhinitis medicamentosa).

Surgical Technique

> **What are some surgical techniques that minimize bleeding during ESS?**
>
> - Prevent unwanted mucosal injury
>   - Precise and strategic placement of endoscope and instruments
>   - Use suction with atraumatic tip
>   - Minimize direct suction of normal tissues
> - Avoid unnecessary mucosal stripping
>   - Use sharp, through-biting or cutting powered instruments
> - Methodical surgical approach
>   - Work quickly to debulk inflammatory tissue; for example, nasal polyps
>   - Where possible work from inferior to superior to avoid blood tracking down the endoscope
> - Avoid potential vascular injury
>   - Recent patient CT scans should be available in the operating theatre
>   - No scans, no surgery

○ Establish intraoperative surgical landmarks
  ■ Level of orbital floor through maxillary antrostomy
  ■ Lateral limit, lamina papyracea
    • Note: gentle pressure on the ipsilateral globe in a pulsatile manner can help identify lamina papyracea dehiscence
  ■ Choana, sphenoid ostium, skull base
○ Confirm with intraoperative navigation
  ■ Consider in revision sinus surgery
  ■ Consider in extensive nasal polyps, allergic fungal rhinosinusitis
  ■ Frontal sinus Draf 3 surgery
  ■ Skull base surgery

MANAGEMENT OF INTRAOPERATIVE BLEEDING

Identify the source of bleeding
• Mucosa
• Bone
• Named vessel

Identifying the source of bleeding is key to obtaining adequate hemostasis. Bleeding from inadvertent vascular injury is often evident immediately because of the onset of sudden and brisk bleeding. Attempts should be made to obtain adequate visualization and to implement vascular control (see Lin G, Bleier B: Surgical management of severe epistaxis, in this issue; Alobaid A, Dehdashti AR: Hemostasis in skull base surgery, in this issue; Gardner PA, Snyderman CH, Fernandez-Miranda JC, et al: Management of major vascular injury during endoscopic endonasal skull base surgery, in this issue; and Valentine R, Padhye V, Wormald P-J: Simulation training for vascular emergencies in endoscopic sinus and skull base surgery, in this issue for more detail on visualization and control of sphenopalatine and internal carotid arteries). With persistent generalized ooze obscuring the visual field, saline irrigation can help identify specific bleeding sites for targeted control.

What are some strategies to control mucosal bleeding in ESS?
• Communicate with the anesthetist   ○ Check hemodynamic parameters
• Topical vasoconstrictors
• Cautery

Bleeding from diseased mucosa generally settles as this is removed, and working quickly to achieve this is helpful. During this time, maintaining good visualization is essential. Communicate with the anesthetist to achieve optimum hemodynamic parameters (MAP and HR). Bleeding from mucosal edges can be managed by topical vasoconstrictors and gentle pressure with pledgets. With nasal polyps, initial application of topical vasoconstrictors may not reach all areas, and reapplication is helpful as the polyps are debulked, exposing fresh mucosa. In addition, cauterization of specific bleeding points with monopolar suction diathermy or bipolar forceps is often sufficient. If using monopolar cautery, care should be taken to limit its use posteriorly to the sphenoid rostrum, and at the level areas below the level of the orbital floor (regions of the root of inferior turbinate, middle turbinate, SPA) to avoid inadvertent skull base or orbital injury.

What are some options for continued mucosal bleeding?

- Hot saline irrigation
- TXA (if not already given)
- Topical hemostatic agents
- DDAVP
- Vasoconstrictor injection or cauterization of major feeding vessels
  - Posterior septal artery
  - Sphenopalatine artery

With continued ooze, TXA can be used either topically (5% TXA) or systemically (1 g of TXA). The beneficial effect of TXA relies on intact patient platelet function and coagulation pathway. Topical hemostatic agents can also be used (for a thorough discussion, see Barham HP, Sacks R, Harvey RJ: Hemostatic materials and devices, in this issue). In unrecognized mild hemophilia A, von Willebrand disease, and congenital or acquired platelet dysfunction such as is caused by aspirin or uremia, DDAVP is helpful. DDAVP has an immediate effect, with 2-fold to 6-fold increase in plasma concentration of coagulation factor VIII, von Willebrand factor, and tissue plasminogen activator, and in platelet adhesiveness.

Another strategy to consider with persistent mucosal bleeding is to reduce blood flow by targeting the major blood supply, by either injecting vasoconstrictor or cauterizing the sphenopalatine artery and its branches, including the posterior septal artery.

Does hot saline irrigation improve the surgical field in ESS?

- What temperature to use? Animal study of sinus mucosal histology after hot water exposure[38]
  - Greater than 52°C, cell necrosis
  - From 48°C to 50°C, moderate mucosal change, no necrosis
  - At 46°C, slight mucosal change, no necrosis
  - From 40° to 44°C, no significant mucosal change

- In ESS, hot saline irrigation at 49°C[39]
  - Improvement in surgical field and blood loss for surgeries of greater than 2 hours' duration

---

Hot water irrigation has been used to successfully treat posterior epistaxis[40–42] and reduce intraoperative bleeding with adenoidectomy.[43] It has been widely used in neurosurgery, skull base surgery, and more recently in sinus surgery. The precise mechanism of hemostasis is not known. Animal studies suggest that the physical characteristics of blood vessels exposed to hot water include vasodilation, followed by interstitial mucosal edema and compression of the blood vessel lumen, and this may reduce mucosal blood flow into the surgical field.[38] The procoagulative activity of hot water, or saline, is also proposed but requires confirmation.

A comparison of the effectiveness of hot (49°C) versus room-temperature (18°C) saline irrigation in patients with polyp and nonpolyp chronic rhinosinusitis undergoing ESS showed that the most benefit with respect to visual field and blood loss occurred after 2 hours of surgery.[39] It is also suggested that, for hemostasis, hot saline irrigation is as effective as topical TXA in ESS.[44] Further studies are required in this area, taking into account the different conditions of sinus disease, anesthesia, and perioperative management.

In addition to the potential independent hemostatic effects, saline irrigation is invaluable in improving the surgical field by clearing the visual field and identifying precise bleeding points for targeted vascular control.

What are Some Strategies to Control Bone Bleeding?

Bleeding from bone is typically encountered when mucosa is stripped or while drilling. If bone bleeding continues despite topical application of vasoconstrictors, this is expected given the microvascular bone anatomy. The intraosseous vessels do not respond well to vasoconstriction and generally rely on clot formation or physical occlusion for hemostasis. The clotting process can be facilitated by topical application of a hemostatic material or TXA, and through physical occlusion by diamond burr or Surgifoam application followed by gentle pressure with a pledget.

What are Some Strategies to Control Named Vessel Bleeding?

Common named vessels and their potential sites for injury are summarised in **Table 1**. During middle or inferior turbinate surgery, exposure of the feeding vessels (branches of the sphenopalatine artery) is common, and can be controlled effectively with focal cautery. Similarly, while performing a sphenoidotomy, if encountered, the posterior septal artery can be cauterized at the sphenoid rostrum. This vessel is found at variable distances below the natural sphenoid ostium during inferior extension of the sphenoidotomy.[45] In conditions requiring resection of the palatine bone posteriorly toward the posterior wall of maxilla (eg, nasal polyps, inverting papilloma [endoscopic medial maxillectomy and variations thereof]) the descending palatine artery may be encountered, and, further posteriorly, the

Table 1 Strategies to control named vessel bleeding	
Vessels at Risk	**Site of Encounter During ESS**
Sphenopalatine artery (see Lin G, Bleier B: Surgical management of severe epistaxis, in this issue) Main trunk Branches to middle and inferior turbinates Posterior septal artery	Extended antrostomy, medial maxillectomy, vidian neurectomy Middle and inferior turbinate surgery Sphenoidotomy
Vidian and posterior pharyngeal artery (see Lin G, Bleier B: Surgical management of severe epistaxis, in this issue; and Snyderman C, Pant H: Endoscopic management of vascular sinonasal tumors including angiofibroma, in this issue)	Vidian neurectomy
Greater palatine artery	Extended antrostomy Medial maxillectomy
Branch to the Little area at incisive foramen (Stensen canal)[47]	Septoplasty, septal flap surgery
Anterior and posterior ethmoid artery (see Lin G, Bleier B: Surgical management of severe epistaxis, in this issue; and Shaftel SS, Chang S-H, Moe KS: Hemostasis in orbital surgery, in this issue)	Ethmoid sinus surgery
ICA (see Gardner PA, Snyderman CH, Fernandez-Miranda JC, et al: Management of major vascular injury during endoscopic endonasal skull base surgery, in this issue)	Sphenoid sinus surgery Onodi cell

sphenopalatine artery. These vessels too can be effectively controlled with monopolar or bipolar cautery. Occasionally excessive bleeding occurs from the greater palatine artery branch coursing through the nasal septum floor, approximately 1 cm posterior to the nasal spine. Topical vasoconstrictors are generally not sufficient, hence requiring cauterization.

The incidence of AEA and ICA injury (reported between 0.1%–0.3%) during routine ESS is low. The ICA is most at risk during sphenoid sinus surgery or posterior ethmoid surgery, the latter most likely to be an unrecognized Onodi cell. The AEA is at risk during anterior ethmoid and frontal recess surgery. Surgeons should be prepared to proficiently and adequately manage these to minimizes or prevent serious patient morbidity and mortality (see Lin G, Bleier B: Surgical management of severe epistaxis, in this issue; Shaftel SS, Chang S-H, Moe KS: Hemostasis in orbital surgery, in this issue; and Gardner PA, Snyderman CH, Fernandez-Miranda JC, et al: Management of major vascular injury during endoscopic endonasal skull base surgery, in this issue).

MANAGEMENT OF POSTOPERATIVE BLEEDING COMPLICATIONS

Only approximately 15% to 25% of postoperative hemorrhage occurs within 24 hours of ESS. A significant bleed can occur up to 6 weeks after ESS and the most common time frame is between 1 and 2 weeks after ESS. Patients should be advised to attend the nearest emergency department for acute management. A thorough assessment for site of bleeding should include a nasal endoscopy to evaluate the source of bleeding, which is most commonly from branches of the sphenopalatine artery (posterior septal artery, and artery to middle and inferior turbinates).

What steps can be taken at the end of surgery to minimize the risk of postoperative bleeding complications?

- Expose persistent bleeding areas:
  - Use saline irrigation to wash away blood clots
  - Request a Valsalva maneuver by the anesthetist

- If operating in the vicinity, ensure that posterior septal artery (sphenoid rostrum), sphenopalatine artery, and vessels at the root of the middle and inferior turbinates are adequately controlled

- If performing a septoplasty, a drainage-hole on 1 mucosal surface suturing the mucosal flaps or temporary septal splints may help reduce the risk of septal hematoma[46]

- Routine generalized nonabsorbable nasal packing is not necessary

- Focal or targeted application of a topical hemostatic agent may be considered

- In select situations, generalized application of a topical antihemostatic agent may be required

> **What are some steps and considerations in the management of post-ESS orbital hematoma (see Shaftel SS, Chang S-H, Moe KS: Hemostasis in orbital surgery, in this issue)?**
>
> AEA bleed into the orbit is a serious complication of sinus surgery. Some immediate management principles are highlighted in the following scenario (developed together with Shaftel SS, Chang S-H, and Moe KS).
>
> ### Scenario
>
> A patient is in recovery after bilateral ESS. Left proptosis and epistaxis are noted. Clinical suspicion is of left AEA injury and retraction into orbit.
>
> Question 1: What are some first steps in the management?
>
> Answer: Remove any intranasal packing.
>
> Check the patient's visual acuity and pupillary responses. Palpate the globe and orbit. If possible, measure intraocular pressure (IOP).
>
> If readily available, immediately start medical management for increased IOP.
>
> Question 2: When should canthotomy and cantholysis be performed? What are the pathophysiologic goals of canthotomy and cantholysis?
>
> Answer: Canthotomy and cantholysis should always be performed without delay for imaging or consultation in the setting of suspected orbital compartment syndrome.
>
> The goal is to reduce the IOP by reducing the compression of the eye by a tight eyelid.
>
> Question 3: Is there enough time to get an ophthalmology colleague to measure IOP?
>
> Answer: Unless IOP can be measured without delay it is not advisable to delay treatment of potential orbital compartment syndrome. Irreversible damage can result in as little as 1 hour and a properly performed canthotomy and cantholysis usually heals well by secondary intention.
>
> Question 4: It was possible to measure IOP within few minutes. Despite some proptosis, the IOP does not show an increase. Should cantholysis be performed?
>
> Answer: There is no benefit of performing cantholysis in the absence of an increased IOP.
>
> The epistaxis has settled. Repeat test shows that the IOP is now elevated. A canthotomy and inferior cantholysis is performed.
>
> Question 5: Is there a risk of rebleeding of the AEA if the tamponade effect is reduced by canthotomy and cantholysis?
>
> Answer: There is a theoretic risk of rebleeding, but the benefit of restoring ocular perfusion significantly outweighs this.
>
> Question 6: Despite inferior cantholysis, the IOP continues to increase. How much time is available, and what should be done next?
>
> Answer: The principal goal is to save vision. If IOP continues to increase, an upper cantholysis can be performed.
>
> If still not adequately reduced, the patient should be returned to the operating theatre emergently. Attempts can then be made to perform orbital wall decompression and identification of active hemorrhages.

Frequent eye monitoring is imperative. Decision for a canthotomy, cantholysis and return to the operating room should be based on clinical assessment and not delayed on the premise of getting further imaging or ophthalmology consultation. Best results for potential orbital compartment syndrome are obtained with treatment within 1 hour.

SUMMARY

The endoscopic approach to sinonasal surgery relies on hemostasis for visualization so that surgical goals can be accomplished without increasing the risk of serious complications or compromising patient outcomes. This article systematically addresses many factors that influence intraoperative and postoperative bleeding, and strategies of bleeding control. These are summarized and a suggested approach to the prevention and management of intraoperative bleeding is presented in **Table 2** and common pitfalls are addressed in **Table 3**. Despite best efforts, if bleeding compromises endoscopic visualization, it is advisable to stop pursuing surgical goals, focus on bleeding control and return at a later date. Proper surgical planning and prevention of bleeding where possible afford the best results. Although major vascular injury such as AEA or ICA bleed is uncommon during ESS, the surgical team and institution should have protocols in place and be prepared to execute proficient management to achieve best patient outcomes.

Table 2
Summary and suggested approach to the prevention and management of intraoperative bleeding

I. Prevention
Preoperative
  Make the correct diagnosis
  Assess preoperative sinus imaging
  Assess and manage:
    Patient comorbid factors
    Medications (off antiplatelet medication where possible)
    No smoking 4 weeks before and after surgery
  Preoperative embolization for vascular tumors
Intraoperative
  Patient position: reverse Trendelenburg 10° to 20°
  Maintain body temperature
  Local topical vasoconstriction: single-agent use
    Suggestion: 1:10,000 adrenaline in 0.75% ropivacaine (1 mL of 1:1000 adrenaline mixed
      with 9 mL of 0.75% ropivacaine, total 10 mL) or oxymetazoline; refer to dosage on the
      preparation
  Maintain favorable intraoperative hemodynamics (HR and blood pressure)
  Talk to anesthetist
  TXA: in patients at high risk of mucosal bleeding
    Nasal polyps, EMCRS, AFRS
  Meticulous surgical technique
II. Management of intraoperative bleeding
Assess site of bleeding: mucosa, bone, named vessel
  Mucosal bleeding
  Communicate with the anesthetist, check hemodynamics (HR, blood pressure)
    Hot saline irrigation (40°–49°C) to clear clots and identify bleeding site, also independent
      hemostatic effect
  Reapply topical vasoconstrictor, inform anesthetist
  Cautery to specific bleeding sites
  Topical hemostatic agents
  TXA (if not given already)
  DDAVP
  Cautery of posterior septal artery or sphenopalatine artery
To prevent postoperative bleeding
  At the end of surgery, Valsalva maneuver to expose and control bleeding sites
  Other measures may be used, such as absorbable nasal packing, Silastic splints; elevation of
    head of bed, and topical oxymetazoline spray

Table 3
Common errors and pitfalls during ESS with some suggestions

Problem	Likely Explanations and Suggestions
Rhinitis medicamentosa	Topical vasoconstrictors may not work effectively TXA can be of benefit intraoperatively
Use of natural or herbal therapies	Many have antiplatelet activity and should be stopped 10 d before surgery Consider DDAVP intraoperatively
Ineffective reverse Trendelenburg position	It might not be a 10°–20° tilt. Confirm with a clinometer
Ineffective topical vasoconstrictor effect	1. Strategic and atraumatic placement of vasoconstrictors at sites of vascular supply 2. Allow time to work: peak vasoconstrictor effect noted ~30 min from application 3. If using adrenaline, do not dilute in alkaline solutions; it reduces its efficacy
Using primary vasodilators to reduce MAP	This reduces SVR and causes reflex tachycardia, which increases rate of blood flow to sinuses and no significant change to surgical field
Blood frequently tracking along the endoscope	Check the mucosa in the area where the endoscope is placed in the nose; this may be traumatized and requiring bleeding control
Bone bleeding not settling with topical vasoconstrictors	Bone vessel hemostasis usually relies on clotting mechanisms. Suggest topical Gelfoam, Surgifoam, or TXA application to facilitate control
Use of room-temperature or lukewarm saline irrigation	Hot irrigation rather than cold is shown to have hemostatic properties
Completely covering eyes with tape or drapes during ESS	This precludes or hinders intraoperative: • Palpation of the ipsilateral globe intermittently to check for lateral lamina bulge or dehiscence • Early detection of potential intraorbital hemorrhage by restricting proptosis, and causing early increase in IOP Suggest keeping eyes within the surgical field protected with copious amounts of lubrication ± consider taping the lateral canthus
Unrecognized Onodi cell	Surgeons may not appreciate that they are working in an area more superior and even lateral to the sphenoid sinus boundaries, hence placing the optic nerve and ICA at risk. This needs to be identified on CT scans pre-operatively
Anterior ethmoid artery on a pedicle below skull base	If not recognised pre-operatively, puts this vessel at risk during ethmoidectomy and frontal recess surgery. If injured, it also risks an intraorbital bleed
Overzealous superior and inferior extension of sphenoidotomy	Superior: • This risks injury to posterior ethmoid artery, and may cause a cerebrospinal fluid leak. Note that the dura dips to a varying extent at the junction of the roof of sphenoid (planum) and ethmoid bones, and a through-biter or rongeur can bite through this fold of dura against the skull base • Suggestion: use a straight curette to gauge the level of skull base immediately behind the sphenoid opening Inferior: • Injury to the posterior septal artery at the inferior limit of sphenoidotomy; this can also bleed postoperatively

Post-Test Questions (Correct answers are in italics)

1. Risk factors for increased mucosal bleeding during nasal/sinus surgery include all of the following except:
   a. Rhinitis medicamentosa
   b. Graves disease
   c. Morbid obesity
   d. *Self-medication with St John's wort*
2. What is the optimal positioning of the patient to decrease venous bleeding?
   a. Trendelenburg position
   b. *Between 10° and 20° of head elevation*
   c. Maximal extension of the neck
   d. Head elevation to 45°
3. What is the best strategy for the use of topical vasoconstrictors?
   a. *Use a single agent*
   b. Combine adrenaline and cocaine for maximum efficacy
   c. Use an agent with selective alpha2 agonist activity
   d. Combine adrenaline with sodium bicarbonate to potentiate its effects
4. Which of the following procedures are at risk for bleeding from the sphenopalatine artery?
   a. Nasal septoplasty
   b. *Sphenoidotomy*
   c. *Vidian neurectomy*
   d. *Medial maxillectomy*
5. Which of the following are effective in decreasing bleeding during ESS:
   a. *TIVA*
   b. Irrigation with saline greater than 52°C
   c. *Topical administration of TXA*
   d. Intravenous administration of adrenaline

SUPPLEMENTARY DATA

Supplementary PDF slides related to this article can be found online at http://www.oto.theclinics.com/.

REFERENCES

1. Makris M, Van Veen JJ, Tait CR, et al. Guideline on the management of bleeding in patients on antithrombotic agents. Br J Haematol 2013;160:35–46.
2. Sargi Z, Casiano R. Endoscopic sinus surgery in patients receiving anticoagulant or antiplatelet therapy. Am J Rhinol 2007;21:335–8.
3. Burger W, Chemnitius JM, Kneissl GD, et al. Low-dose aspirin for secondary cardiovascular prevention - cardiovascular risks after its perioperative withdrawal versus bleeding risks with its continuation - review and meta-analysis. J Intern Med 2005;257:399–414.
4. Mannucci PM, Vicente V, Vianello L, et al. Controlled trial of desmopressin in liver cirrhosis and other conditions associated with a prolonged bleeding time. Blood 1986;67:1148–53.

5. Albu S, Gocea A, Mitre I. Preoperative treatment with topical corticoids and bleeding during primary endoscopic sinus surgery. Otolaryngol Head Neck Surg 2010;143:573–8.
6. Sieskiewicz A, Olszewska E, Rogowski M, et al. Preoperative corticosteroid oral therapy and intraoperative bleeding during functional endoscopic sinus surgery in patients with severe nasal polyposis: a preliminary investigation. Ann Otol Rhinol Laryngol 2006;115:490–4.
7. Ecevit MC, Erdag TK, Dogan E, et al. Effect of steroids for nasal polyposis surgery: a placebo-controlled, randomized, double-blind study. Laryngoscope 2015;125:2041–5.
8. Gunel C, Basak HS, Bleier BS. Oral steroids and intraoperative bleeding during endoscopic sinus surgery. B-ENT 2015;11:123–8.
9. Atighechi S, Azimi MR, Mirvakili SA, et al. Evaluation of intraoperative bleeding during an endoscopic surgery of nasal polyposis after a pre-operative single dose versus a 5-day course of corticosteroid. Eur Arch Otorhinolaryngol 2013; 270:2451–4.
10. Gurr P, Callanan V, Baldwin D. Laser-Doppler blood flowmetry measurement of nasal mucosa blood flow after injection of the greater palatine canal. J Laryngol Otol 1996;110:124–8.
11. Ko MT, Chuang KC, Su CY. Multiple analyses of factors related to intraoperative blood loss and the role of reverse Trendelenburg position in endoscopic sinus surgery. Laryngoscope 2008;118:1687–91.
12. Tankisi A, Rasmussen M, Juul N, et al. The effects of 10 degrees reverse Trendelenburg position on subdural intracranial pressure and cerebral perfusion pressure in patients subjected to craniotomy for cerebral aneurysm. J Neurosurg Anesthesiol 2006;18:11–7.
13. Javer AR, Gheriani H, Mechor B, et al. Effect of intraoperative injection of 0.25% bupivacaine with 1:200,000 epinephrine on intraoperative blood loss in FESS. Am J Rhinol Allergy 2009;23:437–41.
14. Lee TJ, Huang CC, Chang PH, et al. Hemostasis during functional endoscopic sinus surgery: the effect of local infiltration with adrenaline. Otolaryngol Head Neck Surg 2009;140:209–14.
15. Valdes CJ, Al Badaai Y, Bogado M, et al. Does pterygopalatine canal injection with local anaesthetic and adrenaline decrease bleeding during functional endoscopic sinus surgery? J Laryngol Otol 2014;128:814–7.
16. Valdes CJ, Bogado M, Rammal A, et al. Topical cocaine vs adrenaline in endoscopic sinus surgery: a blinded randomized controlled study. Int Forum Allergy Rhinol 2014;4:646–50.
17. Orlandi RR, Warrier S, Sato S, et al. Concentrated topical epinephrine is safe in endoscopic sinus surgery. Am J Rhinol Allergy 2010;24:140–2.
18. Gunaratne DA, Barham HP, Christensen JM, et al. Topical concentrated epinephrine (1:1000) does not cause acute cardiovascular changes during endoscopic sinus surgery. Int Forum Allergy Rhinol 2016;6:135–9.
19. Sarmento Junior KM, Tomita S, Kós AO. Topical use of adrenaline in different concentrations for endoscopic sinus surgery. Braz J Otorhinolaryngol 2009;75(2): 280–9.
20. Dunlevy TM, O'Malley TP, Postma GN. Optimal concentration of epinephrine for vasoconstriction in neck surgery. Laryngoscope 1996;106:1412–4.
21. Shoroghi M, Sadrolsadat SH, Razzaghi M, et al. Effect of different epinephrine concentrations on local bleeding and hemodynamics during dermatologic surgery. Acta Dermatovenerol Croat 2008;16:209–14.

22. Lenders GD, Jorens PG, De Meyer T, et al. Coronary spasm after the topical use of cocaine in nasal surgery. Am J Case Rep 2013;14:76–9.
23. Higgins TS, Hwang PH, Kingdom TT, et al. Systematic review of topical vasoconstrictors in endoscopic sinus surgery. Laryngoscope 2011;121:422–32.
24. Groudine SB, Hollinger I, Jones J, et al. New York State guidelines on the topical use of phenylephrine in the operating room. The Phenylephrine Advisory Committee. Anesthesiology 2000;92:859–64.
25. Latham GJ, Jardine DS. Oxymetazoline and hypertensive crisis in a child: can we prevent it? Paediatr Anaesth 2013;23:952–6.
26. Tobias JD, Cartabuke R, Taghon T. Oxymetazoline (Afrin®): maybe there is more that we need to know. Paediatr Anaesth 2014;24:795–8.
27. Ramesh AS, Cartabuke R, Essig G, et al. Oxymetazoline-induced postoperative hypertension. Pediatric Anesthesia and Critical Care Journal 2013;1:72–7.
28. Beule AG, Wilhelmi F, Kühnel TS, et al. Propofol versus sevoflurane: bleeding in endoscopic sinus surgery. Otolaryngol Head Neck Surg 2007;136:45–50.
29. Eberhart LH, Folz BJ, Wulf H, et al. Intravenous anesthesia provides optimal surgical conditions during microscopic and endoscopic sinus surgery. Laryngoscope 2003;113:1369–73.
30. Yoo HS, Han JH, Park SW, et al. Comparison of surgical condition in endoscopic sinus surgery using remifentanil combined with propofol, sevoflurane, or desflurane. Korean J Anesthesiol 2010;59:377–82.
31. Chaaban MR, Baroody FM, Gottlieb O, et al. Blood loss during endoscopic sinus surgery with propofol or sevoflurane: a randomized clinical trial. JAMA Otolaryngol Head Neck Surg 2013;139:510–4.
32. Yaniv E, Shvero J, Hadar T. Hemostatic effect of tranexamic acid in elective nasal surgery. Am J Rhinol 2006;20:227–9.
33. Alimian M, Mohseni M. The effect of intravenous tranexamic acid on blood loss and surgical field quality during endoscopic sinus surgery: a placebo-controlled clinical trial. J Clin Anesth 2011;23:611–5.
34. Jahanshahi J, Hashemian F, Pazira S, et al. Effect of topical tranexamic acid on bleeding and quality of surgical field during functional endoscopic sinus surgery in patients with chronic rhinosinusitis: a triple blind randomized clinical trial. PLoS One 2014;9:e104477.
35. Ferraris VA, Brown JR, Despotis GJ, et al. 2011 update to the Society of Thoracic Surgeons and the Society of Cardiovascular Anesthesiologists blood conservation clinical practice guidelines. Ann Thorac Surg 2011;91:944–82.
36. Kagoma YK, Crowther MA, Douketis J, et al. Use of antifibrinolytic therapy to reduce transfusion in patients undergoing orthopedic surgery: a systematic review of randomized trials. Thromb Res 2009;123:687–96.
37. Molenaar IQ, Warnaar N, Groen H, et al. Efficacy and safety of antifibrinolytic drugs in liver transplantation: a systematic review and meta-analysis. Am J Transplant 2007;7:185–94.
38. Stangerup SE, Thomsen HK. Histological changes in the nasal mucosa after hot-water irrigation. An animal experimental study. Rhinology 1996;34:14–7.
39. Gan EC, Alsaleh S, Manji J, et al. Hemostatic effect of hot saline irrigation during functional endoscopic sinus surgery: a randomized controlled trial. Int Forum Allergy Rhinol 2014;4:877–84.
40. Stangerup SE, Dommerby H, Lau T. Hot-water irrigation as a treatment of posterior epistaxis. Rhinology 1996;34:18–20.

41. Stangerup SE, Dommerby H, Siim C, et al. New modification of hot-water irrigation in the treatment of posterior epistaxis. Arch Otolaryngol Head Neck Surg 1999;125:686–90.
42. Schlegel-Wagner C, Siekmann U, Linder T. Non-invasive treatment of intractable posterior epistaxis with hot-water irrigation. Rhinology 2006;44:90–3.
43. Ozmen S, Ozmen OA. Hot saline irrigation for control of intraoperative bleeding in adenoidectomy: a randomized controlled trial. Otolaryngol Head Neck Surg 2010;142:893–7.
44. Shehata A, Ibrahim MS, Abd-El-Fattah. Topical tranexamic acid versus hot saline for field quality during endoscopic sinus surgery. Egypt J Otolaryngol 2014;30: 327–31.
45. Zhang X, Wang EW, Wei H, et al. Anatomy of the posterior septal artery with surgical implications on the vascularized pedicled nasoseptal flap. Head Neck 2015;37:1470–6.
46. Quinn JG, Bonaparte JP, Kilty SJ. Postoperative management in the prevention of complications after septoplasty: a systematic review. Laryngoscope 2013;123: 1328–33.
47. Butrymowicz A, Weisstuch A, Zhao A, et al. Endoscopic endonasal greater palatine artery cauterization at the incisive foramen for control of anterior epistaxis. Laryngoscope 2016;126(5):1033–8.

Hemostasis in Skull Base Surgery

Abdullah Alobaid, MD, FRCSC, Amir R. Dehdashti, MD, FACS, FMH*

KEYWORDS

- Hemostasis • Bleeding • Skull base • Pituitary • Coagulation • Hemostatic agents

KEY LEARNING POINTS

At the end of this article, the reader will:

- Understand the importance of hemostasis during endoscopic endonasal approach to skull base and intradural surgery.
- Be able to better understand the techniques for hemostasis in endoscopic endonasal surgery, including pituitary surgery.

INTRODUCTION

Why hemostasis is important

- Bleeding makes visualization difficult, which makes the surgical approach unsafe.
- Increased risk of intraoperative complications and inadvertent neurovascular injury.
- Poor hemostasis is the major leading cause of postoperative hematoma, which is the most common cause for reoperation, and surgical morbidity and mortality.
- The widespread use of antiplatelets and anticoagulation for cardiovascular diseases adds greater challenges for surgeons.
- Increased risk of blood transfusion, which had its own risks:
  - Infection
  - Coagulopathy
  - Fluid overload

Disclosure: The authors have nothing to disclose.
Conflicts of Interest: None.
Department of Neurosurgery, Northshore University Hospital, Northwell Health, 300 Community Drive, Nine Tower, Manhasset, NY 11030, USA
* Corresponding author.
E-mail address: adehdashti@nshs.edu

Otolaryngol Clin N Am 49 (2016) 677–690
http://dx.doi.org/10.1016/j.otc.2016.02.003
0030-6665/16/$ – see front matter © 2016 Elsevier Inc. All rights reserved.

oto.theclinics.com

Skull base surgery, whether transcranial or endoscopic, is based on good exposure and visualization. Surgeons achieve that by better anatomic understanding, appropriate access, generous bone removal, and the adjunct use of neuronavigation. However, visualization can be jeopardized by uncontrolled bleeding. If hemostasis is not achieved, this delays the procedure and puts the patient at risk for intraoperative complications, including inadvertent vascular injury and postoperative hemorrhage. The cause of difficult intraoperative hemostasis in neurosurgical patients is multifactorial.[1] Degree of vascularity of the tumor, thromboplastin released from neural tissues,[2] presence of vascular malformation, intrinsic hemostatic abnormality, or antiplatelet and anticoagulation therapy are all possible causes of difficult hemostasis, in addition to inadequate surgical technique.

PREOPERATIVE WORK-UP AND INTERVENTIONS

Patient history is an important element to detect patients at risk for difficult hemostasis despite normal routine coagulation profile.[3] A suggested list of questions that can be asked in preadmission evaluation can detect those patients at risk (**Box 1**).

In addition to preoperative patient assessment and laboratory tests, review of medical imaging for features of hypervascularity, such as flow void in MRI, and risk for potential vascular injury, such as close proximity to internal carotid artery (ICA) or any of its branches, is essential. Preoperative embolization is an important adjunct that should be considered in some cases. Embolization should be performed 24 to 72 hours before surgery to allow adequate thrombosis and avoid recanalization.[4] The external carotid artery branches can be accessed for embolization, if there is no contraindication, such as direct anastomosis between ophthalmic and middle meningeal arteries. Access through the ICA or vertebral artery is not feasible most of the time and it is limited to balloon test occlusion or complete occlusion if radical

---

Box 1
Preoperative questions to detect patients with bleeding tendency

1. Have you noticed any nose bleeding without obvious trauma?

2. Do you often develop bruises even without bumping into anything?

3. Have you noticed that your gums are bleeding without any obvious cause?

4. Do you develop bleeds or hematomas more than once a week?

5. Do you think that after cuts or abrasion you bleed for longer than usual?

6. Have you ever had prolonged or sever bleeding after an operation?

7. Have you ever had prolonged bleeding after tooth extraction?

8. Have you ever received blood or blood products during an operation?

9. Do you have a family member who had a bleeding problem?

10. Are you taking any pain killer, in particularly antiinflammatory medications?

11. Are you taking any medications, in particularly aspirin or blood thinners?

12 Do you think that you have prolonged menstruation (>7 days) and/or a high frequency of tampon change?

Any affirmative answers require further history, investigation, hematology consult, or postponement of the surgery.
Adapted from Gerlach R, Krause M, Seifert V, et al. Hemostatic and hemorrhagic problems in neurosurgical patients. Acta Neurochir (Wien) 2009;151(8):873–900; with permission.

resection with high-flow bypass is planned. In a study involving 15 patients, the external carotid branches were successfully occluded in most patients, with no adverse effects. A suggested algorithm is presented in (**Fig. 1**).[5]

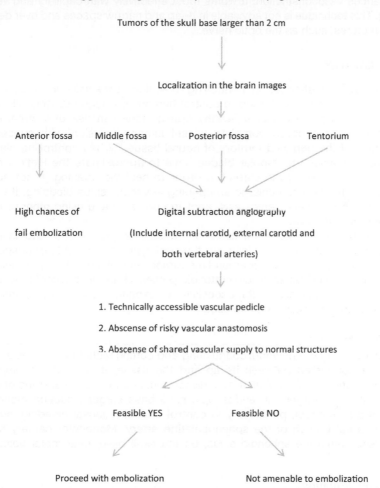

Fig. 1. Suggested algorithm for preoperative embolization. (*Adapted from* Pereza RA, Espinosa-Garcia H, Alcala-Cerra G, et al. Embolization of skull-base hypervascular tumors: description of a series of cases and proposal of a therapeutic algorithm. Bol Asoc Med P R 2013;105(2):20–7.)

Intraoperative hemostatic methods and products
• Mechanical compression: patties, bipolar or monopolar cautery, clips, bone wax, Gelfoam
• Enhance coagulation or platelet aggregation: Surgicel, Avitene
• Introduce coagulation factors topically: fibrin sealants (eg, Tisseel), gelatin-thrombin matrix sealant (eg, Floseal, Surgiflo)
• Multiple mechanisms: warm irrigation
• Systemic agents: tranexamic acid, recombinant factor VII (rFVIIa), prothrombin complex concentrate (PCC), platelets transfusion

MECHANICAL COMPRESSION

Compression with a cottonoid patty over the area of bleeding allows clot formation and enhances vasoconstriction. It works most effectively with capillary and venous bleeding. This technique is not advisable in deep and narrow spaces and over delicate neural structures, such as the optic nerve.

BIPOLAR CAUTERY

Bipolar cautery is effective in controlling bleeding, especially from an arterial source. It is the mainstay method to control hemostasis during surgery. However, this method can place adjacent healthy cranial nerves at risk of thermal injury. Furthermore, it can cause complete vessel lumen occlusion with subsequent compromise of the perfused territory of neural tissue.[1] When controlling bleeding form venous sinuses, the bipolar blades have to approximate the leaflets of the opening before applying the current in order to seal the opening. If not applied correctly, this method can enlarge an opening in venous sinus bleeding. If bipolar cautery does not achieve hemostasis, applying pressure and using other products might be more effective.

Standard bayonet designs are used for transcranial procedures, and there are different types on the market. However, the best types are capable of coagulation and dissect the sylvian fissure or around the tumor using an irrigating tip to decrease eschar adhesion, and can also hold cottonoid patties. However, bayonet bipolars are too large for the endonasal route, especially for expanded endonasal approaches. Instead, a pistol-grip design can be used.[6]

Monopolar Cautery

Monopolar cautery is a powerful coagulating and cutting technique. It uses an electric current conducted between its tip and the tissue. It is used for temporalis muscle dissection, suboccipital muscle dissection, and for the nasal stage of endoscopic skull base surgery. In endoscopic skull base surgery, suction monopolar cautery is a useful tool, particularly to control arterial mucosal bleeding, such as from the septal branch of the sphenopalatine artery. Monopolar cautery should not be used within the sphenoid sinus, on the skull base, near major vessels or nerves.

Warm Saline Irrigation

Warm saline irrigation is used whenever there is diffuse oozing, either from traumatized nasal mucosa, denuded bone surface, or the dissected surface of the tumor or brain.[6] Gentle irrigation of the brain surface with a soft catheter is effective in clearing the field so that bleeding sites can be visualized and selectively cauterized or compressed with a hemostatic material. Care should be taken to avoid excessive irrigation pressure because hydrodissection of the tissues could occur.

Bone Wax

Bone wax consists of beeswax and a softening agent such as paraffin or Vaseline, and is commonly used to stop bleeding resulting from cut bone by physically stopping blood flow from the damaged vessels in the bone.[1] Examples of bone wax applications in the skull base include during sphenoid wing drilling in pterional craniotomy, and during drilling the clivus in the endoscopic approach to the posterior fossa.

Some adverse reactions have been reported, including impeded bone healing, allergic reactions, and granuloma formation.[1]

Conventional Local Hemostatic Adjuncts

Conventional local hemostatic adjuncts tend to work by forming a mesh that encourages clot formation.[1] These agents include various absorbable gelatin sponges (eg, Gelfoam; Baxter, CA), which has the capability to absorb blood up to 10 times its own weight, and which then creates a tamponade over the bleeding site. Microfibrillar collagen (eg, Avitene; Davol, RI) promotes platelet aggregation and adhesion without directly affecting the coagulation cascade. Oxidized regenerated cellulose (eg, Surgicel; Ethicon, NJ) creates an acidic milieu that promotes reaction with blood to precipitate an artificial coagulum that provides a substrate for further clot formation.

An intact patient coagulation cascade with the full spectrum of available clotting factors is required for these products to work effectively, thus they do not work well in the setting of thrombocytopenia.[1]

Fibrin Sealants

The most common example of those is Tisseel (Baxter, IL). It acts by introducing a boost of fibrin locally, so it bypasses the coagulation cascade and induces clot formation.[1] In skull base surgery, open or endoscopic, it has been used mainly for prevention and treatment of cerebrospinal fluid leak.

Gelatin-Thrombin Matrix Sealant

The most common 2 examples are Floseal (Baxter, IL) and Surgiflo (Ethicon, NJ). It had 2 components: bovine gelatin, which works by mechanical tamponade, and thrombin, which converts fibrinogen to fibrin and forms a stable clot in the presence of factor XIII. It does not work in cases of fibrinogen deficiency, which occurs in 1 in 1,000,000 individuals.[1] Because of the cost, it is largely limited to persistent and excessive bleeding that is not amenable to standard techniques of hemostasis. It has major value in the endoscopic approach because of limited space and the ease of applying it over the area of bleeding[1,7,8] (**Fig. 2**).

In a study by Cappabianca and colleagues,[7] out of 65 patients who underwent an expanded endonasal approach, 29 needed Floseal, and all stopped bleeding from 1 application, except 1 with carotid injury, and that patient required repeated application. Caution is required to avoid using an access amount because it may induce brain

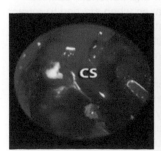 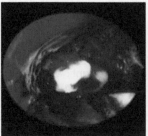 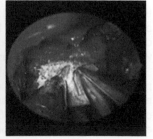

Fig. 2. (*Left*) Bleeding from CS; (*middle*) application of thrombin matrix; (*right*) followed by gentle compression with patty. (*Adapted from* Bedi AD, Toms SA, Dehdashti AR. Use of hemostatic matrix for hemostasis of the cavernous sinus during endoscopic endonasal pituitary and suprasellar tumor surgery. Skull Base 2011;21(3):189–92; with permission.)

edema,[1] and also when applying it over a bleeding vessel because of the risk of complete occlusion, in particular sagittal or transverse sinus.

Systemic Hemostatic Agents

Systemic agents such as antifibrinolytics, rFVIIa, or PCC, or platelet transfusion may be used intraoperatively. Their use needs to be adjusted based on the patient's history and laboratory results preoperatively and intraoperatively, and they should not be used routinely because of cost and possible side effects.

Hemostasis techniques for open skull base surgery

• Multiple open approaches to skull base
• Most common approaches:
  ○ Pterional
  ○ Translabyrinthine-retrosigmoid approach

INCISION AND FLAP

Small branches of superficial temporal artery (STA) are easily controlled with bipolar cautery.[9–11] However, care should be taken to save the main STA to decrease the risk of temporalis muscle atrophy and as a potential donor vessel for bypass. Elevation of temporalis muscle causes some bleeding from bone perforating vessels, which can be quickly controlled with bone wax or monopolar cautery.[9] In cases of interfacial or subfacial dissection of the temporalis muscle, monopolar cautery should be avoided, and only sharp blade dissection and bipolar cautery should be used, to avoid injury to the temporalis branch of the facial nerve.

BONY EXPOSURE

Elevation of a pterional bone flap provides extradural exposure of frontal, temporal, and, if needed, parietal lobes.[9,11] Mild bleeding from the middle meningeal artery (MMA) can be easily controlled by bipolar cautery. Epidural bleeding from the bone edges can be controlled by tack-up sutures, or a strip of Gelfoam packed with 12 × 75 mm (0.5 × 3 inches) cottonoid patties. Bleeding from drilling the greater wing of the sphenoid or from anterior clinoidectomy can be control with bone wax, and, if that does not work, packing with thrombin matrix sealant and cottonoid patties.

During the middle fossa approach, care needs to be taken when starting to retract the temporal dura. The head of the patient needs to tilt laterally toward the ground, to avoid excessive elevation of the temporal lobe, which could cause avulsion to the vein of Labbé. Second, the MMA exit at the foramen spinosum must be found, cauterized with bipolar cautery, and transected (**Fig. 3**).

For complex skull base lesions that might need ICA sacrifice and bypass, finding the petrous carotid during the middle fossa approach is important for proximal control and as a site for high-flow bypass. The petrous ICA is usually found by drilling the Glasscock triangle, between the V3 anteriorly, and greater superior petrosal vein posterolaterally. However, these anatomic landmarks can be difficult to appreciate for a variety of reasons, and using indocyanine green fluoroscopy can be useful.

Drilling the middle fossa can lead to excessive bone bleeding or venous bleeding from the pterygoid plexus. Bone wax can be used first, and if necessary packing it with thrombin sealant and cottonoid patties usually is effective. More anteriorly,

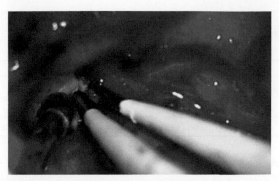

Fig. 3. Left orbitozygomatic craniotomy interdural approach to left cavernous sinus for 56-year-old man with adenocystic carcinoma involving the cavernous sinus. The left MMA coagulated in order to be sectioned to gain access to the cavernous sinuous.

particularly drilling the anterolateral triangle, accessing the pterygomaxillary space often results in significant bleeding from venous and arterial branches of the internal maxillary artery. In this situation, the assistant should hold the suction to clear the field, to find the maxillary artery, and control it with bipolar cautery or hemostatic clip.

TUMOR REMOVAL

Start with extradural dissection of the tumor, whenever possible. This technique achieves less bleeding and better control of tumor blood supply. Cavernous sinus bleeding, if small (likely from a branch site), might be controlled with bipolar cautery. However, heavy bleeding caused by a tear needs tamponade; Gelfoam and cottonoid patties are usually adequate, and, if bleeding persists, thrombin matrix sealant packing can be used (**Fig. 4**). Bipolar cautery should not be used for large tears in the cavernous sinus because it might expand the opening and make the situation worse.

Before attempting removal of an intradural tumor, a thorough inspection of the surrounding neurovascular structures is needed to devise a strategy for dissection and tumor manipulation. Start cauterizing the capsule first and gradually debulk it and then circumferentially dissect it. For large tumors that displace main arterial structures, take great care to avoid pulling the tumor, which could result in catastrophic injury to those vessels (**Tables 1** and **2**).

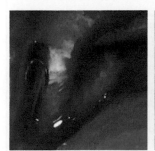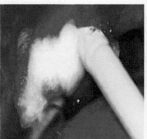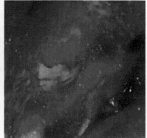

Fig. 4. Left orbitozygomatic craniotomy interdural approach to left cavernous sinus for 56-year-old man with adenocystic carcinoma involving the cavernous sinus. (*Left*) Cavernous sinuous bleeding started around the intercavernous carotid artery; (*middle*) application of thrombin sealant; (*right*) complete control of bleeding.

Table 1
Pterional approach

Surgical Step	Vessels at Risk	Management
Incision and flap	STA	Bipolar
Bony exposure	MMA	Bipolar
	Epidural bleeding	Tack up sutures, Gelfoam
	Bone bleeding	Bone wax
Tumor removal	Tumor and feeding vessels	Bipolar, tamponade, thrombin

INCISION AND FLAP

Following the initial skin incision, the flap is dissected with monopolar cautery in a superior to inferior direction[9] to allow visualization of the mastoid emissary veins; this can be controlled with bipolar cautery extracranially and with bone wax at the foramen. Bleeding from posterior auricular or occipital arteries can be controlled with bipolar cautery.

BONE EXPOSURE

Superior and inferior emissary veins are always opened during mastoid and retrosigmoid bone removal.[9] To avoid a tear at the emissary-sigmoid junction, bone should first be removed from the sinus using a combination of cutting and diamond burrs, a blunt periosteal elevator, and bone rongeurs. The emissary veins can then be bipolar coagulated at their junction with the sigmoid sinus while the distal foramen is bone waxed.

Vigorous bleeding results from inadvertent entry into transverse or sigmoid sinuses. The immediate step is to cover the defect with wet sponge or patty and inform the anesthesiologist to be prepared for possible air embolus. Although tiny lacerations can be controlled with bipolar cautery, management of larger tears requires extraluminal Gelfoam packing. Although there is no evidence for this, the authors do not recommend using thrombin sealant in such situations, because of the potential risk of total occlusion of the sinus.

Before drilling the posterior-inferior aspect of the internal acoustic meatus, preoperative MRI needs to be checked for the possibility of a high-riding jugular bulb. In small

Table 2
Translabyrinthine-retrosigmoid approach

Surgical Step	Vessels at Risk	Management
Incision and flap	Mastoid emissary veins	Monopolar, bipolar, bone wax
	Posterior auricular or occipital arteries	Bipolar cautery
Bony exposure	Superior and inferior emissary veins	Bipolar, bone wax
	Transverse, sigmoid sinus bleeding	Cover defect, bipolar, extraluminal Gelfoam pack
	Jugular vein	Small tear: tamponade with Gelfoam or Surgiflo. Large tear: attempt to suture the defect; if not helpful, intraluminal packing if other measures not effective and if there is a patent contralateral jugular bulb
Tumor removal	Tumor and feeding vessels	Bipolar, tamponade, thrombin
	Petrosal vein	Bipolar

tears, packing with bone wax or Gelfoam is usually adequate. In larger tears with increased bleeding, more aggressing intramural packing is needed, followed by neck exposure for ligation of internal jugular vein.[9]

TUMOR REMOVAL

The petrosal vein is found in the superior and posterior aspect of cerebellum, and is better cauterized with bipolar and sectioned before accessing cranial nerve V for microvascular decompression or large vestibular schwannoma, to avoid bleeding, which can take time to control. If it is injured, direct bipolar coagulation can be tried first, and, if this fails, then packing with Gelfoam or thrombin sealant should be done.

Before starting tumor resection, inspect the surrounding neurovascular structures and build up a dissection strategy. Tumor blood supply can be controlled by sweeping bipolar cautery over the capsule, followed by debulking and tumor dissection.[9]

HEMOSTASIS TECHNIQUES FOR ENDOSCOPIC SKULL BASE SURGERY

Endoscopic endonasal skull base approaches offer a minimal access and some advantages to the patient, including faster recovery and less brain retraction. However, as in the open approaches, any uncontrolled bleeding hinders visualization and increases the risk for further injury. The key is prevention by adequate preoperative preparation, sound anatomic knowledge, proper dissection techniques, and familiarity with hemostatic products.[6] When bleeding happens, teamwork is crucial,[6,12] by having one surgeon offering optimal position of the endoscope, and the other surgeon using the same microsurgical principles when dealing with bleeding (ie, bimanual technique).

Categorization of bleeding during endoscopic skull base surgery

- Arterial, high flow: major feeding arteries, including sphenopalatine, vidian, maxillary, carotid
- Arterial, low flow: perforations in tumor beds, subarachnoid space
- Venous, high flow: cavernous sinus, intercavernous sinus
- Venous, low flow: mucosal ooze

Bleeding can be categorized as arterial or venous, high flow or low flow.[6,12] Venous low-flow bleeding is mostly seen in mucosal ooze, usually controlled by warm irrigation, bone wax for the bone, or packing with a hemostatic product with cottonoid patties. Venous high-flow bleeding is seen in cases of bleeding from cavernous or intercavernous sinus. If it is small (likely a tiny branch site), most are controlled with bipolar cautery. In contrast, large bleeding caused by a tear needs tamponade with Gelfoam and cottonoid patties, and, if bleeding persists, thrombin matrix sealant packing can be used. Bipolar cautery should not be used for large tears in the cavernous sinus because it might expand the opening and make the situation worse. Arterial low-flow bleeding is seen from small perforations in the tumor beds or subarachnoid space. A careful and focal bipolar coagulation should be done, and, in cases of bleeding from important perforations (eg, superior hypophyseal artery), direct bipolar cautery should be avoided, and packing with a small piece of Gelfoam should be done. Arterial high-flow bleeding is seen from big arteries, from the sphenopalatine artery to the ICA. If the artery can be sacrificed (eg, sphenopalatine artery in cases in which there is no need for a flap), suction and direct bipolar cautery or clipping should be used, and blind packing should be avoided.

Endoscopic endonasal surgery for pituitary tumor resection

Preoperative preparation:

- Preoperative corticosteroids in some situations
- Anesthesia and blood pressure; generally greater than 80 mm Hg

Surgical stages:

1. Nasal
2. Sphenoidal
3. Sellar
4. Reconstruction

PREOPERATIVE PREPARATION

Preoperatively, some investigators advocate using steroid to decrease inflammation and have shown improve visualization and better hemostasis.[13] However, in rhinology, steroids are not routinely given, unless there is preoperative evidence of adrenal insufficiency, because they interfere with postoperative serum cortisol levels. Controlled hypotension is commonly used by rhinologists during sinus surgery to improve hemostasis, and a mean arterial pressure (MAP) of 65 to 70 mm Hg has been advocated.[4] However, when dealing with large intradural tumors, it is recommended for MAP to be more than 85 mm Hg to improve brain perfusion.[12]

SURGERY: NASAL STAGE

Patients are placed in the supine position, head neutral to mildly extended, and rotated toward the surgeon. The back of the table is elevated to keep the head above the heart to improve venous return and decrease venous bleeding. The head is fixed with 3 pins with Mayfield clamp and navigation connected. The nasal cavity is packed with patties that are soaked with vasoconstrictor. The authors use 1:1000 epinephrine solution for nasal packing. An endoscope is introduced in the right nostril, and the root of the middle turbinate is identified and injected with lidocaine and 1:200000 epinephrine, and then resected with bipolar cautery and endoscopic scissors. After the removal of the middle turbinate, the sphenoid ostium is identified, and 2 incisions are made: one from the arch of the choana to the base of the nasal septum anteriorly, and the other from the upper border of the sphenoid ostium going through the upper part of the nasal septum and all the way anteriorly to meet the other cut. Those two cuts are made with pointed-tip monopolar cautery. A dissector is used to harvest the septal flap. Caution is needed to avoid injuring the septal branch of the sphenopalatine artery, which supplies the flap. The flap is stored in the nasopharynx. The posterior part of the nasal septum is opened in order to get binostril access, which can be done with dissectors or a drill, and then backward bitter for the mucosa. In cases of bleeding from the posterior edges, suction cautery can be used. In cases of bleeding from the contralateral sphenopalatine artery, suction or bipolar cautery can be used. The face of the sphenoid is exposed now. During this stage, most of the mucosal bleeding can be controlled by warm irrigation, and if any focal bleeding persists, it can be dealt with using bipolar or suction cautery.

SPHENOIDAL STAGE

The sphenoid face is widened with a Kerrison rongeur. At the base of the sphenoid, a drill is used to flatten it and to allow better manipulation of the instruments, and also to shorten the distance for the flap to cover the defect. Bleeding from the bone can be controlled by heat induced by drilling, bone wax, or thrombin sealant. After opening the sphenoid, the mucosa needs to be removed in order to see the anatomic landmarks better, and also to avoid development of mucocele under the septal flap. This condition usually creates diffuse venous bleeding, which can respond well to warm irrigation or, if it persists, thrombin sealant packing. Any septation is removed, and caution is needed not to use this as a landmark of the midline, because it can lead directly to the ICA.

SELLAR STAGE

Usually, the sella floor is thinned out and easy to find; however, with the conchal sphenoid sinus type, the anatomy can be difficult, in which case navigation is helpful. After confirming the position of the carotids anatomically, with navigation and Doppler, the sella floor can be opened. If it is not thin enough, a diamond drill is used to thin it out, and the Kerrison rongeur introduced to remove bone. The sella floor is removed from the medial wall of the cavernous sinus from one side to the other and from the charismatic sulcus above to the base of the sella down. In the cases of incidental sinus injury, a trial with bipolar cautery is started first, but if this does not work, pack the defect with thrombin sealant. The dura is opened in cruciate fashion from the corners, not in a vertical and horizontal fashion, to avoid injuring the intercavernous sinus and the cavernous sinuses. After that, the tumor is exposed, and then the same microsurgical strategies applied: circumferential dissection, no pulling, and no blind dissection.[6,12] Avoid blind dissection over the medial wall of the cavernous sinus, because of the risk of injuring it or even injuring the carotid artery. In order to do this safely, an angled scope can be used. After completion of the resection, the arachnoid membrane herniates down through the diaphragma sellae deficit, and the cavity can be layered with Surgicel.

RECONSTRUCTIVE STAGE

A small piece of DuraGen (Integra, NJ) is applied over the dural defect, then a bigger piece of dura substitute material applied over the bony edges, then the flap is applied over the raw bone surface of the sellar roof. Surgicel is applied over the flap edges; then Tisseel glue used. The nasal mucosa is inspected and irrigated with warm irrigation and any persistent bleeding controlled with bipolar cautery. No packing is needed.

SPECIAL SURGICAL TECHNIQUES FOR EXPANDED ENDONASAL APPROACH

Tumors that involve the anterior cranial base receive most of their blood supply from the anterior and posterior ethmoidal arteries. A complete ethmoidectomy is necessary to expose the roof of the ethmoid sinus. The anterior ethmoid artery crosses the skull base just posterior to the nasofrontal recess. The thin lamina papyracea of the medial orbital wall is fractured and removed up to the plane of the cranial base. Further elevation of the periosteum on the orbital side exposes the vessel where it leaves the orbit, and a hemoclip can be placed.[6,12] The posterior ethmoidal artery is similarly ligated in the roof of the posterior ethmoid air cells.

The anterior intercavernous sinus can limit the exposure to the suprasellar region. In order to get more posterior exposure, and avoid venous bleeding, the dura is opened anterior and inferior to the intercavernous sinus. The sinus can then be coagulated in the middle and sectioned.

CAROTID ARTERY INJURY

Whether using a transcranial or endoscopic approach, this is the ultimate challenge to surgeons and can jeopardize the patient's life. This injury requires the active participation of both surgeons using 2 suctions to maintain visualization, whether under the microscope or the endoscope. The anesthesiologist should be notified immediately to maintain blood pressure and restore intravascular volume. Hypotension should be avoided; the blood pressure should be high enough to maintain cerebral perfusion. In cases of branch bleeding, bipolar cautery can be used to control the bleeding, and the procedure might be continued, provided that there are no changes in the neurophysiologic monitoring. In large tears, bipolar cautery should not be used, and tamponade with Gelfoam should be used, even leaving a cottonoid patty pledget over the tear to achieve bleeding control. At this stage, the procedure should be aborted, and the patient should be rushed to the angiogram suite for consideration of coiling or stent placement if a pseudoaneurysm is identified. If a stent is not an option and adequate collateral circulation is present, carotid occlusion could potentially be considered. If there is no good collateral circulation, a vascular bypass should be planned before carotid sacrifice. As a rule, whether the ICA is occluded or not, any injury to it requires immediate attention and a follow-up angiogram to rule out pseudoaneurysm formation.

SUMMARY

By preparing patients appropriately, studying the preoperative images, understanding the capabilities and limitations of hemostatic products, and careful microsurgical dissection, bleeding can be avoided and controlled.

Post-Test Questions (Correct answers are in italics)

1. Which of the following has more sensitivity and higher predictive value in detecting patients with high risk of intraoperative bleeding:
   a. Bleeding time
   b. International Normalized Ratio and prothrombin time
   c. *Patient history*
   d. Whole-blood impedance aggregometry (Multiplate)
2. Which of the following disorders has a higher chance of successful preoperative embolization:
   a. Medial sphenoid wing meningioma with significant pial blood supply
   b. Olfactory groove meningioma
   c. Pituitary macroadenoma
   d. *Glomus jugulare tumor*
3. Which of the following is considered the least appropriate location to use gelatin-thrombin matrix sealant:
   a. *Bleeding from transverse sinus tear*
   b. Bone bleeding during endoscopic drilling of clivus
   c. Cavernous sinuous bleeding, whether endoscopic or transcranial
   d. Tumor bed resection

SUPPLEMENTARY DATA

Supplementary PDF slides related to this article can be found online at http://www.oto.theclinics.com/.

REFERENCES

1. Yao HH, Hong MK, Drummond KJ. Haemostasis in neurosurgery: what is the evidence for gelatin-thrombin matrix sealant? J Clin Neurosci 2013;20(3): 349–56.
2. Gerald AG. Update on hemostasis: neurosurgery. Surgery 2007;142(Suppl 4): S55–60.
3. Gerlach R, Krause M, Seifert V, et al. Hemostatic and hemorrhagic problems in neurosurgical patients. Acta Neurochir 2009;151(8):873–900 [discussion: 900].
4. Thongrong C, Kasemsiri P, Carrau RL, et al. Control of bleeding in endoscopic skull base surgery: current concepts to improve hemostasis. ISRN Surg 2013; 2013:191543.
5. Pereza RA, Espinosa-Garcia H, Alcala-Cerra G, et al. Embolization of skull-base hypervascular tumors: description of a series of cases and proposal of a therapeutic algorithm [in Spanish]. Bol Asoc Med P R 2013; 105(2):20–7.
6. Kassam A, Snyderman CH, Carrau RL, et al. Endoneurosurgical hemostasis techniques: lessons learned from 400 cases. Neurosurg Focus 2005;19(1):E7.
7. Cappabianca P, Esposito F, Esposito I, et al. Use of a thrombin-gelatin haemostatic matrix in endoscopic endonasal extended approaches: technical note. Acta Neurochir 2009;151(1):69–77 [discussion: 77].
8. Bedi AD, Toms SA, Dehdashti AR. Use of hemostatic matrix for hemostasis of the cavernous sinus during endoscopic endonasal pituitary and suprasellar tumor surgery. Skull Base 2011;21(3):189–92.
9. Leonetti JP, Smith PG, Grubb RL. Control of bleeding in extended skull base surgery. Am J Otol 1990;11(4):254–9.
10. Yasargil MG, Reichman MV, Kubik S. Preservation of the frontotemporal branch of the facial nerve using the interfascial temporalis flap for pterional craniotomy. Technical article. J Neurosurg 1987;67(3):463–6.
11. Yaşargil MG. Microneurosurgery: in 4 volumes. Stuttgart (Germany): Georg Thieme Verlag; 1984.
12. Bhatki AM, Carrau RL, Snyderman CH, et al. Endonasal surgery of the ventral skull base–endoscopic transcranial surgery. Oral Maxillofacial Surg Clin North Am 2010;22(1):157–68.
13. Sieskiewicz A, Olszewska E, Rogowski M, et al. Preoperative corticosteroid oral therapy and intraoperative bleeding during functional endoscopic sinus surgery in patients with severe nasal polyposis: a preliminary investigation. Ann Otol Rhinol Laryngol 2006;115(7):490–4.

SUGGESTED READINGS

Bedi AD, Toms SA, Dehdashti AR. Use of hemostatic matrix for hemostasis of the cavernous sinus during endoscopic endonasal pituitary and suprasellar tumor surgery. Skull Base 2011;21(3):189.
Kassam A, Snyderman CH, Carrau RL, et al. Endoneurosurgical hemostasis techniques: lessons learned from 400 cases. Neurosurg Focus 2005;19(1):1–6.

Leonetti JP, Smith PG, Grubb RL. Control of bleeding in extended skull base surgery. Am J Otol 1990;11(4):254–9.

Lucas JW, Zada G. Endoscopic surgery for pituitary tumors. Neurosurg Clin North Am 2012;23(4):555–69.

Thongrong C, Kasemsiri P, Carrau RL, et al. Control of bleeding in endoscopic skull base surgery: current concepts to improve hemostasis. ISRN Surg 2013;2013: 191543.

Yao HH, Hong MK, Drummond KJ. Haemostasis in neurosurgery: what is the evidence for gelatin-thrombin matrix sealant? J Clin Neurosci 2013;20(3):349–56.

Hemostasis in Airway Surgery

Adult and Pediatric

Diego A. Preciado, MD, PhD

KEYWORDS

- Tracheoinnominate fistula • Subglottic stenosis • Airway hemangiomas
- Recurrent respiratory papillomas • Airway lasers

KEY LEARNING POINTS

At the end of this article, the reader will:

- Know if bleeding is expected in the majority of laryngotracheal procedures.
- Be able to identify which injuries can result in potentially fatal bleeding during tracheal surgery.
- Know the factors that contribute to delayed hemorrhage risk after airway surgery.
- Be able to identify the surgical anatomy of the great vessels around the trachea, and the vascular supply to the larynx.
- Know which endoscopic instruments can be associated with bleeding risk during endoscopic airway surgery.
- Know which techniques can be used to mitigate bleeding in the airway.

INTRODUCTION

Bleeding during airway surgery

- Unlikely, but possibly devastating, early or late complication of tracheal surgery.[1–13]
- Potential trauma during thermal control to important adjacent structures (ie, recurrent laryngeal nerve).
- Medical morbidities include:
  - Potential for added morbidity owing to airway obstruction when bleeding into the airway;
  - Hypoxia; and
  - Transfusion of blood products.

Pediatric Otolaryngology, Children's National Health System, 111 Michigan Avenue Northwest, Washington, DC 20010, USA
E-mail address: dpreciad@childrensnational.org

Otolaryngol Clin N Am 49 (2016) 691–703
http://dx.doi.org/10.1016/j.otc.2016.02.007
0030-6665/16/$ – see front matter © 2016 Elsevier Inc. All rights reserved.

oto.theclinics.com

Surgical bleeding is an unlikely, but potentially devastating, event during the surgical management of pediatric and adult laryngotracheal disorders. As such, an intimate knowledge of the anatomy of the large vessels coursing in the vicinity of the airway is imperative. A frequently cited, albeit rare, complication while approaching the trachea either during resection techniques or tracheotomy tube placement is injury to the innominate artery. It is normal for the innominate artery to ride over the trachea in the region of the suprasternal notch, usually at the level of tracheal rings 7 to 9 (**Fig. 1**). However, in some cases, the innominate artery may be "high riding" and cross the anterior trachea as high as tracheal ring 2. In cases where neck extension is not possible or feasible during tracheotomy surgery there is an increased risk of innominate artery injury. For this reason, it is important to be cognizant of the position of the innominate artery when performing dissection of tissues over the anterior tracheal wall surface, lower in the neck. In most cases, however, injury to the innominate artery is delayed after tracheotomy tube placement, and does not occur during the surgical procedure itself. This situation is discussed elsewhere in this paper.

Bleeding when dissecting circumferentially around the trachea, lifting it off of the esophagus, frequently results in persistent slow oozing in the posterolateral aspects of the airway wall. The tracheoesophageal party wall is a hypervascular area with a plethora of small venocapillary vessels that contribute to slow bleeding in this location. Overzealous use of cautery techniques to control this bleeding can result in thermal injury to the recurrent laryngeal nerves, because they course just lateral to the trachea in the tracheoesophageal grooves. It is essential to be meticulous with hemostasis in this location, and to avoid random, continuous, and widespread use of electrocautery. Pledgets soaked in oxymetazoline can help tremendously in reducing the esophageal party wall ooze during pediatric tracheal surgery.

When making incisions into the laryngotracheal airway during a reconstructive procedure (see details in the later discussion), slow bleeding is invariably encountered from the incised airway mucosal edges. This bleeding can be an annoyance in completing the reconstructive maneuvers (either resection or insertion of free grafts), but more importantly can create a persistent bloody drip into the lower tracheobronchial tree. Use of gentle bipolar cautery on the mucosal edges can be helpful, but again, its indiscriminate use is discouraged. It is especially useful to inject the posterior

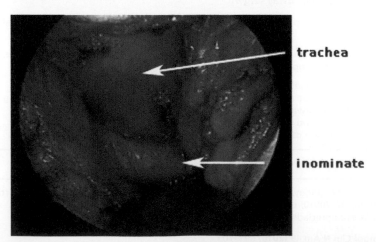

trachea

inominate

Fig. 1. Intraoperative photograph demonstrating course of innominate artery over the distal third of the cervicothoracic trachea.

mucosal wall overlying the posterior cricoid plate with 1:100,000 epinephrine containing local anesthesia, before incising it during a posterior cricoid split. Finally, continual soft suction catheter aspiration of the lower tracheal segment and main bronchi while the airway is open intraoperatively is of paramount importance to prevent bloody mucosal plugs in the tracheobronchial tree, and to minimize the risk of bronchiectasis with resultant hypoxia in the postoperative recovery period.

SURGICAL MANAGEMENT OF ADULT AND PEDIATRIC LARYNGOTRACHEAL PATHOLOGIES

What are the common respiratory and airway lesions requiring open and endoscopic surgical management, during which hemostasis is vital?

- Laryngotracheal stenosis.
- Airway hemangiomas.
- Recurrent respiratory papillomas.

Laryngotracheal stenosis

- Direct laryngoscopy and bronchoscopy is required for determining the site of stenosis.
- Stenosis grade: Myer-Cotton scale.
- Based on endotracheal tube sizes: grade I, less than 50% obstruction.
- Grade II, 51% to 70% obstruction.
- Grade III, 71% to 99% obstruction.
- Grade IV, no detectable lumen.
- Acquired laryngotracheal stenoses are much more frequent than congenital and most often a consequence of intubation injury.
- Children with great vessel anomalies will have complete tracheal rings with congenital tracheal stenosis up to 50% of the time.
- Symptomatic acquired soft subglottic stenotic lesions can be treated with endoscopic techniques with balloon dilation and/or laser treatment.
- Congenital or more severe acquired stenoses are generally treated with open airway surgical reconstruction.
- Laryngotracheoplasty.
- Partial cricotracheal resection.
- Tracheoplasty.
- Tracheotomy may be required to bypass the stenosis in some cases.

Although lateral and anteroposterior radiographs may suggest glottic, subglottic, and tracheal narrowing, direct laryngoscopy and bronchoscopy are needed to adequately diagnose laryngotracheal stenosis. The stenosis is graded by the Myer-Cotton scale (originally intended for subglottic narrowing only) is based on endotracheal tube sizes: grade I, less than 50% obstruction; grade II, 51% to 70% obstruction; grade III, 71% to 99% obstruction; grade IV, no detectable lumen. Congenital stenoses are less common, and are associated with failure of normal embryologic recanalization of the larynx, or owing to complete tracheal rings. Children with Down syndrome frequently have a mild degree of congenital subglottic stenosis (SGS). Children with great vessel anomalies, most frequently pulmonary artery sling, will have complete tracheal rings with congenital tracheal stenosis up to 50% of the time. Acquired laryngotracheal stenoses are much more frequent than congenital and most often a consequence of intubation injury. Symptomatic acquired soft subglottic stenotic lesions can be treated with endoscopic techniques with balloon dilation and/or laser treatment. Congenital or more severe acquired stenoses are treated with open airway surgical reconstruction either through laryngotracheoplasty airway expansion or with partial cricotracheal resection for laryngeal lesions, and slide tracheoplasty for congenital tracheal stenosis. In some cases, a tracheotomy may also be needed to bypass the stenotic lesions.

The management of pediatric laryngotracheal stenosis in children and adults poses multiple challenges for treating clinicians. In general, multidisciplinary expertise in anesthesia, surgery, pulmonology, gastroenterology, intensive care management, and general medicine is requisite to adequately manage these patients.

DEFINITION AND CLASSIFICATION

With the improved survival of premature neonates, the use of prolonged intubation and ventilatory support has increased. Although a heightened awareness of the potential damage to the subglottis related to intubation has led to a decrease in acquired SGS, the incidence remains 1% to 2% of neonates. The grading scale most universally used to categorize SGS was proposed by Myer and Cotton in 1994 and describes grade 1 SGS as 0% to 50% narrowing, grade 2 SGS as 50% to 75% narrowing, grade 3 SGS as 75% to 99% narrowing, and grade 4 SGS as no identifiable lumen. This grading scheme is important in outcomes assessment, for planning therapy, and in discussing objective disease severity among parents and colleagues. The nature of the stenosis can be further qualified as soft, firm, or a combination.

EVALUATION

Preoperative radiographic imaging plays little to no role in surgical planning except to help characterize and determine the length of a stenotic airway segment. Undoubtedly the gold standard in the preoperative airway evaluation and SGS characterization is a rigid direct microlaryngoscopy and bronchoscopy procedure under general anesthesia. Almost universally, the anesthetic management for this evaluation can be accomplished in children with spontaneous ventilation with oxygen insufflation using a combination of inhalational agents and propofol for induction. This approach allows for a dynamic assessment of the laryngotracheobronchial tree while manipulating the airway without needing intubation or ventilation through a rigid bronchoscope.

SURGICAL MANAGEMENT OF LARYNGOTRACHEAL STENOSIS

What are the goals of surgical treatment for laryngotracheal stenosis?

- Avoid or remove tracheotomy tube.
- Minimize morbidity.
- Preserve voice and function.

The ideal timing of laryngotracheal reconstructive surgery remains somewhat ill-defined. Although some have demonstrated that children younger than 24 months have higher rates of reconstruction failure despite lesser degrees of stenotic pathology when compared with older children, recent large series have shown that although younger children have a higher rate of reintubation after single stage procedures, eventually they are able to extubate, and that age alone is not a predictor for reconstructive failure (defined as failure to decannulate or avoid tracheotomy). In children with existing tracheotomies, any timing decisions must consider the fact that severe SGS managed with tracheotomy, where reconstruction is deferred, is potentially life threatening because yearly tracheotomy-specific mortality in children owing to tracheotomy tube obstruction is 1% to 3.4%. Tracheotomy tube associated morbidity also includes delayed speech and language development, feeding difficulties, and infection. Therefore, many authors propose reconstruction as early as possible to avoid tracheotomy.

What are the surgical options for stenotic lesions?

- Endoscopic.
- Cricoid split.
- Laryngotracheoplasty.
- Cricotracheal resection.
- Slide tracheoplasty.

Endoscopic Treatment

- Better suited for acquired stenoses than for congenital.
- CO_2 is workhorse in airway owing to low tissue penetration; however, hemostasis is modest at best. A cycle of multiple, serial endoscopic treatments should generally be avoided.
- The potassium-titanyl-phosphate (KTP) and YAG lasers maintain better vessel coagulation properties than the CO_2 laser.
- A rare anatomic variant of the superior laryngeal artery, with it piercing the thyroid cartilage through an aberrant thyroid foramen, may be associated with bleeding risk during endoscopic airway procedures.

In general, endoscopic treatment is limited to acquired (and not congenital) airway stenoses. Classically, endoscopic treatment has taken the form of laser ablation of lesions that narrow the airway, and is mostly useful for nonmature, noncircumferential, short soft lesions that comprise mild stenoses (grades 1 or 2). Recent small case series have also described the use of balloon dilating catheters as potential tools that can successfully treat some patients with SGS, even if severe, but larger confirmatory studies are necessary to validate this approach. In any circumstance, dilation may certainly help to temporize obstructive symptoms. Multiple, serial dilations may eventually weaken the airway lateral walls, effectively making the pathology worse.

Intraoperative hemorrhage and bleeding is rare with the use of lasers in the airway. The CO_2 laser has remained the workhorse laser system for laryngotracheal ablative interventions, especially when dealing with stenosis. The CO_2 laser operates in the wavelength of 10,600 nm. The radiant energy is absorbed strongly by water at this wavelength, and as such there is good tissue precision of the cutting function of the laser, with minimal surrounding tissue damage. Hemostasis with this laser, however, is modest at best, and really only good for small venocapillary vessels of less than 0.5 mm. Until recently, the CO_2 laser could only be delivered through a rigid system of suspension, but flexible fibers for CO_2 laser delivery are now readily available. The flexible fiber consists of a mirror surrounding a hollow core. The mirror reflects CO_2 laser energy along the hollow core of the fiber. Inert gas, usually helium, is funneled through the fiber to ensure a clear pathway through its core.

The YAG lasers can also be delivered through flexible fibers and possess a smaller light wavelength of 1064 nm. This wavelength allows for better tissue absorption and vessel coagulation. The tissue thermal dispersion, however, is greater than with CO_2, at 200 to 300 μm. Hemostasis is better than the CO_2 laser, and as such this laser is better suited for coagulation of vascular lesions in the airway.

The KTP laser has a smaller wavelength of 532 nm, placing it in the visible range and allowing for preferential absorption by hemoglobin, making the KTP laser the best option for the ablation of vascular lesions in the airway. Indeed, CO_2 laser coagulative properties are inferior to those of the KTP laser and there has been a shift in airway surgery from CO_2 to KTP laser application for the treatment of airway vascular lesions such as hemangiomas. Both the YAG and KTP lasers have deeper tissue penetration and can be associated with greater cartilage injury; therefore, they must be used with extreme caution and precision in the airway.

The vascular supply to the larynx is relatively constant and comes from the superior laryngeal artery, a branch off the superior thyroid artery. The superior laryngeal artery typically pierces the thyrohyoid membrane to enter the larynx, where it branches into 4 sections (superior, anterior, posterior, and inferior) to irrigate the supraglottis. In typical anatomy, the vocal cords are devoid of major arteries, and the propensity for major bleeding during procedures on the glottis and subglottis is quite small. However, an anatomic variation of the superior laryngeal artery has been described, with it piercing the thyroid cartilage through an aberrant thyroid foramen to reach the vocal cords and subglottis. In these rare cases, brisk and severe bleeding can be encountered when using a laser or cold instrument in the airway endoscopically. Getting arterial bleeding at these levels of the larynx under control during endoscopic laryngeal surgery can be quite challenging and, although rare, the surgeon must be prepared for these complications.

Anterior Cricoid Split

> - Alternative to tracheotomy in the failing to extubate neonate when SGS/edema is the primary source of extubation failure.
>
> - Premature neonates should have matured enough—to a weight at least 1.5 kg, have required no assisted ventilatory support for 10 days, and require minimal supplemental oxygen requirement of less than a fraction of inspired oxygen (Fio_2) of 35%, and be without congestive heart failure.

The anterior cricoid split procedure was introduced by Cotton and Seid in 1980. This was an alternative approach to tracheotomy in the failing to extubate premature neonates with healthy lungs but had laryngeal obstruction owing to edema and early stenosis. To qualify for this procedure, laryngeal obstruction should be the primary reason for extubation failure. Additional characteristics include a neonatal weight of at least 1.5 kg, no assisted ventilatory support for 10 days, supplemental oxygen requirement of less than an Fio_2 of 35%, and no evidence of congestive heart failure. The procedure consists of making an anterior vertical split through the first tracheal ring, cricoid cartilage, and lower thyroid cartilage followed by nasotracheal intubation for 10 to 14 days in the neonatal intensive care unit. Hemostasis is generally not a major issue during these cases.

Laryngotracheoplasty with Cartilage Grafting

- Aims to expand a narrowed glottic/subglottic airway with grafting (typically autologous cartilage).
- In single stage procedures, tracheotomy is avoided postoperatively; in double stage surgery, a tracheotomy is left postoperatively.
- Great care should be taken when grafting near the innominate artery. In a rare but devastating complication, infection around the graft could contribute to innominate artery fistula in the recovery period.

Laryngotracheoplasty with interposition of cartilage graft was introduced by Fearon and Cotton in 1972, as a means to expand a segment of narrowed subglottic airway. The principle of the procedure is to distract the cricoid cartilage either anteriorly or posteriorly or both by suturing cartilaginous grafts in place over an appropriately sized luminal stent. In single stage laryngotracheoplasty procedures, the stent is an endotracheal tube that is left in place, while the child is nasotracheally intubated and sedated in the pediatric intensive care unit for a period of 5 to 14 days. In double stage procedures, a tracheotomy tube is left in place after the surgery. A sutured indwelling suprastomal stent is left in place postoperatively while the grafts heal. Usually the stents are left in place for a period of 2 to 4 weeks. Double stage approaches are necessary when the child has a need for prolonged stenting, more complex airway lesions, concomitant airway pathology (such as tracheomalacia, impaired vocal cord mobility, or tongue base obstruction), or in revision surgeries. In cases when the reconstructed tracheal walls are flaccid, or there is poor graft stability, or a highly distorted anatomy owing to previous multiple reconstruction attempts, longer stenting periods of more than 6 weeks are warranted. Traditionally in adults the most commonly used long-term laryngotracheal stent has been the Montgomery T-tube.

Especially in revision cases, great care should be taken when grafting low on the anterior airway, near the innominate artery. A rare but devastating complication of infection around a 'low' graft is innominate artery fistula in the recovery period.

Cricotracheal Resection

- Involves laryngotracheal resection of involved stenotic segment, with thyrotracheal anastomosis.
- Well-suited for severe grades 3 or 4 stenoses.
- Ideally, there should be a 3-mm margin between the membranous vocal cord margin and the stenotic site. Chin-to-chest sutures are mandatory in the early postoperative stage.

Resection of a narrowed laryngotracheal airway segment was first introduced in adults by Conley in 1953, and later popularized in children by Monnier in the 1990s. Multiple reports have since demonstrated that this procedure is more likely to achieve decannulation or avoid a tracheotomy tube in children with severe, grades 3 or 4 stenoses, where success rates of greater than 90% have been reported. The concept of this procedure is to resect the narrowed subglottic airway, including the anterolateral cricoid cartilage ring, sparing the posterior cricoid cartilaginous plate which maintains functional cricoarytenoid joints. As with the laryngotracheoplasty procedures, CTR can be done in a single or double stage. Added postoperative considerations include the usage of chin-to-chest sutures for 7 to 10 days postoperatively to prevent neck extension and anastomotic dehiscence.

Slide Tracheoplasty

- Workhorse technique for congenital tracheal stenosis.
- Shortens the trachea in half, but increase the luminal diameter 2-fold.
- Surgery is typically carried out under cardiopulmonary bypass with requisite anticoagulation. Careful, bloodless dissection is critical.

Originally introduced by Tsang in 1998 and popularized by Grillo in 2002, slide tracheoplasty has become the workhorse surgery for the treatment of congenital tracheal stenosis owing to complete tracheal rings. In this surgical technique, the stenotic tracheal segment is transected at its midpoint, the upper and lower stenotic segments are incised vertically anteriorly in 1 segment and posteriorly in the other, the corners of these splayed segments are then trimmed, and the 2 are slid together and sutured. In doing so, the length of the stenotic trachea is halved and the luminal cross-sectional diameter is quadrupled. Tracheotomy tube placement is typically avoided after these procedures.

This procedure is almost universally done under cardiopulmonary bypass with requisite intraoperative anticoagulation. As such, great care must be taken to perform the surgical steps without violating any major blood vessels. Careful dissection around the trachea is an absolute must.

Bleeding complications after laryngotracheal reconstructive procedures

- Early (first 48 hours):
  - Anterior jugular vessels.
  - Thyroid vessels.
- Late (2–3 weeks):
  - Innominate artery injury (0.1%–0.5%).

Tracheoinnominate fistula

- Presents as delayed bleeding, either luminally or in neck.
- Reported to occur in 0.1% to 0.5% of open tracheal surgery cases.
- Survival rate is only 10% to 30%. Risk factors include: infection, excessive cuff pressures, revision tracheal surgery, excessive movement of tracheotomy tube, and poor nutritional state.

Tracheoinnominate Fistula Complication

Delayed bleeding (2–3 weeks) must be regarded as possible injury to the innominate artery. Injury to the innominate artery can occur in 0.1% to 0.5% of open tracheal procedures and often results from infection in the area, after revision reconstructive surgery, or owing to damage from the tip of a tracheotomy tube. In most cases, there is some bleeding before onset of the hemorrhage. Given that the onset is sudden and there is massive bleeding, the prognosis is poor, with a reported survival rate of 10% to 30%. Factors associated with risk of innominate artery fistula are excessive movement of the tracheostomy tube, pressure exerted by the cuff of the tracheostomy tube, tracheostomy at lower levels, and the fragility of blood vessels and the trachea owing to previous surgeries, steroids, or malnutrition. Other factors include extratracheal shifting of the trachea and major blood vessels owing to congenital kyphoscoliosis or thoracic deformity.

The treatment of innominate artery bleeding focuses initially on stopping the hemorrhage into the airway and from the artery by instituting pressure maneuvers. A cuffed endotracheal tube should be immediately placed into the trachea with the balloon overinflated. If this is not sufficient, direct digital pressure in the pretracheal space, to compress the bleeding artery onto the posterior face of the sternum can be helpful. Immediate proximal control of the distal and proximal segments of the injured artery is mandatory. This control can be achieved through a median sternotomy or through percutaneous intraarterial placement of a balloon. The risk of stroke after clamping the artery is greater in adults than in children. Repair of the damaged artery can be considered subsequently with an interposition vascular graft.

HEMANGIOMAS, PAPILLOMAS, AND OTHER AIRWAY NEOPLASMS
Infantile Hemangiomas

- Are benign congenital vascular malformations.
- May present in the airway as subglottic hemangiomas.
- Proliferative phase: presents in the first 6 months of life with inspiratory or biphasic stridor.
- Undergoes an involution phase at 12 to 18 months of life.
- Associated skin congenital hemangiomas are present in 50% of patients, especially in a "beard" facial distribution.

Infantile hemangiomas (IH) may present in the airway at birth as small, red macular lesions without stridor. As the infant grows, IH will undergo a proliferative phase around the first 3 to 6 months of life, and variable symptoms of stridor with airway obstruction will ensue depending on the size of the lesion (**Fig. 2**). If the child is having significant symptoms and as such is under consideration for tracheotomy tube placement, one should consider treatment to avoid the need for the tracheotomy.

Classic surgical treatment has entailed endoscopic laser ablation with steroid injection, and more recently open surgical excision. The advent of propranolol as an effective systemic therapy for IH has changed radically the treatment of these airway lesions. It has become standard to start these children on the medical regimen of propranolol and only consider surgical management for those who fail to respond. Open, submucosal excision of IH in the subglottis was popularized by Cotton in 2006. The lesion is approached by elevating submucosal flaps via an anterior airway split approach. Local anesthetic with epinephrine is infiltrated around the hemangioma to reduce bleeding. The mucosa is incised over the hemangioma, and the hemangioma is dissected out in a submucosal plane. The subglottic mucosa is preserved and draped over the cricoid lamina after removal of the lesion. A plane of dissection

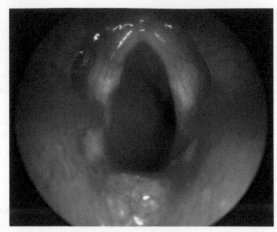

Fig. 2. Typical endoscopic photograph of a subglottic airway hemangioma.

between the lesion and the mucosa of the subglottis may be quite difficult to establish in patients who have undergone extensive laser surgery in the past. In general, precise and meticulous dissection in the correct plane will avoid significant bleeding during removal of these vascular lesions.

Subglottic Cysts

- Subglottic cysts often mimic the presentation of subglottic hemangiomas.
- These are composed of obstructed submucosal glands that expand and form fluid-filled cysts.
- Subglottic cysts most frequently occur in infants with a history of prematurity and intubation, and as such frequently coexist with SGS.
- Endoscopic techniques are used to excise subglottic cysts, but these have a high tendency to recur.

Recurrent Respiratory Papillomas

- Recurrent respiratory papillomatosis is the most common benign neoplasm of the larynx in children.
- Recurrent respiratory papillomatosis occurs owing to the human papilloma virus, most frequently subtypes 6 and 11, and tend to initiate in zones of epithelial transition such as the laryngeal glottis.
- Children usually present in the second to third year of life with dysphonia.
- Younger presentation is typically associated with more severe and aggressive recurrent respiratory papillomatosis where children often may also present with stridor and airway obstruction.

Recurrent respiratory papillomas can occur at different sites within the upper aerodigestive tract, with a predilection to sites of epithelial transition. As such, the most commonly involved site is the larynx. A wide array of treatment methodologies has been suggested for these lesions, all aiming to maintain the airway caliber, maintain vocal quality, and minimize scar trauma to the vibrating margin of the membranous vocal cords and larynx. Surgical eradication for cure is not possible. Traditionally, the CO_2 laser has been the most widely used instrument to ablate and vaporize the lesions while minimizing collateral healthy mucosal damage and scarring. More recently, powered instrumentation in the form of microdebriding instruments have been introduced for the larynx and are now also widely used for debridement of pedunculated, bulky laryngeal lesions. The use of microdebriders allows for rapid debulking with no associated fire risk. However, limitations of powered instrumentation in airway surgery compared with the lasers include hemostasis and less fine control.

Both the microdebrider and the laser can be associated with significant bleeding in the airway while debulking these highly vascular lesions. Clearly, the topical application of vasoconstrictive medications while working on the lesions is mandatory. Most usually this in the form of topical oxymetazoline for children or 1:10,000 epinephrine in adults. In the past 4% topical cocaine has also been used.

SUMMARY

Surgical bleeding is an unlikely, but potentially devastating, event during the surgical management of pediatric and adult laryngotracheal disorders. As such, an intimate knowledge of the anatomy of the large vessels coursing in the vicinity of the airway is imperative. Anatomic variants in the position of the innominate artery or the superior thyroid artery can place individuals with these variations at particular risk in these cases. Delayed bleeding from an innominate artery fistula is a particularly devastating complication from open airway surgery. A high index of suspicion is necessary to allow for early identification and aggressive treatment of this potential complication.

Post-Test Questions (Correct answers are in italics)

1. Which of these factors does not increase the risk of tracheoinnominate fistula after airway reconstructive surgery?
   a. Wound infection.
   b. Revision surgery.
   c. Low tracheotomy.
   d. *Use of cartilage grafts.*
2. What is the more likely source of brisk bleeding from the neck 2 to 3 weeks after laryngotracheal surgery, especially when a tracheotomy tube has been left in place?
   a. Carotid artery.
   b. *Innominate artery.*
   c. Superior thyroid artery
   d. Anterior jugular vein.
3. Which of these lasers is more effective for airway vascular coagulation?
   a. CO_2 laser.
   b. YAG laser.
   c. *KTP laser.*
   d. Holmiuim laser.
4. Which of the following is not a recommended intraoperative hemostasis strategy?
   a. *Aggressive cautery lateral to the trachea.*
   b. Topical application of oxymetazline.
   c. Injection of 1:100,000 before incisions in the airway.
   d. Bipolar cautery on cut mucosal edges.

5. Which of the following statements is true?
   a. The CO_2 laser is a preferred modality for controlling airway bleeding endoscopically.
   b. Transfusion, and other blood-sparing techniques, are often required during open laryngotracheal reconstruction.
   c. *Persistent oozing is frequently encountered when dissecting in the tracheoesophageal party wall.*
   d. An aberrant entry of the superior laryngeal artery into the larynx may be associated with endoluminal arterial bleeding during endoscopic airway surgery.

SUPPLEMENTARY DATA

Supplementary PDF slides related to this article can be found online at http://www.oto.theclinics.com/.

REFERENCES

1. Cotton RT. Management of laryngotracheal stenosis and tracheal lesions including single stage laryngotracheoplasty. Int J Pediatr Otorhinolaryngol 1995;32(Suppl):S89–91.
2. El-Bitar MA, Zalzal GH. Powered instrumentation in the treatment of recurrent respiratory papillomatosis: an alternative to the carbon dioxide laser. Arch Otolaryngol Head Neck Surg 2002;128:425–8.
3. Grillo HC, Wright CD, Vlahakes GJ, et al. Management of congenital tracheal stenosis by means of slide tracheoplasty or resection and reconstruction, with long-term follow-up of growth after slide tracheoplasty. J Thorac Cardiovasc Surg 2002;123:145–52.
4. Howell RJ, Solowski NL, Belafsky PC, et al. Microdebrider complications in laryngologic and airway surgery. Laryngoscope 2014;124:2579–82.
5. Leschber G. Management of tracheal surgery complications. Thorac Surg Clin 2014;24:107–16.
6. Maresh A, Preciado DA, O'Connell AP, et al. A comparative analysis of open surgery vs endoscopic balloon dilation for pediatric subglottic stenosis. JAMA Otolaryngol Head Neck Surg 2014;140(10):901–5.
7. Maruti Pol M, Gupta A, Kumar S, et al. Innominate artery injury: a catastrophic complication of tracheostomy, operative procedure revisited. BMJ Case Rep 2014;2014.
8. Ogawa K, Nitta N, Sonoda A, et al. Tracheo-brachiocephalic artery fistula after tracheostomy associated with thoracic deformity: a case report. J Med Case Rep 2011;5:595.
9. Rameau A, Zur KB. KTP laser ablation of extensive tracheal hemangiomas. Int J Pediatr Otorhinolaryngol 2011;75:1200–3.
10. Rutter MJ, Hartley BE, Cotton RT. Cricotracheal resection in children. Arch Otolaryngol Head Neck Surg 2001;127:289–92.
11. Vijayasekaran S, White DR, Hartley BE, et al. Open excision of subglottic hemangiomas to avoid tracheostomy. Arch Otolaryngol Head Neck Surg 2006;132:159–63.

12. Weingarten TN, Bojanic K, Scavonetto F, et al. Management of delayed hemorrhage after partial vocal cord cordectomy. J Clin Anesth 2013;25:666–8.
13. Whigham AS, Howell R, Choi S, et al. Outcomes of balloon dilation in pediatric subglottic stenosis. Ann Otol Rhinol Laryngol 2012;121(7):442–8.

SUGGESTED READINGS

El-Bitar MA, Zalzal GH. Powered instrumentation in the treatment of recurrent respiratory papillomatosis: an alternative to the carbon dioxide laser. Arch Otolaryngol Head Neck Surg 2002;128:425–8.
Leschber G. Management of tracheal surgery complications. Thorac Surg Clin 2014; 24:107–16.

Hemostasis in Laryngeal Surgery

Theodore Athanasiadis, MBBS, PhD, FRACS[a],*, Jacqui Allen, MBChB, FRACS[b]

KEYWORDS

- Larynx • Hemostasis • Epinephrine • Topical • Neck • Laryngeal artery

KEY LEARNING POINTS

At the end of this article, the reader will:

- Have a good understanding of the major vessels supplying the larynx.
- Appreciate why hemostasis is critical in laryngeal surgery.
- Be able to describe methods of applying topical agents to the larynx.
- Be able to discuss the properties and appropriate use of various surgical tools used in hemostasis.
- Understand the indications for preoperative embolization.
- Review the general guidelines on perioperative management of anticoagulant medication.

INTRODUCTION

- Types of laryngeal surgery
  - Endoscopic, external, and combined approach
- Endoscopic approach
  - Hemostasis critical to microsurgery of superficial lamina propria and postoperative voice outcomes
- External approach
  - May require control of the following vessels
    - Internal carotid artery
    - External carotid artery (ECA)
    - Common carotid artery
    - Internal jugular vein (IJV)

[a] Adelaide Voice Specialists, 191 Wakefield Street, Adelaide, South Australia 5000, Australia;
[b] Voice and Swallow, Auckland, New Zealand
* Corresponding author.
E-mail address: theoathans@gmail.com

Otolaryngol Clin N Am 49 (2016) 705–714
http://dx.doi.org/10.1016/j.otc.2016.03.009   oto.theclinics.com

Laryngeal surgery has continued to evolve over the last century with a multitude of endoscopic and external procedures commonly performed. In recent times technology has allowed an increasing number of procedures to be performed under local anesthesia. An improved understanding of the phonatory mechanism and microstructure of the vocal fold has also led to an increased awareness of the important role the superficial lamina propria plays in phonation. Consequently, protection of this layer is paramount in laryngeal microsurgery; hemostasis is essential for visualization and ensuring protection of the delicate microstructure.

External laryngeal procedures, such as total laryngectomy, often in combination with neck dissection may result in exposure, resection, or injury to major vessels. When possible this should be planned before surgery with the availability of blood products anticipated in some situations.

VASCULAR SUPPLY OF LARYNX

- Superior and inferior laryngeal arteries supply most of the larynx.
  - Superior laryngeal artery (SLA): branch of the superior thyroid artery from the ECA
  - Inferior laryngeal artery (ILA): branch of the inferior thyroid artery arising from the thyrocervical trunk of the subclavian artery
- SLA supplies most of tissues of larynx from epiglottis down to the vocal folds.
- ILA supplies the region around the cricothyroid and posterior cricoarytenoid.
- There are multiple anastomoses between the ipsilateral and contralateral laryngeal arteries.
- Superior and inferior laryngeal veins run parallel to the arteries and drain into the superior and inferior thyroid veins.

The blood supply of the larynx is derived mainly from the SLA and ILA. The SLA branches off the superior thyroid artery as the latter passes down towards the upper pole of the thyroid gland. Rarely SLA may arise directly from the ECA. The SLA courses towards the larynx, with the internal branch of the superior laryngeal nerve lying above it. It enters the larynx by penetrating the thyrohyoid membrane and divides into several branches that supply the larynx from the tip of the epiglottis down to the inferior margin of thyroarytenoid. It anastomoses with the contralateral SLA as well as the ILA.

The ILA is smaller than the SLA, supplies the area around the cricothyroid, and has a small branch travelling back to the region of the posterior cricoarytenoid muscle. It is a branch of the inferior thyroid artery that arises from the thyrocervical trunk of the subclavian artery. It ascends on the trachea with the recurrent laryngeal nerve entering the larynx at the lower border of the inferior constrictor, just behind the cricothyroid joint. It also anastomoses with the contralateral ILA as well as the SLA.

There is also a cricothyroid artery that arises from the superior thyroid artery and follows a variable course either superficial or deep to the sternothyroid muscle anastomosing with the ILA.

Venous return from the larynx occurs via the superior and inferior laryngeal veins, which run parallel to the SLA and ILA. They drain into the superior and inferior thyroid veins, respectively. The superior thyroid vein then drains into the IJV and the inferior thyroid vein into the left brachiocephalic vein.

LARYNGEAL PROCEDURES

In general, hemostasis in laryngeal surgery can be achieved is straightforward to control, particularly when it is anticipated by the Surgeon with good anatomical knowledge and correct instrumentation available (**Fig. 1**). It is preferable to avoid blood in the airway as it may lead to airway compromise, distal migration for example, clot, alveolar irritation and coughing and laryngospasm during emergence from anesthesia. The risk of hemorrhage may be predicted by assessing the pathology being treated, the method of surgery, medication use and level of anesthesia.

Endoscopic approach

- Benign lesions (excision or ablation)
  - Cysts, polyps, nodules, papillomas, fibrous masses, polypoid corditis (Reinke edema), vocal fold granuloma, sulcus vocalis
  - Injection laryngoplasty

- Premalignant or malignant lesions (excision? biopsy?)
  - Leukoplakia
  - Partial laryngectomy
  - Airway stenosis: supraglottic, glottic, subglottic, tracheal (airway reconstruction?)

External approach

- Laryngeal framework surgery, thyroid surgery, laryngocele, laryngeal fracture, partial and total laryngectomy

---

Laryngeal surgery may be performed endoscopically, externally, or combined external and endoscopic approaches. The advent of robotic surgery with microinstrumentation and laser surgery may well alter the breadth of procedures conducted endoscopically in the future.[1] Increasingly many procedures are now being performed under local anaesthesia,[2] which presents new challenges to the surgeon and can make bleeding more intrusive in awake patients and challenging to control because of limited access, patient discomfort or intolerance, and labile blood pressures.

Microlaryngeal surgery uses a magnified view via an operating microscope to optimize preservation of delicate vocal fold microstructure. Because the field of view is narrow, just a few milliliters of blood will obscure anatomic detail and limit safe surgery.

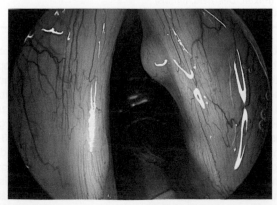

Fig. 1. Vocal fold cyst with prominent microvessels.

Particularly when resecting or dissecting the epithelium or superficial lamina propria zones, visualization is critical. Even minute amounts of blood can impair visualization and adversely affect surgical outcomes. If bleeding occurs, then dissection should be temporarily ceased and the bleeding controlled before proceeding. Not only does this improve visualization but it also prevents dispersion of blood (and its subsequent inflammatory hemolytic cascade) within the pliable vibratory tissues, which translates to better functional preservation and improved vocal outcomes. Vocal fold hemorrhage results in a stiff, bulky vocal fold that does not vibrate because of excess fluid within the superficial compartment and, if a large volume is present, even a convexity to the vocal fold that may result in early contact and glottal gapping. Marked dysphonia to complete aphonia may ensue, and recovery of normal mucosal wave and contact can take weeks as proteolysis occurs and vocal fold mass returns to normal.

During external procedures on the larynx there is often retraction or disruption of multiple tissue layers, including the muscles and vessels of the neck as well as reconstruction of these structures. Large vessels, such as the common carotid, internal or external carotid, the IJV, and their tributaries, may be encountered. If traumatized or resected, then large-volume blood loss may occur. The surgeon will need to be prepared to establish vascular control, which may require appropriate vascular instrumentation, surgical ties, titanium clips, or electrocautery. Blood loss is managed by consultation with the anesthetic staff and includes fluid replacement (colloid and/or crystalloid) and in some cases blood transfusion. In addition there is the possibility of air embolus when the IJV is transected. The surgeon and anesthetist should be alert to this possibility and use surgical vessel control and patient positioning to minimize this risk. Effective communication between the surgeon and anesthetist is vital. Large-vessel trauma requires appropriate exposure, control with pressure, vascular clips and ties, and consideration of reanastomosis in specific cases.

Role of topical hemostatic agents

- Topical or subepithelial infusion
  Epinephrine
  - α1 receptor vasoconstrictor
  - 1:1000 to 1:10,000

- Thrombin-based products
  - Floseal (Baxter, Deerfield, Illinois)
  - TachoSil (Baxter, Deerfield, Illinois)

With many endoscopic laryngeal procedures, such as removal of cysts, polyps, or nodules, minimal bleeding is encountered. In these circumstances topical application of epinephrine either 1:1000 or 1:10,000 on a cotton neuro pattie and allowing 2 to 3 minutes for effect will control the bleeding effectively. Sterile cotton neuro patties ranging from 4 to 10 mm in size can be used depending on the size of the area of the larynx affected, with smaller patties indicated for fine microsurgery. The key in this type of hemostasis is to allow appropriate time of at least 2 to 3 minutes for the topical epinephrine to work before removing the neuro pattie. In addition, the use of a fine microlaryngeal sucker of 3F to 5F gauge without obstruction of the thumb port will allow removal of blood without trauma to the surrounding tissue.

Topical application of thrombin-based products both endolaryngeal and to external wounds has been described with varying success. Although these products are powerful in effect, they have several detractors, including the risk of scar formation or allergic reaction.[3]

Subepithelial infusion may be used for certain laryngeal lesions, such as polyps, papilloma, scar, sulcus, and some premalignant or malignant lesions. Using a solution of 1 mL 1:1000 epinephrine with 9 mL normal saline and infiltrating with a 30-gauge needle causes vasoconstriction as well as delineating the lesion from the underlying vocal ligament. In some circumstances, such as excision of small cysts, infiltrating with epinephrine will assist with vasoconstriction but may make delineation of the lesion more difficult.

Infiltration of epinephrine can also be used in combination with local anesthetic agents for external laryngeal surgery. This capability is useful for the skin incision as well as deeper structures making surgery more efficient and precise.

SURGICAL INSTRUMENTATION

- Electrocautery
  - ○ Bipolar
  - ○ Monopolar
- Radiofrequency, for example, Coblation
- Surgical hemoclips

Occasionally during endolaryngeal surgery larger blood vessels are encountered that do not settle with topical epinephrine. In these situations it is useful to judiciously apply electrocautery to assist with hemostasis. The type of instrument used and settings applied will vary depending on the region of concern. Bipolar instruments that reach the supraglottis, glottis, and subglottis are readily available and have the advantage of less surrounding thermal trauma than monopolar devices (**Fig. 2**). When combined with suction (eg, suction monopolar) these devices are highly effective at controlling endolaryngeal bleeding and should be available for any significant partial laryngeal resection procedure (**Fig. 3**). Care should be taken, however, to limit collateral trauma from electrocautery. The risk of airway fire with diathermy is a possibility and largely depends on the type of anesthesia being used. Caution is required with high oxygen concentrations (fraction of inspired oxygen [F_{IO_2}] >35%) and when ventilating without an endotracheal tube. Previous investigators have recommended using only room air or airway control by intubation with the endotracheal cuff being placed distal to the area of surgery.[4]

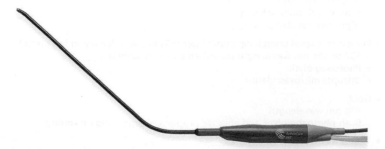

Fig. 2. Coblation Laryngeal Wand (Smith & Nephew). (*Courtesy of* Smith & Nephew ENT, Austin, TX; with permission.)

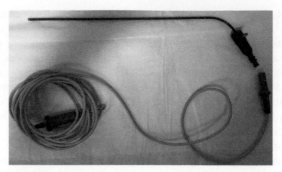

Fig. 3. Suction Monopolar.

With external laryngeal surgery, hemostasis is obtained in similar fashion to most external neck procedures with the use of combination electrocautery and clipping and tying named vessels or feeding arteries. Care should be taken in the region of nerves, such as the recurrent laryngeal nerve, where electrocautery to associated vasa nervorum may result in collateral neural injury. In the case of larger vessels, monopolar diathermy can induce trauma due to electrical conductivity and dispersion, thermal transmission to surrounding structures, or by arcing through tissues.[5]

In recent times the use of radiofrequency Coblation (Smith & Nephew, Austin Texas) has been recommended for some laryngeal procedures, such as airway stenosis treatment.[6] Anecdotal reports suggest some hemostatic benefit; however, the laryngeal Coblation wand does have a bipolar diathermy application at its tip that allows control of small vessels below the glottis. This wand is used by direct application to the area of interest and a foot pedal control used to activate the bipolar diathermy.

Finally the use of surgical hemoclips has been reported in the larynx by several investigators, including robotic application.[1] They are reported to be effective; during the healing process, it is thought that the clips are coughed out by patients.

LASER

- Delivery system: fiber-based versus direct line of site
- Wide range of properties influence laser-tissue interactions and, therefore, coagulation, vaporization, or a combination of both
- Carbon dioxide (CO_2)
  - 10,600 nm wavelength (absorbed by water)
  - Ablative: cutting tool
  - Seals vessels up to 0.5 mm
  - High thermal conductivity
- Potassium-titanyl phosphate crystal laser (KTP)/pulsed dye liquid laser (PDL)
  - 532 to 585 nm wavelength (absorbed by hemoglobin)
  - Photoangiolytic
  - Disrupts microvasculature
- Gold
  - 980 nm wavelength
  - Both photoangiolytic and ablative properties depending on settings
- Thulium
  - 2103 nm (absorbed by water)
  - Ablative

Laser use in laryngeal surgery is common, with a variety of lasers used for different indications. Delivery of laser light may be through a handpiece, fiber, or by direct line of site depending on the laser and its engineering. Each laser has different properties that influences its tissue effects, including hemostasis. The surgeon should be familiar with the settings and fluence (joules per square centimeter) that each laser delivers to tissues in order to maximize the beneficial effect of the laser tool and to minimize unwanted collateral damage. Key laser settings include the power output, pulse width, and pulse separation. Laser energy delivered to tissue gives rise to heat by diffusion. A heat sink absorbs heat and takes it away from the laser target site. Typically the surrounding vasculature provides the greatest protection by absorbing energy into the blood flow and removing heat from the immediate penumbra of the laser target site. When a high power output is used, more time is needed between laser pulses to enable blood flow to dissipate heat energy; therefore, the pulse width should be short and pulse separation large. If increased thermal effect or vaporization of tissue is desired, then reducing the pulse separation or increasing the pulse width (effectively increasing the on time of the laser) will achieve increased fluence. In some circumstances the laser might be used on continuous mode, wherein there is no pulsing at all but a steady beam of laser light. This creates a cutting tool analogous to an electrocautery device. Surgeons must be familiar with individual laser properties, spectra, and power settings in order to optimize the utility of the laser and minimize side effects.

The CO_2 gas laser is the most commonly used laser in laryngeal surgery. Light is produced in the far infrared spectrum (nonvisible); therefore, these lasers also contain an aiming beam (usually a diode laser light). It provides hemostasis, cutting, and ablative properties. Traditionally the CO_2 laser was a free beam laser, needing a direct line of site to the target or delivered by a small, articulated arm handpiece. Latterly a CO_2 laser with fiber delivery system has been developed to take advantage of fiber benefits. With regard hemostasis, the CO_2 laser results in thermal coagulation down to a depth of about 0.5 mm. Its effect is, thus, limited to microcirculation. Some investigators suggest defocussing the CO_2 beam in order to achieve hemostasis.[7]

The KTP and PDL yield a visible light at 532 nm and 585 nm, respectively. Both are preferentially absorbed by oxyhemoglobin with some studies suggesting there is slightly more collateral damage with the PDL than the pulsed KTP laser because of the rupture of the microvasculature seen with PDL treatment.[8] Because of their wavelengths, they are ideal for the treatment of vascular lesions, including varices and ectasias of the vocal fold, papillomata, neoangiogenesis of early carcinoma, hemangiomata, and microvascular polyps. However, once bleeding occurs, the laser effect is significantly hampered as blood absorbs the laser light and prevents the tissue from receiving energy. The result can be appearance of char and incomplete treatment of target lesions. Bleeding should, therefore, be controlled before proceeding further with laser use.

The Gold laser (Medical Energy Inc, Pensacola, FL) is a combination laser with a wavelength of 980 nm, in the near infrared spectrum. Chromophore targets are dark pigments and water depending on laser settings. Gold laser studies demonstrate hemostatic and coagulative effects; but at increasing fluence, the laser performs as an excellent ablative or cutting instrument.

The thulium laser (2013 nm) has also been reported to have anecdotally improved hemostasis when compared with other ablative lasers when it was used via a fiber-based delivery system.[9]

EMBOLIZATION

> - Case reports only
> - Rare
> - Large vascular lesions
> - Branches of ECA, superior thyroid artery can be targeted

There are very few indications for embolization of laryngeal vessels. However, large vascular lesions involving the larynx, including cavernous hemangiomas, arteriovenous malformations particularly between the pyriform fossa and supraglottis and potentially congenital subglottic hemangiomata, may benefit from preoperative embolization. When these lesions require surgical intervention, then embolization of the SLA as well as the ILA is possible. Case reports of embolization of the SLA and ILA before thyroid surgery exist[10] as does one case report for treatment of adult giant hemangioma. It seems that hemostasis is improved in these reported cases.[11]

ANESTHETIC CONSIDERATIONS

> - Patient position
> - Cardiovascular parameters
>   - Heart rate
>   - Blood pressure
>   - End-tidal CO_2

In other areas of otolaryngologic surgery, including otologic and sinus surgery, there is good evidence for improvement in the surgical field when heart rate and blood pressure are controlled within certain limits. Although such studies are scarce in laryngeal surgery, based on first principles, it would be reasonable to expect the beneficial effects of heart rate and blood pressure control in laryngeal surgery. Patient position is usually constrained by the procedure; however, with external laryngeal surgery, it may be possible to position patients head up in order to improve hemostasis a little.

ANTICOAGULATION

> - Aspirin
> - Low-molecular-weight heparins
> - Platelet inhibitors, for example, clopidogrel
> - Warfarin, dabigatran
> - Natural medications: St Johns Wort, *Echinacea*

It is the authors' practice not to cease any anticoagulant medication for laryngeal surgery of any type, however in cases where there is malignancy, a regional or free tissue transfer or an expected vascular lesion reversal of anti-coagulation or bridging to a heparin-based anticoagulant that may be stopped at short notice, can be appropriate. It is important to note that many newer agents do not have readily available or reliable reversal agents, for example, dabigatran (Boehringer Ingelheim - Ingelheim, Germany), and that stopping medication may result in a very long nonprotected period for patients following surgery. When there is doubt or substantial risk of thrombotic complications, discussion with a hematologist is recommended.

SUMMARY

Successful laryngeal microsurgery, including phonosurgery, and external laryngeal procedures require excellent hemostasis. Surgeons have a variety of tools at their disposal, which will allow good hemostasis, the choice of which depends on the procedure performed and the amount of bleeding encountered or expected. Hemostasis in laryngeal surgery ensures optimal views and minimizes tissue impact and, therefore, facilitates good surgical outcomes.

Post-Test Questions (Correct answers are in italics)

1. The larynx derives its blood supply from
   a. Superior laryngeal artery
   b. Inferior laryngeal artery
   c. Cricothyroid artery
   d. *All of the above*
2. Subepithelial infusion of adrenalin may help delineate all of the following except
   a. Papilloma
   b. Vocal fold scar
   c. Sulcus vocalis
   d. *Small cysts*
3. The CO_2 laser is useful in sealing and coagulating vessels smaller than
   a. *0.5 mm*
   b. 0.8 mm
   c. 5.0 mm
   d. 1.5 mm
4. All of the following are useful in preventing airway fire except
   a. Low power laser settings
   b. Reduce F_{IO_2} less than 35%
   c. *Jet ventilation*
   d. Good communication between surgeon and anesthesiologist
5. Preoperative embolization for endoscopic laryngeal surgery has been described for
   a. Vocal fold polyps
   b. Subglottic stenosis
   c. *Hemangioma*
   d. Paraganglioma

SUPPLEMENTARY DATA

Supplementary PDF slides related to this article can be found online at http://www. oto.theclinics.com/.

REFERENCES

1. Hockstein NG, Weinstein GS, O'Malley BW Jr. Maintenance of hemostasis in transoral robotic surgery. ORL J Otorhinolaryngol Relat Spec 2005;67: 220–4.
2. Rosen CA, Amin MR, Sulica L, et al. Advances in office-based diagnosis and treatment in laryngology. Laryngoscope 2009;119(Suppl 2):S185–212.
3. Ujam A, Awad Z, Wong G, et al. Safety trial of Floseal ((R)) haemostatic agent in head and neck surgery. Ann R Coll Surg Engl 2012;94:336–9.
4. Roy S, Smith LP. Surgical fires in laser laryngeal surgery: are we safe enough? Otolaryngol Head Neck Surg 2014;152(1):67–72.
5. Zohar Y, Sadov R, Strauss M, et al. Ultrastructural study of peripheral nerve injury induced by monopolar and bipolar diathermy. Ann Otol Rhinol Laryngol 1996; 105:673–7.
6. Chan CL, Frauenfelder CA, Foreman A, et al. Surgical management of airway stenosis by radiofrequency coblation. J Laryngol Otol 2015;129(Suppl 1):S21–6.
7. Yan Y, Olszewski AE, Hoffman MR, et al. Use of lasers in laryngeal surgery. J Voice 2010;24:102–9.
8. Zeitels SM, Akst LM, Burns JA, et al. Office-based 532-nm pulsed KTP laser treatment of glottal papillomatosis and dysplasia. Ann Otol Rhinol Laryngol 2006;115: 679–85.
9. Zeitels SM, Burns JA, Akst LM, et al. Office-based and microlaryngeal applications of a fiber-based thulium laser. Ann Otol Rhinol Laryngol 2006;115:891–6.
10. Tazbir J, Dedecjus M, Kaurzel Z, et al. Selective embolization of thyroid arteries (SETA) as a palliative treatment of inoperable anaplastic thyroid carcinoma (ATC). Neuro Endocrinol Lett 2005;26(4):401–6.
11. Kawakami M, Hayashi I, Yoshimura K, et al. Adult giant hemangioma of the larynx: a case report. Auris Nasus Larynx 2006;33:479–82.

SUGGESTED READINGS

Yan Y, Olszewski AE, Hoffman MR, et al. Use of lasers in laryngeal surgery. J Voice 2010;24:102–9.

This article contains a good summary of the various lasers used in laryngeal surgery, their safety profile, as well as hemostatic properties.

Zeitels SM, Akst LM, Burns JA, et al. Office-based 532-nm pulsed KTP laser treatment of glottal papillomatosis and dysplasia. Ann Otol Rhinol Laryngol 2006;115: 679–85.

This article contains a summary of the properties of the KTP laser compared with other lasers and its use in treatment of respiratory papilloma.

Hockstein NG, Weinstein GS, O'Malley BW Jr. Maintenance of hemostasis in transoral robotic surgery. ORL J Otorhinolaryngol Relat Spec 2005;67:220–4.

This article contains a good description of robotic laryngeal surgery as well as hemostatic techniques.

Hemostatic Options for Transoral Robotic Surgery of the Pharynx and Base of Tongue

Julia A. Crawford, MBBS[a], Ahmed Yassin Bahgat, MD[b],
Hilliary N. White, MD[c], J. Scott Magnuson, MD[d],*

KEYWORDS

- TORS • Oropharyngeal malignancy • Hemostasis

KEY LEARNING POINTS

At the end of this article, the reader will:

- Know the vascular anatomy that is relevant to transoral robotic surgery (TORS).
- Know the techniques for intraoperative hemostasis during TORS.
- Know the risk factors for postoperative hemorrhage following TORS.
- Know the techniques for gaining hemostasis in secondary hemorrhage following TORS.

INTRODUCTION

Transoral robotic surgery (TORS) is an emerging technique in the management of both benign and malignant neoplasms of the head and neck.[1,2] Following the first feasibility study by Hockstein and colleagues[1] in 2005 and subsequent approval from the US Food and Drug Administration (FDA) in 2009, the use of this minimally invasive technology for resection of lesions of the upper aerodigestive tract has flourished.[2] There is a growing body of literature to support the functional and oncologic outcomes of TORS in malignant lesions of the oropharynx, hypopharynx, supraglottis, and glottis and also for its use in resection of benign tongue base conditions such as obstructive sleep apnea. It is likely that the applications for TORS in the head and neck will continue to grow and be further refined with increasing experience.

[a] Department of Otolaryngology - Head and Neck Surgery, St Vincent's Hospital Sydney, 390 Victoria St, Darlinghurst, NSW 2010, Australia; [b] Department of Otorhinolaryngology, Faculty of Medicine, Alexandria Hospital, Alexandria, Egypt; [c] Head and Neck Surgery Center of Florida, 410 Celebration Place, Suite 305, Celebration, FL 34747, USA; [d] Department of Otolaryngology - Head and Neck Surgery, University of Central Florida College of Medicine, Orlando, FL 32827, USA
* Corresponding author.
E-mail address: scott.magnuson.md@flhosp.org

Otolaryngol Clin N Am 49 (2016) 715–725
http://dx.doi.org/10.1016/j.otc.2016.03.002
0030-6665/16/$ – see front matter © 2016 Elsevier Inc. All rights reserved.

Compared with traditional open surgical techniques, robotic surgery has a different anatomic perspective. Transoral surgeons approach the anatomy from the inside out and this change in perspective can initially be disorientating, potentially increasing the complications of surgery.[3] One such complication is bleeding from major branches of the external carotid artery. When considering hemostasis in TORS it is essential to have an adequate understanding of this different anatomic perspective in order to minimize complications.

RELEVANT ANATOMY

> - It is important to have an understanding of the inside-out anatomy, which is significantly different from the anatomy of an open approach
> - The parapharyngeal fat is an important landmark for the internal carotid artery
> - The styloid muscular diaphragm is a guide to the vasculature because the major vessels lie lateral to this

The oropharynx extends from the superior surface of the soft palate to the superior surface of the hyoid bone. It is composed of the soft palate and the uvula, anterior and posterior tonsillar pillars, palatine tonsils, glossotonsillar sulci, base of tongue, and the posterior and lateral pharyngeal walls. There is a rich vascular supply to this region from the external carotid artery with multiple anastomoses between various branches of this major arterial system. An understanding of the vascular anatomy and the relation of this to the surrounding muscular anatomy is important for minimizing the risk of significant bleeding during TORS surgery (**Fig. 1**).

The first muscular landmark of importance is the superior pharyngeal constrictor muscle with the underlying buccopharyngeal fascia. Deep to this buccopharyngeal fascia lies the medial pterygoid superiorly and parapharyngeal space more inferiorly. The internal carotid artery is protected in the region of the parapharyngeal space only by a layer of parapharyngeal fat and pulsations can often be appreciated in this region. Surgeons should avoid dissecting lateral to the pharyngeal fat pad so as not to encounter the internal carotid artery and so that this fat provides protection to the carotid arterial system postoperatively.

The next important landmarks are the stylopharyngeus and styloglossus; these form the styloid diaphragm and most vascular structures lie lateral to these muscles. The stylopharyngeus muscle spans from the base of the styloid process lateral to the superior constrictor before passing between the superior and middle constrictor muscles to attach onto the posterior border of the thyroid cartilage and the palatopharyngeus muscle. The styloglossus muscle is positioned more superficially and laterally to the stylopharyngeus and arises from the inferior and lateral edge of the styloid process, broadening out as it descends to insert into the lateral aspect of the tongue. Following identification of these muscles, surgeons typically encounter the tonsillar branch of the glossopharyngeal nerve, which often courses between these two muscles.[4]

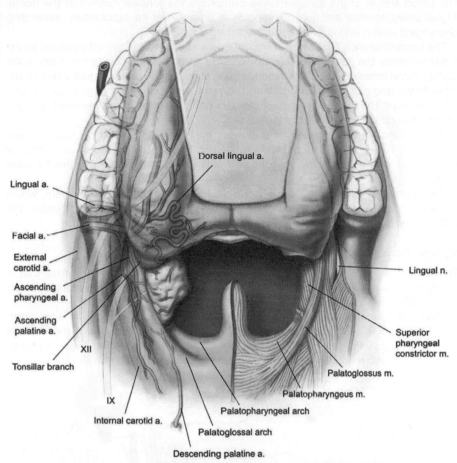

Fig. 1. The vascular and neural anatomy and its muscular relationships as most commonly encountered during TORS. a, artery; m, muscle; n, nerve. (*From* Moore EJ, Janus J, Kasperbauer J. Transoral robotic surgery of the oropharynx: Clinical and anatomic considerations. Clin Anat 2012;25:136; with permission.)

Vascular Supply of the Tonsillar Fossa

The tonsillar fossa receives supply from the:

- Lingual artery
  - Tonsillar branch of dorsal lingual artery

- Facial artery
  - Tonsillar branch
  - Ascending palatine branch

- Ascending pharyngeal artery

- Internal maxillary artery

The blood supply of the tonsillar fossa comprises the tonsillar branch of the dorsal lingual artery, tonsillar and ascending palatine branches of the facial artery, ascending pharyngeal artery, and internal maxillary artery (**Fig. 2**).

The tonsillar branch of the dorsal lingual artery approaches from inferolateral to the tonsil to pierce the superior constrictor muscle laterally and provide the main blood supply to the tonsillar fossa. The ascending palatine branch of the lingual artery arises close to the origin of the facial artery and ascends between the styloglossus and stylopharyngeus. The tonsillar branch of the ascending palatine artery pierces the superior constrictor muscle to supply the fossa.

The ascending pharyngeal artery divides into pharyngeal and neuromeningeal branches. The pharyngeal branch divides into superior, middle, and inferior pharyngeal arteries and the middle and inferior branches supply the tonsillar fossa.

The internal maxillary artery supply is from the descending palatine artery, which travels through the lesser palatine canal to reach the tonsillar fossa and anastomose with the ascending palatine.

Vascular Supply of the Base of Tongue

The pharyngeal part of the tongue is covered by lymphoid tonsillar tissue that is contiguous with the palatine tonsil at the glossotonsillar sulcus. Immediately deep to this tissue lies the intrinsic tongue musculature.

The main issue when considering the vasculature of the base of tongue is to understand the course of the lingual artery and its branches. It arises from the external carotid artery at the level of the hyoid bone and continues lateral to the middle constrictor muscle until the hypoglossal nerve crosses it. From here it passes deep

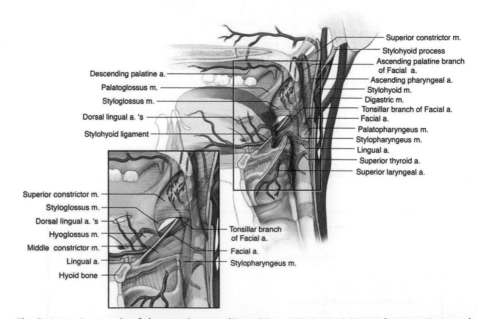

Fig. 2. Vascular supply of the oropharynx. (*From* Moore EJ, Janus J, Kasperbauer J. Transoral robotic surgery of the oropharynx: clinical and anatomic considerations. Clinical Anatomy 2012;25:138; with permission.)

to the hyoglossus muscle and runs along the superior surface of the hyoid bone. It is in this position that it is most likely to be encountered during TORS. Here it divides into 4 branches, with the most important branch for consideration in TORS being the dorsal lingual artery, which supplies the base of tongue.

PREVENTION OF SIGNIFICANT INTRAOPERATIVE AND POSTOPERATIVE BLEEDING

- Bleeding rates after surgery range from 1.5% to 11.5% in the literature
- Targeted ligation of branches of the external carotid artery may decrease intraoperative and postoperative bleeding

---

Posttransoral hemorrhage can be unpredictable and may have potentially serious complications for the patient. The highly morbid effects come from asphyxiation secondary to the bleeding with subsequent brain hypoxia, or from aspiration of blood with secondary respiratory failure rather than from exsanguination. Bleeding rates from 1.5% to 11.5%[5] have been documented following transoral resection of upper aerodigestive tract malignancies, which corresponds with established postoperative tonsillectomy bleeding rates. It is likely that previous oncologic treatment via either surgery or radiotherapy will increase the risk of postoperative hemorrhage, although this has not been established with statistical significance. What also remains clinically unproved is whether targeted external carotid artery ligation can help to decrease both intraoperative and postoperative bleeding.

Within the available TORS literature to date there is some disagreement on the timing of operative procedures, with some groups performing concurrent transoral and neck dissection surgery and other groups performing staged procedures. There is also variation as to whether, in the staged procedures, the primary surgery is performed before or after the neck dissection surgery. One of the potential benefits of performing the neck dissection before the primary resection is that it allows for preoperative ligation of appropriate tumor feeding vessels.

The practice of the senior author is to perform a neck dissection 1 week before the TORS surgery. At the time of the neck dissection either the facial artery, lingual artery, or dorsal lingual branch of the lingual artery is ligated. The rationale behind this lies in not only aiming to decrease postoperative bleeding but also in decreasing the amount of intraoperative bleeding during the primary resection. In a series of 50 consecutive patients treated under this protocol, there have been 2 episodes of minor postoperative hemorrhage (Magnuson, unpublished data, 2015). In a recently published article from the University of Pittsburgh Medical Center, the rate of bleeding in patients with prophylactic ligation was similar to the rate in those without; however, the severity of the postoperative bleeding was diminished.

Similarly, data published from the Mayo Clinic group did not show any statistically significant decrease in postoperative hemorrhage in patients who had carotid system vessel ligation versus those who did not. However, it was noted that of the 10 patients who developed severe bleeding postoperatively, only 1 had had the external carotid vessel system tied off. In addition, those with higher primary T stages were more likely to bleed, whereas those who had previous treatment, whether surgical or radiotherapy, did not have an increased risk of bleeding. Again, of the 5 patients who bled in this salvage group, 3 had severe bleeding. This finding led the investigators to recommend that ligation of the carotid vessel system should be undertaken in higher-T-stage tumors and those patients undergoing revision surgery.

MANAGEMENT OF SIGNIFICANT BLEEDING
Intraoperative Prevention and Management of Bleeding

- The management of vessels during surgery typically depends on their caliber
- Larger vessels encountered during surgery should be clipped using endovascular clip appliers
- Smaller vessels may be controlled with monopolar or bipolar cautery
- Hemostatic agents may be used as an adjunct to achieve hemostasis

---

The best principle in maintaining hemostasis is avoidance of bleeding. The high-definition, three-dimensional optics available with the robotic system allow precise dissection of tissues, aiding in the identification and dissection of vessels from surrounding muscles and fascia (**Fig. 3**). The management of vessels encountered during the surgery varies depending on their caliber. For smaller vessels it is possible to apply cautery to control the bleeding. Low-flow vascular bleeding can also be controlled using a suction monopolar or bipolar cautery instrument manipulated by the bedside assistant.

For larger caliber vessels, vascular clips can be used. The options available for this are the EndoWrist clip-applying instruments (**Fig. 4**) or the endoscopic clip applier (**Fig. 5**). The difficulty with the EndoWrist clip appliers is that they are only available as 8-mm instruments. If a surgeon typically uses the 5-mm EndoWrist instruments, then the cannula along with the EndoWrist instrument has to be exchanged at the time of use. In the event of significant hemorrhage this may be too time consuming and may take control of the robotic arms away from the console surgeon. The endoscopic clip appliers allow application of Ligaclips by the bedside assistant. There is a right-angled and left-angled clip and the console surgeon can use the robotic arms to display the vessel so that multiple clips can

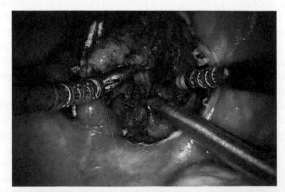

Fig. 3. Intraoperative picture during a right lateral pharyngectomy showing the precision of view that can be obtained with the da Vinci Surgical robot. (*Courtesy of* J Scott Magnuson, MD, Celebration, FL.)

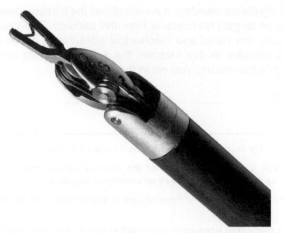

Fig. 4. EndoWrist clip applicator. (*Courtesy of* Intuitive Surgical, Sunnyvale, CA; with permission.)

be applied to the distal end and 1 to the proximal end before transecting the vessel.

A useful technique that may be used for significant bleeding at the tongue base is to have either the nurse or the bedside surgical assistant apply external neck pressure just above the ipsilateral greater cornu of the hyoid bone, which puts pressure on the lingual artery and slows the bleeding enough for the console surgeon to find and pick up the bleeding branch in preparation for clip application. At the end of the procedure, the surgeon may use hemostatic agents such as Tiseel (Baxter Healthcare, Hayward, CA) or FloSeal Hemostatic Matrix (Baxter Healthcare, Hayward, CA) to cover the mucosal defect.

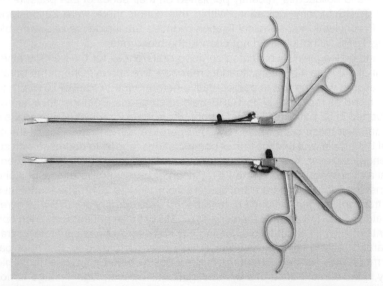

Fig. 5. Endoscopic clip applier. (*Courtesy of* J Scott Magnuson, MD, Celebration, FL.)

In the event of significant bleeding, it is critical that the surgeon does not remove the robot in an attempt to gain hemostasis from the bedside. The best way to control bleeding is by using the visual and mechanical advantages of the robot. If it is not possible to stop bleeding in this manner, the surgeon should use a transcervical approach and ligate the feeding vessels in the neck.

Delayed Bleeding

- Risk factors for delayed bleeding include the use of antithrombotic medication
- Prophylactic ligation of branches of the external carotid artery (lingual and facial) may decrease the incidence or severity of bleeding
- Management of secondary hemorrhage is performed without the surgical robot
- Securing the airway is the most important element of surgical management

Risk factors

At present there are limited published data for the postoperative complications of TORS and specifically the risk of secondary hemorrhage. A pertinent study by Asher and colleagues[6] from the University of Birmingham, Alabama, specifically assessed the bleeding rate of 145 patients undergoing transoral robotic-assisted surgery for any indication. Of these patients, 11 (7.5%) developed some degree of postoperative hemorrhage, with 9 (6%) requiring reoperation for examination and/or control of bleeding. The most consistent risk factor in those patients who bled was that they were on antithrombotic medication, either anticoagulants or antiplatelet agents, for other medical comorbidities. There was also a high bleeding rate in salvage surgery as opposed to primary surgery; however, this did not reach statistical significance.

Mandal and colleagues[7] recently published on their series of 224 patients who underwent TORS for any indication. Within this cohort there were 22 postoperative bleeds. Prophylactic transcervical ligation reduced the incidence of severe bleeding following TORS, although it did not change the bleed rate.

Chia and colleagues[8] investigated surgeon preferences for the perioperative management of TORS in a multi-institutional retrospective survey. One of the parameters they measured was the risk of postoperative hemorrhage. A total of 2015 procedures were included as reported by 35 TORS-trained surgeons. Postoperative hemorrhage was reported in 62 patients (3.1%). Of note, there were 7 patient deaths in the survey period and 4 of these were caused by postoperative hemorrhage. One of the conclusions of this article was that the rate of complications tended to decrease with surgeon experience; however, this was not specifically related to postoperative hemorrhage.

Pollei and colleagues[9] conducted a multicenter retrospective review of a single institutions' experience with transoral surgery from 1994 to 2012. The techniques used for the transoral surgery included both transoral laser surgery and TORS. There was a bleed rate of 5.4% (49 of 906 patients) with 67.3% of these patients requiring operative intervention. The investigators did not find any statistically significant role for transcervical carotid system ligation; however, it was only performed in 15.6% of patients. Furthermore, they noticed a trend toward reduced postoropharyngectomy bleeding severity in the context of carotid system ligation. However, high-T-stage tumors had a higher bleeding rate.

Management

The management of delayed postoperative bleeding depends on the severity of the bleed. As with posttonsillectomy hemorrhage, conservative measures may be applied and, if these fail, then operative intervention becomes necessary. Surgical management is performed without the use of the robot. Although the surgical robot is an excellent tool to improve visualization and instrumentation in the upper aerodigestive tract, it is not an ideal measure to gain control of hemorrhage in the postoperative setting. The setup of the robot requires trained ancillary staff, additional equipment, and a longer preparation time. None of this may be available at the time of an acute postoperative hemorrhage.

The most critical element of the management is securing the airway and this must be performed expediently. Depending on the clinical scenario, the airway may be secured by the anesthesia team in the operating room via traditional direct laryngoscopy after a rapid sequence induction or by awake transnasal intubation over a flexible fiberoptic scope. If all these techniques fail, the surgeon must be prepared for an emergency tracheotomy to secure the airway. Once the airway is appropriately established, access to the point of hemorrhage can be obtained either with a typical tonsil gag, such as a Boyle-Davis or Crowe-Davis for more tonsillar-based issues, or with a laryngoscope for base of tongue hemorrhage. Once visualization of the clinically indicated area is obtained, suction monopolar cauterization controls most hemorrhage points. If the bleeding cannot be stopped intraorally, the neck can be accessed for ligation of either the external carotid artery or an appropriate branch of this artery.

SUMMARY

Surgery with TORS offers significant advantages compared with traditional open surgical approaches and can potentially minimize the long-term side effects of organ preservation therapy with chemoradiation. The use of angled telescopes and wristed instruments allows visualization and access to areas of the pharynx that are difficult to reach with line-of-sight instrumentation. Although the application of TORS in head and neck surgery has expanded considerably since FDA approval in 2009, there are still only limited data available on the postoperative complications and their management. As further data become available, it is likely that further risk factors and treatment strategies will become available.

Post-Test Questions (Correct answers are in italics)

1. The main arterial supply of the tonsillar fossa comes from
   a. *The facial artery*
   b. The lingual artery
   c. The ascending pharyngeal artery
   d. The internal maxillary artery
2. Where is the lingual artery most at risk during TORS surgery?
   a. At the origin from the external carotid artery
   b. *Along the superior border of the hyoid deep to the hyoglossus muscle*
   c. Medial to the hypoglossal nerve
   d. Lateral to the hypoglossal nerve
3. What risk factors are associated with postoperative hemorrhage following TORS?
   a. Stage of the primary tumor

> b. Experience of the primary surgeon
> c. Use of antithrombotic therapy
> d. *All of the above*
> 4. In the event of significant bleeding, mortality is most often caused by
>   a. Electrolyte abnormalities secondary to fluid shift
>   b. Exsanguination
>   c. *Asphyxiation with subsequent hypoxic brain injury*
>   d. Physician error

SUPPLEMENTARY DATA

Supplementary PDF slides related to this article can be found online at http://www.oto.theclinics.com/.

REFERENCES

1. Hockstein NG, O'Malley BW, Weinstein GS. Assessment of intraoperative safety in transoral robotic surgery. Laryngoscope 2006;116(2):165–8.
2. Weinstein GS, O'Malley BW Jr, Magnuson JS, et al. Transoral robotic surgery: a multicenter study to assess feasibility, safety, and surgical margins. Laryngoscope 2012;122(8):1701–7.
3. Hockstein NG, Weinstein GS, O'Malley BW. Maintenance of hemostasis in transoral robotic surgery. ORL J Otorhinolaryngol Relat Spec 2005;67:220–4.
4. Goyal N, Atmakuri M, Golderberg D. Anatomy of the oropharynx: the robotic perspective. Operat Tech Otolaryngol 2013;24:70–3.
5. Salassa JR, Hinni ML, Grant DG, et al. Postoperative bleeding in transoral laser microsurgery for upper aerodigestive tract tumors. Otolaryngol Head Neck Surg 2008;139(3):453–9.
6. Asher SA, White HN, Kejner AE, et al. Hemorrhage after trans-oral robotic-assisted surgery. Otolaryngol Head Neck Surg 2013;149(1):112–7.
7. Mandal R, Duvvuri U, Ferris R, et al. Analysis of post-transoral robotic assisted surgery hemorrhage: Frequency, outcomes and prevention. Head Neck 2015. [Epub ahead of print].
8. Chia SH, Gross NH, Richmon JD. Surgeon experience and complications with transoral robotic surgery (TORS). Otolaryngol Head Neck Surg 2013;149(6):885–92.
9. Pollei TR, Hinni ML, Moore EJ, et al. Analysis of post-operative bleeding and risk factors in transoral surgery of the oropharynx. JAMA Otolaryngol Head Neck Surg 2013;139(11):1212–8.

SUGGESTED READINGS

Asher SA, White HN, Kejner AE, et al. Hemorrhage after trans-oral robotic-assisted surgery. Otolaryngol Head Neck Surg 2013;149(1):112–7.

This study examined the postoperative bleeding complications encountered at 1 tertiary referral institution to determine the risk factors for this complication and the management options. The medical records of 147 consecutive patients undergoing TORS were reviewed. Eleven (7.5%) of the patients developed postoperative hemorrhage. Eight of these were on antithrombotic medication for other medical comorbidities. Typically, these postoperative bleeds can be controlled with nonrobotic means.

Mandal R, Duvvuri U, Ferris R, et al. Analysis of post-transoral robotic assisted surgery hemorrhage: frequency, outcomes and prevention. Head Neck 2015. [Epub ahead of print].

This study classified and reviewed postoropharyngectomy hemorrhage rates and associated risk factors from a single-institution, multicenter, retrospective medical chart review analysis of 906 patients who underwent transoral surgery for oropharyngeal carcinoma from 1994 to 2012. The total postoperative bleed rate was 5.4% with 67.3% of these patients requiring return to surgical intervention. The recommendation was that patients with higher-T-stage tumors, primary tonsil tumors, and patients undergoing revision surgery should have ligation of feeding vessels performed.

Pollei TR, Hinni ML, Moore EJ, et al. Analysis of post-operative bleeding and risk factors in transoral surgery of the oropharynx. JAMA Otolaryngol Head Neck Surg 2013;139(11):1212–8.

This study provided an analysis of a single institution's experience with hemorrhage after TORS. All 224 patients were operated on by one of 3 experienced TORS surgeons. There were 22 postoperative bleeds. The conclusion was that prophylactic arterial ligation may reduce the incidence of severe bleeding after TORS. In addition, TORS patients who have a preoperatively difficult airway should be considered for prophylactic tracheostomy.

Thyroidectomy Hemostasis

Russell B. Smith, MD[a,b], Andrew Coughlin, MD[a,b,*]

KEYWORDS

- Thyroidectomy • Hemostasis • Harmonic Scalpel • LigaSure • Hemorrhage

KEY LEARNING POINTS

At the end of this article, the reader will:

- Understand the risk of bleeding in thyroid surgery.
- Have a good knowledge of the neck vessels that can lead to significant perioperative bleeding and describe the management of post-thyroidectomy hemorrhage.
- Be able to compare conventional techniques to newer technologies for hemostasis.
- Understand the role of hemostatic agents as adjuncts in thyroid surgery.
- Be able to discuss the role of a drain in the prevention and management of bleeding and hematoma formation after thyroid surgery.

INTRODUCTION

How has the risk of bleeding in thyroid surgery evolved over time?

- Abu al-Qasim
  - In 952 AD, Islam's legendary medieval surgeon performs first goiter excision.
  - His report states that the patient "just avoided exsanguination."[1]

- Diffenbach
  - In 1848, he stated this was "one of the most thankless, most perilous undertakings which, if not altogether prohibited, should at least be restricted."[2]

- Theodor Billroth
  - In 1860, 8 of his first 20 patients with goiter died perioperatively leading to cessation of the surgery.
  - In 1866, with improved anesthesia, asepsis, and hemostasis, his death rate dropped to less than 10%.

- Emil Theodore Kocher
  - In 1909, he won the Nobel Prize for work in decreasing thyroidectomy mortality to less than 1%.
  - With close attention to hemostasis, he achieved 0.5% mortality in 5000 thyroidectomies by 1912.[3]

Neither author has any disclosures.
[a] Department of Otolaryngology – Head and Neck Surgery, 981225 Nebraska Medical Center, Omaha, NE 68198-1225, USA; [b] Nebraska Methodist Hospital, Estabrook Cancer Center, 8303 Dodge Street, Omaha, NE, USA
* Corresponding author.
E-mail address: acoughlin82@gmail.com

The first total thyroidectomy for goiter was reported in 952 AD by Islam's legendary medieval surgeon, Abu al-Qasim. In his initial report, he stated that the patient "just avoided exsanguination."[1] Diffenbach further described thyroid surgery as "One of the most thankless, most perilous undertakings which, if not altogether prohibited, should at least be restricted."[1] Despite European sentiment that thyroid surgery was a terrible procedure, Theodor Billroth took on the challenge of the operation. However, in 1860, 8 of his first 20 patients died perioperatively. Emil Theodore Kocher, a trainee of Billroth, was the first to use precise surgical technique and meticulous hemostasis to reduce the mortality rate to 0.5% in more than 5000 thyroidectomies.[3] His work in thyroid surgery led to a Nobel Prize in 1909.

VASCULAR ANATOMY: ARTERIES
Superior Thyroid Artery

- Branch off the external carotid artery
- Associated with the external branch of the superior laryngeal nerve (SLN)
  - SLN lies less than 1 cm from the superior pole vessels[4] in about 37% of patients and below the upper border of the gland in 20%, thereby putting the nerve at significant risk of injury during thyroid surgery
- Lateral traction on superior pole can be helpful to prevent injury
- **Fig. 1** shows superior pedicle with lateral traction using an Allis or Babcock clamp

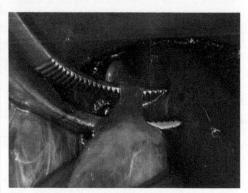

Fig. 1. Superior pole pedicle retracted inferolaterally to protect the SLN.

The superior thyroid artery is the first branch of the external carotid artery and descends inferomedially into the central neck (see **Fig. 1**). Care should be taken when dividing the artery to avoid injury to the external branch of the SLN given that it is less than 1 cm from the superior pole vessels in 37% of patients and below the upper border of the gland in 20%.[4] The latter puts the nerve at particularly high risk. Lateral and inferior traction on the superior pole can help identify and avoid the nerve while opening the avascular plane.

Inferior Thyroid Artery

The inferior thyroid artery arises as a branch from the thyrocervical trunk that arises from the subclavian artery (see **Fig. 2**). In addition to supplying the thyroid gland, these vessels are the main blood supply for both the superior and inferior parathyroid glands. The artery travels posterior to the common carotid artery and has a variable relationship to the RLN. In 10% of cases, the artery will run between branches of the RLN, putting the nerve at particularly high risk during ligation.[5] An attempt should be made to ligate the artery distal to the parathyroid branches to prevent hypoparathyroidism (**Fig. 3**).

- Branch of the thyrocervical trunk
- Main vascular supply to the parathyroid glands
- Travels posterior to the common carotid artery to enter central neck
  - Artery and its branches have variable relationship to recurrent laryngeal nerve (RLN)
- In 10% of cases, the RLN lies between branches of the artery[5]
- Attempt to ligate distal to parathyroid branches
- **Fig. 2** shows inferior artery posterior to the common carotid artery

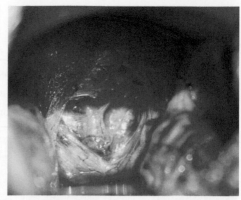

Fig. 2. Inferior thyroid coursing posterior to the common carotid artery.

Thyroidea Ima Artery

- Arises from the brachiocephalic trunk and ascends in front of the trachea to supply the lower portion of the thyroid gland
- Uncommonly encountered but can cause significant bleeding if not identified and controlled

Perforating Tracheal Blood Vessels

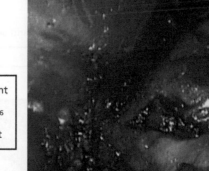

- Small vessels around Berry ligament that can significantly put the RLN at risk when cauterization is attempted[6]
- **Fig. 3** shows vessels at Berry ligament

Fig. 3. Perforating vessels near the Berry ligament have been cauterized meticulously to prevent postoperative bleeding.

VASCULAR ANATOMY: VEINS
Anterior Jugular Veins

- Identify near the midline raphe at the beginning of surgery to prevent injury
- Understand that there may be bridging vessels in the midline
- **Fig. 4** shows anterior jugular veins and bridging vessels

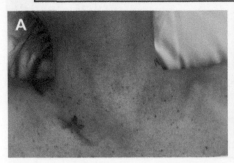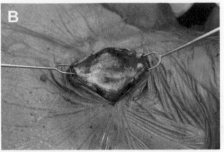

Fig. 4. (A) Anterior jugular veins are identified before skin incision. (B) These are then identified just lateral to the midline raphe.

Superior Thyroid Veins

- Smaller and within the superior pedicle
- Superior veins also associated with the SLN

Inferior Thyroid Veins

- Usually associated with inferior parathyroid glands
- Anterior to the inferior thyroid artery
- Drain directly into the innominate vein and are usually easily ligated

Middle Thyroid Veins

- Found laterally during dissection of the strap muscles off of the gland
- Course superficial to common carotid artery to enter internal jugular vein
- Can be multiple branches
  - **Fig. 5** shows middle thyroid veins

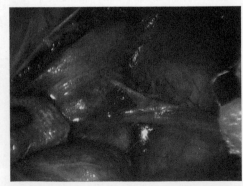

Fig. 5. Middle thyroid vein extending medially from the carotid sheath and branching into 2 separate veins.

Intrathyroidal Capsular Veins

- Can cause significant bleeding and can be quite prominent in large goiters[6]
- Bipolar cautery is generally enough to control the bleeding
  - **Fig. 6** shows control of intrathyroidal capsular veins

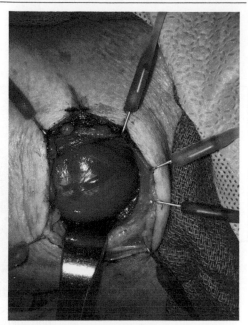

Fig. 6. Intrathyroidal or capsular blood vessels in a patient with Graves disease.

The anterior jugular veins are the first encountered during thyroid surgery (see **Fig. 4**). These should be carefully visualized during division of the midline raphe to prevent injury. Because the fascia is released superiorly and inferiorly, understand that bridging veins can be present. The superior and inferior thyroid veins are much smaller. The superior vein runs within the superior pole pedicle whereas the inferior vein drains directly into the innominate vein and is anterior to the inferior thyroid artery. These vessels are easily identified and ligated during capsular dissection. The middle thyroid veins are found during lateral dissection and multiple branches may be present (see **Fig. 5**). These should be divided just outside the capsule. In general, no nerves or parathyroid tissue are associated with the middle veins. Intrathyroidal or capsular veins can be quite prominent in patients with large goiters (see **Fig. 6**).[6] If injured, these vessels can generally be controlled with bipolar electrocautery.

WHY IS HEMOSTASIS IMPORTANT?

Hemostasis is of the utmost importance during thyroid surgery. Minimizing intraoperative blood loss is the goal but meticulous hemostasis as described by Kocher with capsular dissection is critical. Bleeding during thyroidectomy blurs operative planes thus putting the RLN and parathyroid glands at significant risk of injury. Ultimately, meticulous hemostasis is also important to prevent the dreaded complication of postoperative hematoma (see **Fig. 7**).

- To maintain a low intraoperative blood loss and avoid transfusion
- To avoid inadvertent injury of the laryngeal nerves and parathyroid glands
- To prevent postoperative hematoma causing airway compromise
  ○ **Fig. 7** shows a post-thyroidectomy hematoma

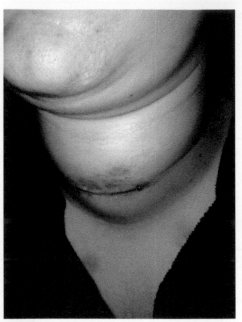

Fig. 7. Figure showing a patient presenting with postoperative hematoma. Note the ecchymotic skin differentiating this from a seroma.

Postoperative Hematoma

- Incidence of 0.1% to 1.1%[7]
- Most occur within first 6 hours of operation
- Causes include
  ○ Loosening of the surgical knot
  ○ Opening of the cauterized vessel due to hypertension, retching, or Valsalva during recovery
  ○ Oozing from cut edges of the thyroid
- Prevention
  ○ Perform Valsalva before closing
  ○ Consider closing strap muscles loosely to prevent airway obstruction
    ■ Described by Terris[8] in 2009
- Treatment
  ○ Most hematomas need to be evacuated and re-explored
  ○ If patient is stable without air hunger it is acceptable to intubate before opening the neck
    ■ The most experienced team member should intubate because marked edema of the epiglottis and arytenoids can be present
- Postoperative care proceeds no differently than primary thyroid surgery
- **Fig. 8** shows the strap muscles being approximated loosely

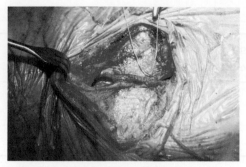

Fig. 8. Midline stitch to approximate the strap muscles.

Postoperative hematoma occurs at a rate of about 0.1% to 1.1%.[7] Almost all cases occur in the first 6 hours after surgery and can be the result of several surgeon or patient factors. Several studies have shown that only around 20% of hematomas occur between 6 and 24 hours postoperatively and virtually no hematomas occur afterwards.[9] Prevention of symptomatic or life-threatening hematoma can also be achieved by avoiding tight reapproximation of the strap muscles as described by Terris[8] in 2009 (see **Fig. 8**). Although this will not prevent hematoma, it should allow earlier recognition of the process and delay the lymphatic outflow blockage that leads to laryngeal edema and dyspnea. Performing a Valsalva can also be effective to identify potential sources of bleeding before closing. Treatment of hematomas really depends on the symptomatology. Most hematomas need to be evacuated and re-explored but only an unstable or progressively worsening hematoma in a patient requires immediate evacuation at the bedside. Often, reintubation in a controlled operating room (OR) environment is possible. The most senior endoscopist should perform the intubation because significant epiglottis and arytenoid edema may be present. Postoperative care generally does not change after an evacuation.

SURGICAL HEMOSTASIS
Clamp, Tie, and Cut

- Traditional form of vessel control
- Requires meticulous capsular dissection
- Requires larger incision and does require more time to perform
- Surgical clips are an alternative

Electrocautery

- Good for small vessels
- Thermal energy is up to 150 to 400°C
- Monopolar cautery causes more heat dispersion
- Bipolar cautery is more pinpoint and defined

Harmonic Scalpel

- Cut and coagulate at lower temperatures of 50 to 100°C[10]
- Less dispersion of heat energy

LigaSure

- A form of bipolar electrocautery that seals vessels
- Direct pressure also required for vessel sealing
- **Fig. 9** shows LigaSure (Medtronic, New Haven, CT), clamp, tie, cut, bipolar electrocautery, and Harmonic Scalpel (Ethicon Inc., Sommerville, NJ, USA)

Several options exist for intraoperative ligation of blood vessels. Conventional techniques include clamp, tie, and cut methods with or without cautery. Some surgeons use monopolar cautery; however, this form causes a significant amount of heat dispersion, putting adjacent structures at risk for injury. Bipolar cautery is more pinpoint and allows less dispersion of heat. Newer techniques include use of the Harmonic Scalpel and LigaSure tissue sealer (see **Fig. 9**). Electrocautery is exceptionally good with smaller vessels; however, heat energy can be up to 150 to 400°C, whereas the Harmonic Scalpel operates at around 50 to 100°C.[10] This lower temperature theoretically creates less dispersion of heat and thus prevents peripheral injury of adjacent structures.

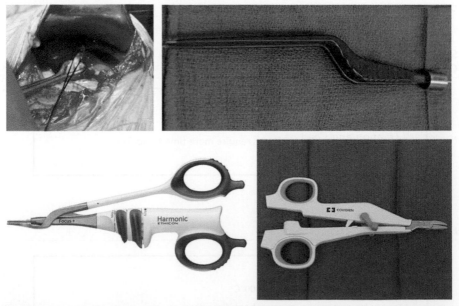

Fig. 9. Four techniques to perform surgical hemostasis. (*A*) Suture ligation of the superior pole vessels. (*B*) Bipolar electrocautery. (*C*) Harmonic scalpel. (*D*) LigaSure. (*Courtesy of* Medtronic, New Haven, CT; with permission.)

Harmonic Scalpel

- Three parts[11]
  - Generator
  - Hand piece
  - Scalpel
- Ultrasonic energy creates vibrations at 55,000 Hz
- Disrupts hydrogen bonds and produces an endovascular coagulum
- Up to 5 mm vessels

The Harmonic Scalpel has 3 parts, including the generator, the hand piece, and the scalpel itself. Mechanical energy, in the form of ultrasonic vibrations at the rate of 55,000 Hz, is created and disrupts tissue hydrogen bonds to create an endovascular coagulum, thus sealing off the vessel. Vessels up to 5 mm in diameter can be controlled with this method.[10]

LigaSure

- Bipolar heat denatures collagen and elastin in vascular walls thus merging vessels with[11]
  - Electrical head
  - Direct pressure
- The tissues are then divided in the middle with a blade
- Up to 7 mm vessels

The LigaSure uses a closed loop bipolar electrocautery system that denatures collagen and elastin in the vascular walls, thus merging vessels with surrounding soft tissue. Both the electrical head and direct pressure are involved with vessel sealing. Older models required division with scissors or a separate blade but newer models have the blade included. Division of vessels up to 7 mm can be controlled. Because it is a closed loop system, virtually no heat dispersion occurs.[11]

Standard Ligation and Coagulation Versus Harmonic Scalpel

- Meta-analysis of 12 randomized controlled trials (RCTs) including 1153 subjects[12]
- Included benign and malignant disease
- Decreased operative time by 22.67 minutes (25%) $P<.00001$
- Decreased blood loss by 20.03 mL $P<.00001$
- Pain decreased by 0.86 points $P = .02$
- Length of stay, wound drainage, and rate of complications were not significantly different
- **Table 1** shows significant differences found with Harmonic Scalpel

In 2010 Ecker and colleagues performed a meta-analysis of 12 RCTs, including 1153 subjects to compared standard ligation techniques to the Harmonic Scalpel. Surgery was performed for both benign and malignant disease; however, benign disease dominated the series. Operative time was significantly shorter by 22.67 minutes ($P<.00001$), intraoperative blood loss was decreased by 20.03 mL ($P<.00001$), and in a few studies postoperative pain was decreased by 0.86 points on a 1 to 10 scale ($P = .02$) in favor of the Harmonic Scalpel (see **Table 1**). Length of hospital stay, wound drainage, and rate of complications were not significantly different between the groups.[12]

Standard Ligation and Coagulation Versus LigaSure

- Meta-analysis of 9 prospective trials (4 randomized, 5 nonrandomized)[13]
- Most studies were for benign disease (0%–26% malignant)
- Operative time studied in 6 trials and 586 subjects
  - Decreased operative time by average of 20.32 minutes $P<.003$
- Hospital stay studied in 7 trials
  - No difference in hospital stay $P = .31$
- No differences blood loss or complications
- **Table 2** shows significant results of this study

Table 1 Results from trial comparing Harmonic Scalpel with conventional hemostasis techniques	
Harmonic Scalpel vs Conventional Hemostasis	
Operative time	Decreased by 22.67 min $P<.00001$[a]
Blood loss	Decreased by 20.03 mL $P<.00001$[a]
Pain	Decreased by 0.86 points $P = .02$[a]

No significant difference in (1) Length of stay, (2) Wound drainage, (3) Wound infection, (4) Postoperative complications (ie, nerve injury or hypoparathyroidism).
[a] In favor of Harmonic Scalpel.
Data from Ecker T, Carvalho AL, Choe JH, et al. Hemostasis in thyroid surgery: Harmonic Scalpel versus other techniques—a meta-analysis. Otolaryngol Head Neck Surg 2010;143(1):17–25.

Similarly, in 2009, Yao and colleagues[13] performed a meta-analysis of standard ligation techniques compared with the LigaSure tissue sealing system. The study included 9 prospective trials, 4 of which were randomized. Most of the disease was benign goiter. Operative time was decreased with the LigaSure by 20.32 minutes ($P<.003$). Hospital stay, blood loss, and complications were no different between the 2 techniques (see **Table 2**).

Standard Ligation and Coagulation Versus LigaSure Versus Harmonic Scalpel

All 3 techniques were combined in a smaller RCT in which 20 subjects were enrolled in each arm. Only benign thyroid disease was evaluated. Operative time was significantly less in both LigaSure and Harmonic Scalpel groups compared with conventional techniques by 37 minutes ($P<.001$) and 8 minutes ($P<.001$), respectively. Blood loss and

- RCT of 60 subjects, 20 in each arm[11]
- Excluded cancer subjects
- Mean operative time differences were
  - 29 minutes longer for suture ligation compared with LigaSure (P<.001)
  - 37 minutes longer for suture ligation compared with Harmonic Scalpel (P<.001)
- Blood loss was significantly less compared with suture ligation
  - LigaSure decreased blood loss by 18 mL (P<.005)
  - Harmonic Scalpel decreased blood loss by 16 mL (P<.01)
- Pain medication consumption was significantly less with LigaSure and Harmonic scalpel (P = .016 and P = .02, respectively)
- No significant difference in hospital stay, seroma formation, drain output, hypocalcemia, or nerve injury
- **Table 3** shows significant differences between the groups

pain medication consumption were also significantly less with Harmonic Scalpel and LigaSure techniques (see **Table 3**). Again no differences in hospital stay, seroma formation, drain output, or other perioperative complications were identified.[11]

Table 2
Results from trial comparing LigaSure with conventional hemostasis techniques

LigaSure vs Conventional Hemostasis	
Operative time	Decreased by 20.32 min P<.003[a]

No significant difference in (1) Length of stay, (2) Blood loss, (3) Postoperative complications (ie, nerve injury or hypoparathyroidism).
[a] In favor of LigaSure.
Data from Yao HS, Wang Q, Wang WJ, et al. Prospective clinical trials of thyroidectomy with LigaSure vs conventional vessel ligation: a systematic review and meta-analysis. Arch Surg 2009;144(12):1167–74.

Table 3
Results from trial comparing Harmonic Scalpel and LigaSure with conventional hemostasis techniques

Harmonic Scalpel vs LigaSure vs Conventional Hemostasis	
Operative time	Decreased by 37 min P<.001[a] Decreased by 29 min P<.001[b]
Blood loss	Decreased by 16 mL P<.01[a] Decreased by 18 mL P<.005[b]
Pain medication consumption	Significantly less with both Harmonic Scalpel P<.02[a] and LigaSure P = .016[b]

No significant difference in (1) Length of stay, (2) Wound drainage, (3) Seroma formation, (4) Postoperative complications (ie, nerve injury or hypoparathyroidism).
[a] In favor of Harmonic Scalpel.
[b] In favor of LigaSure.
Data from Pons Y, Gauthier J, Ukkola-Pons E, et al. Comparison of LigaSure vessel sealing system, harmonic scalpel, and conventional hemostasis in total thyroidectomy. Otolaryngol Head Neck Surg 2009;141:496–501.

Harmonic Scalpel Versus LigaSure

- 400 subjects, mostly benign but some malignant cases[14]
- Drain left in all cases to assess blood loss
- No significant difference in operative time Harmonic 65 minutes versus LigaSure 75 minutes ($P = .27$)
- Postoperative bleeding or drainage was similar Harmonic Scalpel 50 cc versus LigaSure 55 cc ($P = .32$)
- Hospital stay was similar in both groups
- No difference in hypocalcemia, vocal cord paralysis, infection, hematoma, or seroma
- **Box 1** shows results from study

In 2014, Ruggiero and colleagues[14] performed a larger RCT of 400 subjects comparing the LigaSure system to the Harmonic Scalpel. A drain was left in all cases to assess postoperative blood loss. There was no significant difference in blood loss ($P = .27$), postoperative drain output or bleeding ($P = .32$), hospital stay, or complications. They concluded that no differences existed between the systems and that surgeon preference and comfort should drive use of a particular device (see **Box 1**).

Box 1
Results from trial comparing Harmonic Scalpel with LigaSure.

No significant differences seen in

- Operative Time
- Length of stay
- Wound drainage
- Wound infection
- Postoperative complications (ie, nerve injury or hypoparathyroidism)

Data from Ruggiero R, Gubitosi A, Conzo G, et al. Sutureless thyroidectomy. Int J Surg 2014;12:S189–93.

Harmonic Scalpel Versus LigaSure in Papillary Thyroid Cancer

- RCT evaluating 320 subjects[15]
  - 164 in the Harmonic Scalpel group
  - 156 in the LigaSure group
- Single surgeon
- Only subjects with papillary thyroid cancer were enrolled
- There were no significant differences identified in
  - Operative time, hospital stay, amount of total postoperative day (POD) 1 drain output, or perioperative complications such as hypoparathyroidism, hematoma, or RLN injury
- **Box 2** shows statistically significant differences in the study

Although most previous studies included both benign and malignant cases, almost all subjects were treated for benign disease. In 2013, Kwak and colleagues[15] performed a single-surgeon RCT comparing Harmonic Scalpel to the LigaSure system for papillary thyroid cancer. They found no significant difference in operative time, hospital stay, postoperative wound drainage, or perioperative complications. They concluded that both instruments are safe and effective for use in thyroid surgery and that no differences exist for thyroid cancer patients (see **Box 2**).

SURGICAL TECHNIQUE SUMMARY

- Surgeon comfort with the instrument is paramount
- Strong consideration for incorporating Harmonic Scalpel or LigaSure in thyroid surgery to decrease OR time and cost
- A combination of methods that include advanced technologies as well as more traditional techniques will likely be used in most cases
- **Fig. 10** shows Harmonic Scalpel plus bipolar electrocautery plus suture equals happy surgeon and patient

Based on the review of all these studies, it seems that either the Harmonic Scalpel or LigaSure system significantly decrease operative times (see **Fig. 10**). When choosing a system to use, surgeon comfort with the respective instrument is paramount and should take precedent because no single instrument has been found to be better than the other in thyroid surgery. Although products like the LigaSure and Harmonic Scalpel may be useful for larger vessels at the inferior and superior pole, more precise vessel ligation with clamp, cut, and tie, surgical clips, or bipolar electrocautery may be the method of choice for control of vessels immediately adjacent to the nerve, parathyroid glands, or on the Berry ligament.

HEMOSTATIC AGENTS

All surgeons have encountered the situation of minimal but persistent ooze from the superior pedicle or from the area directly adjacent to the nerve during thyroid surgery. Use of any of the previously described techniques to control this type of bleeding can markedly increase the risk of nerve injury. Several studies have assessed the use of adjunctive hemostatic agents during thyroidectomy. These agents are reviewed in the following section.

Box 2
Harmonic Scalpel versus LigaSure in subjects with papillary thyroid cancer

No significant differences seen in

- Operative time
- Length of stay
- Wound drainage as assessed by drain on POD 1
- Postoperative complications (ie, nerve injury or hypoparathyroidism)

Data from Kwak HY, Chae BJ, Park YG, et al. Comparison of surgical outcomes between papillary thyroid cancer patients treated with the harmonic ACE scalpel and LigaSure precise instrument during conventional thyroidectomy: a single-blind prospective randomized controlled trial. J Surg Res 2014;187(2):484–9.

- Plant extract containing *Urtica dioica, Vitis vinifera, Glycyrrhiza glabra, Alpinia offcinarum,* and *thymus vulgaris*[16]
- 55 subjects randomized to
  - 29 conventional hemostasis (CH)
  - 26 Ankaferd Blood Stopper (ABS)
- Randomized and blinded until envelope opened in the OR
- Drain volumes in first 24 hours
  - Significantly lower in ABS (12.0 mL) compared with HC (24.6 mL) group *P*<.001
- No impact on length of stay
- No difference in morbidity or formation of hematoma
- **Table 4** shows statistically significant differences in the study

Ankaferd Blood Stopper

The study evaluated a unique plant extract called the ABS, which previously has been evaluated for use with post-tonsillectomy bleeding. Guler and colleagues[16] performed an RCT using this extract in the neck postoperatively; 55 subjects were randomized to either CH (n = 29) or to the ABS (n = 26). They found that drain volumes were significantly less in subjects treated with ABS (12.0 mL) compared with CH (24.6 mL) in the first 24-hour period (*P*<.001). Length of stay and postoperative morbidity was not different between the 2 groups. Although they were able to show a significance difference, the study enrollment was small and the difference in drain output would not likely change drain management or even the need to place a drain because drain outputs were less than most institutions' threshold for drain removal (see **Table 4**).

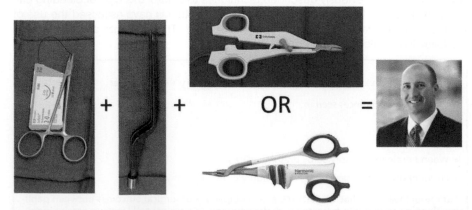

Fig. 10. Traditional hemostatic techniques of suture ligation and bipolar electrocautery when necessary plus the Harmonic Scalpel or LigaSure makes a happy surgeon. (*Courtesy of* Medtronic, New Haven, CT; with permission.)

Surgicel

- Prospective RCT of 190 subjects[17]
  - 92 in the CH treatment group
  - 98 in the CH plus Surgicel (Ethicon Inc., Sommerville, NJ, USA) group
- Postoperative bleeding was no different between groups
- Total drain output, time to drain removal and hospital stay were all significantly more in the Surgicel group versus CH group
- **Table 5** shows statistically significant differences in the study

Table 4
Results from trial comparing the Ankaferd Blood Stopper with conventional hemostasis techniques

ABS vs Conventional Hemostasis	
24 h drain output	Decreased by 12.6 mL $P<.001$[a]

No significant difference in (1) Length of stay, (2) Wound drainage, (3) Wound Infection.
[a] In favor of ABS.
Data from Guler M, Maralcan G, Kul S, et al. The efficacy of Ankaferd Blood Stopper for the management of bleeding following total thyroidectomy. J Invest Surg 2011;24(5):205–10.

Table 5
Results from trial comparing Surgicel to conventional hemostasis techniques

Surgicel vs Conventional Hemostasis	
Drain output	Significantly more for Surgicel 40 mL $P<.001$
Time to drain removal	Significantly longer for Surgicel 0.47 d $P<.001$
Hospital stay	Significantly longer for Surgicel 1.1 d $P = .001$

No significant difference in postoperative bleeding or seroma.
Data from Amit M, Binenbaum Y, Cohen JT, et al. Effectiveness of an oxidized cellulose patch hemostatic agent in thyroid surgery: a prospective, randomized, controlled study. J Am Coll Surg 2013;217(2):221–5.

Surgicel is an oxidized cellulose mesh that adheres to tissue especially in areas of bleeding and helps form a hemostatic clot. In 2013, Amit and colleagues[17] performed an RCT of 190 consecutive subjects undergoing total thyroidectomy. They placed a 2 by 2 cm patch of Surgicel in the thyroid bed and avoided placement on the RLN. There was no significant difference in hematoma rate between groups; however, they found significantly higher postoperative drain output (133 mL vs 93 mL, $P<.001$), increased time to drain removal (1.87 vs 1.4 days, $P<.001$), and longer hospital stay (2.7 vs 1.8 days, $P<.001$) in the Surgicel group compared with CH group (see **Table 5**).

FloSeal

Testini and colleagues[18] performed an RCT comparing conventional surgery alone to conventional surgery with the addition of FloSeal or a standard cellulose patch intraoperatively. They evaluated 155 subjects treated by a single surgeon, 49 who had surgery alone, 52 who had placement of a cellulose patch, and 54 who had FloSeal applied. Operative times ($P<.0001$ and $P<.0003$), time to drain removal ($P<.006$ and

- Prospective randomized control study with 155 subjects by a single surgeon[18]
  - 49 surgery alone
  - 52 surgery and Tabotamp (Ethicon Inc., Sommerville, NJ, USA) cellulose patch
  - 54 surgery and 5 mL FloSeal (Baxter Healthcare Corporation, Freemont, CA, USA)
- Operative time
  - Surgical hemostasis (133 minutes) and Tabotamp (122 minutes) were significantly longer than FloSeal (105 minutes) $P<.0001$ and $P<.0003$ respectively.
- Drain removal
  - Significantly longer in surgical hemostasis (39.7 h) and Tabotamp (39.7 h) groups compared with FloSeal (32.4 h) $P<.006$ and $P<.008$, respectively
- Hospital stay
  - Significantly longer in surgical hemostasis (49.8 h) and Tabotamp (47.5 h) groups compared with FloSeal (42.2 h) $P<.002$ and $P<.02$, respectively
- No significant difference in postoperative mortality
- **Table 6** summarizes the results of study

$P<.008$), and hospital stay ($P<.002$ and $P<.02$) were all significantly longer in subjects treated with surgery alone and surgery with cellulose patch, respectively. There were, however, no differences in postoperative hematoma or other complications related to thyroid surgery between the 3 groups (see **Table 6**).

Table 6
Results from trial comparing FloSeal with Tabotamp and conventional hemostasis techniques

FloSeal vs Tabotamp vs Conventional Hemostasis	
Operative time	Decreased by 28 min with FloSeal $P<.0001$
Time to drain removal	Decreased by 7.3 h with FloSeal $P<.006$
Hospital stay	Decreased by 7.6 h with FloSeal $P = .002$

No significant difference in hematoma.
Data from Testini M, Marzaioli R, Lissidini G, et al. The effectiveness of FloSeal matrix hemostatic agent in thyroid surgery: prospective, randomized, control study. Langenbecks Arch Surg 2009;394: 837–42.

Harmonic Scalpel Plus FloSeal

- 165 subjects[19]
  - 100 Harmonic Scalpel plus FloSeal
  - 65 standard ligature and cauterization
- Primary endpoint was 24-hour drain output
  - Significantly lower in the harmonic plus FloSeal group 48.1 mL versus 97.9 mL in the standard ligation and cauterization group $P<.00001$
- Confounded by no comparison of Harmonic Scalpel versus FloSeal
- **Table 7** shows results of study

Another study compared the Harmonic Scalpel with the addition of FloSeal to conventional techniques. It evaluated 165 subjects with a primary endpoint of 24 hour drain output. The group treated with the Harmonic Scalpel and FloSeal showed significantly lower volumes of drain output in the first 24 hours compared with the conventionally treated group 48.1 mL versus 97.9 mL (P<.00001).[19] Unfortunately, no comparison was made to subjects treated only with the Harmonic Scalpel, thus making it difficult to interpret whether the decreased drain output was from the use of the instrument or the hemostatic product (see **Table 7**).

POSTSURGICAL DRAINS

Almost all studies assessing the impact of different approaches to hemostasis during thyroid surgery have measured postoperative blood loss with the use of a drain. The question remains, however, "Are drains even necessary in thyroidectomy to prevent life-threatening hematomas?" Two meta-analyses have been completed to attempt to address that question (**Fig. 11**).

Cochrane Review Database

- Thirteen eligible studies with 1646 subjects[20]
- Drain versus no-drain in 11 studies with 1436 subjects
  - Showed no difference in reoperation rates, risk of respiratory distress or wound infections
  - Significantly decreased seroma in drain subjects P = .04 but this disappeared with the high-quality studies
  - Significantly shorter hospital stay without a drain by 1.18 days P<.003
  - Significantly increased postoperative pain with a drain in 2 studies
  - **Table 8** presents results of the study

Table 7
Results from trial comparing the Harmonic Scalpel plus FloSeal with conventional hemostasis techniques

	FloSeal vs Conventional Hemostasis
24 h drain output	Decreased by 49.2 mL with Harmonic Scalpel plus FloSeal P<.00001

No significant difference in hematoma.
Data from Docimo G, Salvatore T, Ruggiero R, et al. Total thyroidectomy with Harmonic Scalpel combined to gelatin-thrombin matrix hemostatic agent: is it safe and effective? A single-center prospective study. Int J Surg 2014;12:S209–12.

In 2007, a Cochran Review was performed by Samraj and Gurusamy[20] evaluating 1646 subjects in 13 eligible studies. When comparing drain versus no drain after a total thyroidectomy, subjects showed no significant difference in reoperation rates, risk of respiratory distress, or wound infections. Subjects without drains did have significantly higher rates of seroma (P = .04). However, when only high-quality studies were evaluated, this difference was no longer noted. Subjects with drains had significantly longer hospital stays by 1.18 days (P<.003) and increased postoperative pain. Overall, drains did not seemed to improve surgical outcomes. Even with a higher rate of seroma formation in the no-drain group, this did not lead to increased morbidity such as wound infection (see **Table 8**).

Meta-Analysis

- Total of 2939 subjects in 25 RCTs[21]
  - 1493 in the drain group
  - 1446 in the no-drain group
- Pain was assessed in 938 subjects and 6 studies on POD 1
  - Lower pain scores with no drain with mean difference of 1.46 $P<.001$
- Hospital stay assessed in 2192 subjects and 18 studies
  - Longer hospitalization in subjects with a drain with mean difference of 1.26 days $P<.001$
- No difference in wound infection rate, hematoma, reoperation rate, or seroma as assessed by POD1 ultrasound
- **Table 9** summarizes results from study

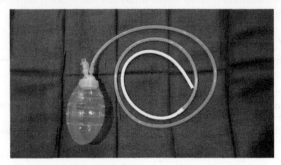

Fig. 11. Drain. "To Drain or Not To Drain?"

Table 8
Results from Cochran Review comparing drain versus no drain after thyroid surgery

Drain vs No-drain Cochran Review	
Hospital stay	Decreased by 1.18 d without a drain $P<.003$
Pain	Significantly lower in no-drain group

No significant difference in (1) Seroma formation (when looking only at high quality studies), (2) Reoperation rates, (3) Respiratory distress, (4) Wound infection.
Data from Samraj K, Gurusamy KS. Wound drains following thyroid surgery. Cochrane Database Syst Rev 2007;4:CD006099.

In 2014, a second meta-analysis was completed which included 25 RCTs. These studies assessed 2939 subjects evenly distributed between drain versus no-drain groups. Postoperative pain was assessed in 6 studies (938 subjects) showing significantly lower pain scores by 1.46 on a 10 point scale ($P<.001$). Hospital stay was evaluated in 18 studies (2192 subjects) with significantly longer hospital stay by 1.26 days in the postoperative drain group ($P<.001$). Wound infection rates were actually increased in the drain group when 17 studies were evaluated (2035 subjects) with a relative risk increase of 2.53 ($P = .01$); however, this fell out after sensitivity analysis was performed. Finally no difference in hematoma, reoperation rate, or seroma as assessed by POD 1 ultrasound was observed.[21] Once again, no obvious benefit to drain usage could be identified (see **Table 9**).

WHAT ARE THE COST SAVINGS?

- OR dollars per minute
  - $43 per minute of OR time times 22.67 minutes equals $974.81
- Cost of the instrument
  - LigaSure: $393.60
  - Harmonic: $550.87

If operative time is significantly decreased with the use of the Harmonic Scalpel or Liga-Sure device, then what is the cost breakdown to using these new technologies? For hospital costs alone, if an average of 22.67 minutes is saved for each case, it is a net cost savings to use the Harmonic Scalpel or the LigaSure rather than CH methods.

Table 9 Results from meta-analysis comparing drain with no drain after thyroid surgery	
Drain vs No-Drain Meta-analysis	
Hospital stay	Decreased by 1.26 d without a drain $P<.003$
Pain	Decreased by 1.46 points without a drain $P<.001$

No significant difference in (1) Seroma formation (assessed by U/S POD 1), (2) Reoperation rates, (3) Hematoma, (4) Wound infection.
   Data from Woods RS, Woods JF, Duignan ES, et al. Systematic review and meta-analysis of wound drains after thyroid surgery. Br J Surg 2014;101(5):446–56.

SUMMARY

- Hemostasis in thyroid surgery, although preserving vital structures, continues to be the most Important goal.
- The Harmonic Scalpel and LigaSure systems have been shown to significantly decrease operative times without increasing costs or complications.
- Adjunctive hemostatic agents have shown equivalent differences when added to standard methods from a clinically significant perspective. Surgicel has actually shown increases in drain output making its use less desirable.
- Postoperative drain use plays no role in thyroid surgery because it increases hospital stay and pain without improving patient outcomes.

Post-Test Questions (Correct answers are in italics)

1. Which of the following developments most significantly improved hemostasis and morbidity rates in thyroid surgery?
   a. The use of oxidized cellulose mesh
   b. The use of monopolar and bipolar electrocautery
   c. *Meticulous capsular dissection and ligation of vessels*
   d. Postoperative drain
2. With respect to the inferior thyroid artery, which of the following is incorrect?
   a. It courses posterior to the common carotid artery
   b. *It is reliably always anterior to the RLN*
   c. If generally gives blood supply to inferior and superior parathyroid glands
   d. It is a branch off of the thyrocervical trunk

3. Which of the following statements regarding vessel control techniques is correct?
   a. The traditional clamp, tie, and cut method is superior to newer devices
   b. The Harmonic Scalpel is significantly faster and more effective than the Liga-Sure system during surgery
   c. The Harmonic Scalpel system causes more heat dispersion than other devices.
   d. *The Harmonic Scalpel and LigaSure systems significantly decrease operative times compared with traditional methods*
4. Adjuncts such as Surgicel to prevent postoperative oozing when used in thyroid surgery
   a. Lead to significantly fewer hematomas
   b. *Lead to significantly more drain output*
   c. Lead to significantly more neck infections
   d. Lead to more voice related complaints
5. Use of a drain postoperatively has been shown to
   a. Decrease postoperative pain due to decreased fluid accumulation
   b. Decrease the risk of wound infection
   c. *Increase hospital stay*
   d. Improve the reoperation rate

SUPPLEMENTARY DATA

Supplementary PDF slides related to this article can be found online at http://www.oto.theclinics.com/.

REFERENCES

1. Hannan SA. The magnificent seven: a history of modern thyroid surgery. Int J Surg 2006;4:187–91.
2. Diffenbach JF. Die operative chirurgie II. Leipzig (Germany): FA Brockhaus; 1848. p. 331.
3. McGreevy PS, Miller FA. Biography of Theodor Kocher. Surgery 1969;65:990.
4. Cernea CR, Ferraz AR, Nishio S, et al. Surgical anatomy of the external branch of the superior laryngeal nerve. Head Neck 1992;14(5):380–3.
5. Tang W, Sun S, Wang X, et al. An applied anatomical study on the recurrent laryngeal nerve and inferior thyroid artery. Surg Radiol Anat 2012;34:325–32.
6. Bhargav PRK. Salient anatomical landmarks of thyroid and their practical significance in thyroid surgery: a pictorial review of thyroid surgical anatomy (revisited). Indian J Surg 2014;76(3):207–11.
7. Shaha AR, Jaffe BM. Practical management of post-thyroidectomy hematoma. J Surg Oncol 1994;57:235–8.
8. Terris DJ. Novel surgical maneuvers in modern thyroid surgery. Op Techn Otolaryngol Head Neck Surg 2009;20:23–8.
9. Terris DJ, Snyder S, Carneiro-Pla D, et al. American Thyroid Association statement on outpatient thyroidectomy. Thyroid 2013;23(10):1193–202.

10. Bandi G, Wen CC, Wilkinson EA, et al. Comparison of blade temperature dynamics after activation between the Harmonic Ace Scalpel and the Ultracision Harmonic Scalpel LCS-K5. J Endourol 2008;22:333–6.
11. Pons Y, Gauthier J, Ukkola-Pons E, et al. Comparison of LigaSure vessel sealing system, Harmonic Scalpel, and conventional hemostasis in total thyroidectomy. Otolaryngol Head Neck Surg 2009;141:496–501.
12. Ecker T, Carvalho AL, Choe JH, et al. Hemostasis in thyroid surgery: Harmonic Scalpel versus other techniques–a meta-analysis. Otolaryngol Head Neck Surg 2010;143(1):17–25.
13. Yao HS, Wang Q, Wang WJ, et al. Prospective clinical trials of thyroidectomy with LigaSure vs conventional vessel ligation: a systematic review and meta-analysis. Arch Surg 2009;144(12):1167–74.
14. Ruggiero R, Gubitosi A, Conzo G, et al. Sutureless thyroidectomy. Int J Surg 2014;12:S189–93.
15. Kwak HY, Chae BJ, Park YG, et al. Comparison of surgical outcomes between papillary thyroid cancer patients treated with the harmonic ACE scalpel and LigaSure precise instrument during conventional thyroidectomy: a single-blind prospective randomized controlled trial. J Surg Res 2014;187(2):484–9.
16. Guler M, Maralcan G, Kul S, et al. The efficacy of Ankaferd Blood Stopper for the management of bleeding following total thyroidectomy. J Invest Surg 2011;24(5):205–10.
17. Amit M, Binenbaum Y, Cohen JT, et al. Effectiveness of an oxidized cellulose patch hemostatic agent in thyroid surgery: a prospective, randomized, controlled study. J Am Coll Surg 2013;217(2):221–5.
18. Testini M, Marzaioli R, Lissidini G, et al. The effectiveness of FloSeal matrix hemostatic agent in thyroid surgery: prospective, randomized, control study. Langenbecks Arch Surg 2009;394:837–42.
19. Docimo G, Salvatore T, Ruggiero R, et al. Total thyroidectomy with Harmonic Scalpel combined to gelatin-thrombin matrix hemostatic agent: Is it safe and effective? A single-center prospective study. Int J Surg 2014;12:S209–12.
20. Samraj K, Gurusamy KS. Wound drains following thyroid surgery. Cochrane Database Syst Rev 2007;(4):CD006099.
21. Woods RS, Woods JF, Duignan ES, et al. Systematic review and meta-analysis of wound drains after thyroid surgery. Br J Surg 2014 Apr;101(5):446–56.

SUGGESTED READINGS

Hannan SA. The magnificent seven: a history of modern thyroid surgery. Int J Surg 2006;4:187–91.

Excellent review of thyroid surgery and its complications including the pioneers that revolutionized the field.

Ecker T, Carvalho AL, Choe JH, et al. Hemostasis in thyroid surgery: Harmonic Scalpel versus other techniques–a meta-analysis. Otolaryngol Head Neck Surg 2010;143(1):17–25.

This is the largest meta-analysis comparing the Harmonic Scalpel to CH techniques. It clearly shows the operative time benefit compared with conventional camp, tie and cut methods but also shows its safety with no increase in complication rates.

Ruggiero R, Gubitosi A, Conzo G, et al. Sutureless thyroidectomy. Int J Surg 2014;12: S189–93.

This is a good study showing no statistical difference between the Harmonic Scalpel and LigaSure system when used for thyroid surgery.

Woods RS, Woods JF, Duignan ES, et al. Systematic review and meta-analysis of wound drains after thyroid surgery. Br J Surg 2014;101(5):446–56.
This meta-analysis was a revision of the previous Cochran review in 2007 with updated information. They showed significantly increased hospital stay and postoperative pain in subjects treated with postoperative drains without any clear benefit in preventing postoperative hematoma and seroma formation.

Hemostasis in Otologic and Neurotologic Surgery

Asmi Sanghvi, DO[a], Brad Bauer, BS[b], Pamela C. Roehm, MD, PhD[b],*

KEYWORDS

- Hemostasis • Bleeding • Middle ear • Mastoid • Lateral skull base

KEY LEARNING POINTS

At the end of this article, the reader will:

- Understand the factors that make a hemostatic agent more ideal for use in different situations.
- Appreciate the patient factors that limit use of topical agents.
- Review the blood supply for paragangliomas of the middle ear and jugular foramen.

INTRODUCTION

> **Why is bleeding during otologic and neurotologic surgery a problem?**
>
> - The combination of a small surgical field and very small critical structures increases the risk of injury due to poor visualization.
>
> - Incomplete surgery due to poor visualization can easily occur.
>
> - Postoperative bleeding can negatively impact
>   - Tympanic membrane graft take
>   - Positioning of middle ear prosthesis
>   - Brain function/brainstem position in the case of neurotologic procedures and may lead to emergent surgery to control bleeding
>
> - Wound hematomas can lead to
>   - Postoperative discomfort
>   - Short term inability to wear glasses
>   - Wound Infection
>   - Device removal may ultimately follow wound infection in the case of cochlear implants.
>   - Wound infection can lead to meningitis in neurotologic procedures.

Disclosure Statement: The authors have nothing to disclose.
[a] Department of Medicine, Crozer-Keystone Health System, Drexel Hill, PA 19026, USA;
[b] Department of Otolaryngology, Head and Neck Surgery, Temple University School of Medicine, 3509 North Broad Street, Philadelphia, PA 19140, USA
* Corresponding author.
E-mail address: pamela.roehm@tuhs.temple.edu

Otolaryngol Clin N Am 49 (2016) 749–761
http://dx.doi.org/10.1016/j.otc.2016.03.010
0030-6665/16/$ – see front matter © 2016 Elsevier Inc. All rights reserved.

oto.theclinics.com

SURGICAL STRATEGIES

> **What are the strategies for control of bleeding during otologic and neurotologic surgery?**
>
> - Initial injection of vasoconstrictive medications along incision line
> - Cautery (monopolar and bipolar)
> - High-speed otologic drill with diamond burr
> - Topical use of vasoconstrictive medications
> - Topical hemostatic agents
> - Angiography and embolization
> - Angiography and stenting (internal carotid)
> - Arterial ligations of branches of the external carotid artery

For most otologic surgeries, the most critical component of hemostasis is the initial injection of diluted epinephrine into the ear canal and any planned postauricular or pinna incision sites. Subsequent control of bleeding for these procedures often involves cautery. Use of the otologic drill with an appropriately sized diamond burr and irrigation is an effective means of controlling bleeding from the mastoid bone (**Fig. 1**). Topical agents should be used when cautery or drilling with a diamond burr would otherwise not be indicated, for example, when the bleeding process is adjacent to or on nerves or other delicate structures that would be damaged by heat transfer. Topical agents are also useful for control of bleeding in areas that are too small for introduction of the cautery.

Topical agents should be used cautiously in the sigmoid sinus and jugular bulb because of the potential for thrombosis. Careful use is also recommended in areas where excessive compression on nerves or other critical structures could occur. For otologic or neurotologic procedures involving vascular tumors, such as paragangliomas, preoperative angiography and embolization should be considered if possible. Emergent control of bleeding due to trauma or large tumors of the skull base may require embolization, stenting, or arterial ligation.

> **What are the goals of treatment?**
>
> - Removal of disease
> - Repair of hearing
> - Minimization of morbidity

 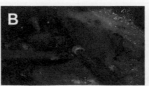 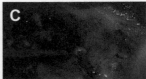

Fig. 1. Use of high-speed drill for hemostasis. (*A*) Bleeding from bony surfaces is common in surgery for chronic otitis media. (*B, C*) Use of a high-speed otologic drill with a diamond bur without irrigation can effectively control bleeding in this context.

Removal of chronic infection or tumor is often the goal in otologic surgery for those conditions. However, a significant portion of otologic surgery is directed at improvement of hearing, particularly in the setting of otosclerosis or severe-profound sensorineural hearing loss. Control of bleeding particularly in these procedures is critical because morbidity resulting from damage to surrounding structures is unacceptable in elective hearing improvement surgery.

OPTIONS FOR HEMOSTASIS

What factors should be considered when evaluating hemostatic agents?

- Source of bleeding
- Amount of bleeding
- Speed of hemostasis
- Risk of injury
- Impact on inflammation and healing
- Risk of infection
- Risk of systemic complications
- Origin
- Cost

The most critical factors to consider include the source and amount of bleeding. The use of certain agents can be inappropriate in some contexts and can cause severe morbidity. Another critical factor is the speed of hemostasis. Other factors to consider include impact on inflammation and healing, risk of infection, and risk of systemic complications in light of the patient comorbidities. Also important to consider are origin (plant, animal, human), cost, and available forms (sponge, fabric, powder, paste, and liquid).

INJECTION OF VASOCONSTRICTING MEDICATIONS

Given the small size of the surgical field, a small amount bleeding from incision lines can obscure the field within seconds. Injectable vasoconstricting agents are used initially during otologic procedures to ensure adequate hemostasis from incision lines, particularly in the external auditory canal (**Fig. 2**). Systemic complications are dose dependent.

Vasoconstrictors

- Types: diluted epinephrine; lidocaine + epinephrine
- Mechanism: vasoconstriction of blood vessels
- Advantages: inexpensive, can provide hemostasis throughout surgery if appropriately applied, lidocaine + epinephrine can also provide analgesia in addition to hemostasis
- Complications
  - Lidocaine
    - Systemic neurologic excitation followed by depression, convulsions, respiratory depression and arrest, bradycardia, hypotension, and cardiovascular collapse
    - Temporary facial nerve paralysis if facial nerve is dehiscent in the middle ear (if applied in the external auditory canal or middle ear)
  - Epinephrine
    - Systemic effects: hypertension and tachycardia
    - Local effects: tissue ischemia

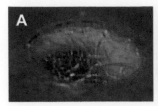
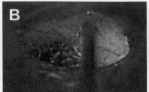
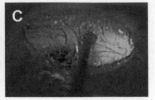

Fig. 2. Injection of diluted epinephrine into the external auditory canal. This critical step can influence hemostasis throughout the remainder of surgery on the middle ear. (*A*) Initial view of the left external auditory canal through the operating microscope. The speculum is positioned to allow visualization of the bony-cartilaginous junction. (*B*) The needle is advanced through the hair-bearing skin of the region, and the tip is positioned on the bone of the external auditory canal. A small amount (<1 mL for the entire canal) of diluted epinephrine (1:100,000 solution in sterile saline) is injected slowly to avoid formation of blebs. Proper positioning of the needle tip on bone is confirmed by the presence of frost along the needle. (*C*) With adequate injection, blanching of both the external auditory canal and tympanic membrane are observed (tympanic membrane not shown in this view).

CAUTERY

Both monopolar and bipolar cautery are useful in controlling bleeding from small blood vessels of the scalp, pinna, and from scalp incision lines (**Fig. 3**).[1]

- Forms: bipolar and monopolar
  - Bipolar cautery current passes through the tissues between the 2 electrodes of the instrument. Monopolar cautery current passes through patients to a grounding pad.
- Mechanism: (coagulation setting) Interrupted high-voltage current is dispersed over the surface, allowing superficial heating of tissue that causes protein denaturation and dehydration.
- Advantages: low cost, wide availability
- Complications
  - Generation of areas of carbonization and necrotic tissue
    - Increased likelihood of infection
    - Delayed wound healing
  - Generation of potentially toxic or infectious smoke that could potentially harm patients, surgeon, or operating staff

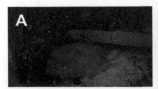
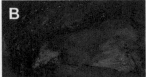
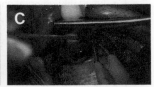

Fig. 3. Monopolar and bipolar cautery. (*A*) Use of monopolar cautery to control bleeding from the medial edge of the postauricular skin flap. (*B*) Use of monopolar cautery to control bleeding from vessels within the mastoid bone and from the attachments of the lateral portion of the sternocleidomastoid muscle to the mastoid tip. (*C*) Use of bipolar cautery to control bleeding from the temporalis muscle and soft tissues superior to the external auditory canal. Bipolar cautery should be used in areas in which current spread from monopolar cautery will harm soft tissues, including the anterior external auditory canal skin flap and in areas neighboring nerves.

TOPICAL VASOCONSTRICTING AGENTS

Both epinephrine and cocaine are vasoconstricting agents that can be used topically to control bleeding in the middle ear and mastoid. Cocaine is exclusively used topically, whereas epinephrine can be used both topically and as an injected agent, as noted earlier.

- Forms: 4% and 10% solutions of cocaine hydrochloride
- Mechanism: local vasoconstriction through the inhibition of noradrenaline reuptake
- Advantage
  - Low cost
  - Topical analgesia
- Disadvantages
  - Risk of misuse by medical providers and staff
  - Heavy bureaucratic regulation
  - Need for cardiac monitor and pulse oximetry
- Complications
  - Dizziness
  - Nausea
  - Restlessness
  - Hypersensitivity reactions
  - Severe side effects like seizures, cardiac arrhythmias, and death have been reported

BONE WAX

Bone wax is a topical agent that is useful for controlling bleeding from bone surfaces. Because of the potential for embolization, it should not be directly applied to larger vessels, such as the sigmoid sinus or jugular bulb.[1]

- Origin: beeswax based, contains white beeswax (88%) + isopropyl palmitate (12%) with or without paraffin wax
- Form: stick
- Mechanism: physically plugs channels containing emissary veins
- Advantages
  - Low cost
  - Inert
  - Immediacy of action
  - Ease of preparation
- Complications
  - Foreign body granulomatous reactions
  - Wound infection

ABSORBABLE GELATIN (GELATIN MATRIX)

One of the more useful agents for middle ear surgery, absorbable gelatin, can not only be used as a hemostatic agent on its own but can also be used to apply epinephrine topically to a confined surface and can serve as a supportive scaffold for tympanic membrane and ossicular reconstruction (**Fig. 4**).[1,2]

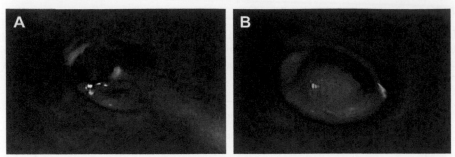

Fig. 4. Absorbable gelatin sponge with epinephrine. Although initial injection of diluted epinephrine caused blanching, often other hemostatic agents are necessary in revision tympanoplasty, particularly in the setting of chronic or acute on chronic infection. Within the external auditory canal, absorbable gelatin sponge soaked with epinephrine (1:10,000 in sterile saline) can efficiently affect hemostasis. (*A*) Initial tympanomeatal incision leads to bleeding, despite adequate external auditory canal injection. (*B*) Placement of absorbable gelatin sponge soaked with diluted epinephrine quickly leads to control of bleeding.

- Origin: porcine-derived hydrocolloids
- Forms: sponge or powder
- Absorption time: 4 to 6 weeks
- Mechanism: forms a matrix for platelet adherence and aggregation, which provides the foundation for clotting
- Advantages
  - Nonadherent to gloves, instruments, or gauze
  - Rapid hemostatic action
  - Can also serve as a scaffold for tympanic membrane reconstruction or ossiculoplasty
- Complications
  - Infection
  - Abscess
  - Granuloma formation
  - Fibrosis
  - Clot disruption if removed

INTENTIONAL HYPOTENSION

Initially used in the middle of the last century for control of bleeding during otologic surgery, intentional hypotension fell out of favor after reports of mortality following use of this modality. However, notable increases in bleeding during otologic and neurotologic procedures occur with elevated blood pressure; so lowering elevated pressure can help control excessive bleeding, as can elevating the head. Recently, the use of otoendoscopy for visualization of entire otologic procedures has increased interest in this modality for hemostasis.[3]

- Mechanism: It lowers blood pressure through the combined use of multiple anesthetic agents.
- Mechanism: Decreased systemic vascular resistance leads to decreased blood pressure.
- Advantages: It does not require use of agents that would block a small surgical field.
- Disadvantages
  - It may not be possible in all patients.
  - Extreme hypotension is associated with morbidity and mortality.
  - Tolerance of hypotension varies greatly between individual patients.

THROMBIN/GELATIN PREPARATIONS

These agents are often useful for control of bleeding during neurotologic procedures when working around delicate neural structures and the brainstem. They can also be useful in controlling bleeding from the jugular bulb and sigmoid sinus during otologic or neurotologic surgery.[1]

- Origin: bovine or porcine derived
- Forms: liquid/colloid
- Mechanism
  - Provides a matrix for platelet adhesion and accelerates formation of platelet plugs that ultimately become a mature clot
  - Also decreases the pH to allow localized vasoconstriction
  - Absorption time: 6 to 8 weeks
- Advantages
  - Readily available in most centers performing neurosurgical procedures
  - Does not adhere to surgical instruments, gloves, or sponges
- Complications
  - Formation of granulation tissue and adhesions
  - Prolongation of prothrombin time and inhibition of coagulation due to antithrombin antibody development by patients

TOPICALLY APPLIED HYDROGEN PEROXIDE

Utility of this method is limited to neurotologic cases for control of bleeding near the brainstem and cerebellum because of its debated ototoxicity.[2] Although this method is not effective at controlling large amounts of bleeding from injury to larger vessels, it can be used to control bloody ooze from multiple areas as well as to clear blood and clot to identify the site of rapid active bleeding. Hydrogen peroxide should be cautiously used in the middle ear or in the setting of a perforation, as it has been associated with hearing loss in laboratory animals.[4]

- Origin: inorganic chemical
- Form: liquid, diluted to 35%
- Mechanism
  - Liberates reactive oxygen species allowing control of minor bleeding during procedures
  - Absorption time: immediate
- Advantages: low cost, allows visualization of source of bleeding
- Complications
  - Formation of venous emboli
  - Postoperative pneumocephalus
  - Cardiac arrhythmias

MICROFIBRILLAR COLLAGEN

Mainly used during neurotologic procedures to control bleeding from oozing surfaces of the brainstem and cerebellum, these agents can effectively control bleeding without causing a large mass effect on critical structures.[1]

- Origin: bovine dermis derived
- Forms: sheets or powder
- Mechanism
  - Acts as a framework for platelet aggregation
  - Activates the intrinsic coagulation pathway through factor XII
  - Absorption time: 14 to 84 days
- Advantages
  - Rapid onset of hemostasis
- Complications
  - Granuloma formation
  - Allergic/hypersensitivity reactions
  - Adhesions
  - Foreign body reactions

OXIDIZED REGENERATED CELLULOSE

Similar to microfibrillar collagen, these agents are typically used during neurotologic procedures to control bleeding from oozing surfaces of the brainstem and cerebellum and can effectively control bleeding without causing a large mass effect on critical structures.[1]

- Origin: plant derived (cotton)
- Form: mesh
- Mechanism
  - Provides a physical meshwork for clot formation
  - Activates intrinsic and extrinsic clotting pathways
  - Lowers pH, leading to small vessel vasoconstriction
- Advantages
  - Bacteriostatic action against gram-positive and gram-negative bacteria
  - Relatively rapid reabsorption (14 days)
- Complications
  - Foreign body reaction
  - Infection
  - Adhesions

FIBRIN SEALANTS

These agents have limited utility for control of bleeding at the end of neurotologic procedures, when they are often applied to materials used for repair of the dura or bony defects of the skull base.[1]

- Origin: human based

- Form: liquid

- Mechanism: concentrated fibrinogen and factor XIII combined and form a clot along with the patients' platelets.

- Advantages
  o Immediate action
  o Useful in fully anticoagulated and heparinized patients
  o Do not require application of pressure or vasoconstriction for action

- Disadvantages
  o Cost
  o Potential exposure to blood-borne viruses

OTOLOGIC AND NEUROTOLOGIC VASCULAR EMERGENCIES

- Emergencies requiring immediate hemostasis can arise from many causes, including the following:
  o Blunt and penetrating trauma
  o Iatrogenic damage from surgery, radiation therapy, endovascular procedures
  o Tumors
  o Pseudoaneurysms

- Frequently implicated vessels include the following:
  o Petrous carotid artery
  o Jugular bulb
  o Ascending pharyngeal artery and other vessels supplying large glomus jugulare tumors (particularly when they have grown outside of the pinna)

- Methods of hemostasis include the following:
  o Endovascular stenting of embolization
  o Surgical ligation

The petrous segment of the internal carotid artery runs deep to the floor of middle ear and may send branches to supply to tympanic cavity. Occasionally, this vessel can be dehiscent within the middle ear cavity and subject to potential trauma during middle ear procedures.[5] The jugular bulb or even the sigmoid sinus may also be dehiscent within the middle ear space.[5,6] All of the aforementioned methods of hemostasis may be appropriate on occasion to control bleeding in these emergent situations, in addition to the methods listed earlier.[7,8]

INTERVENTIONAL ENDOVASCULAR TECHNIQUES

- Stenting
  o Requires subsequent anticoagulation

- Embolization
  o Detachable coils (platinum, stainless steel)
  o Liquid (cyanoacrylates)
  o Particle (polyvinyl alcohol)

- Risks
  o Minor complications: fever, localized pain, and puncture site hematomas
  o Failure to occlude targeted vessels
  o Tissue necrosis
  o Stroke or death from particle or coagulant migration into the internal carotid artery or vertebral artery
  o Facial nerve and lower cranial nerve paralysis if their blood supply is inadvertently embolized

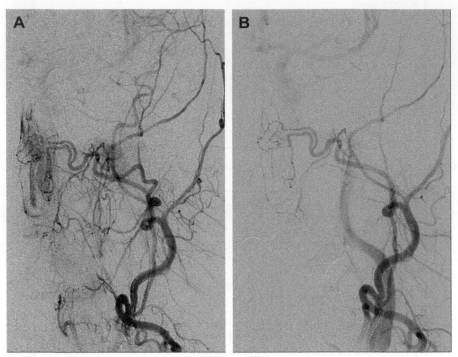

Fig. 5. Embolization of glomus jugulare. Before resection, embolization of the vasculature originating from the external carotid should be considered, as this can drastically decrease blood loss and operating time. (*A*) Pre-embolization angiogram of large glomus jugulare. (*B*) Postembolization view of the same tumor.

There are 2 major options for stopping a bleeding vessel via the endovascular approach: reconstructive (stenting) and deconstructive (embolization) (**Fig. 5**). Reconstructive approaches aim to maintain the patency of the damaged vessel and restore its function. Deconstructive hemostasis closes the vessel to stop the bleeding. To perform these procedures, catheters are often introduced through the femoral artery; but other entry points can be used.[7,9]

LIGATION OF BLEEDING VASCULATURE

Surgical ligation of the bleeding vessel can be used when necessary to control bleeding within the temporal bone and lateral skull base. In an emergent setting this may involve ligation of the external carotid within the neck, rather than the subsequent arborization of this vessel.

- Risks
  - Recurrent hemorrhage may occur because of collateralization
  - Delayed tissue ischemia

- Advantages
  - Rapid control of bleeding is possible
  - Often more widely and readily available than endovascular approaches

GLOMUS TYMPANICUM AND GLOMUS JUGULARE TUMORS

Although many of the pathologies treated during otologic and neurotologic procedures are associated with bleeding, none are associated with as much blood loss as paragangliomas of these surgical areas. Adequate exposure, readily accessible hemostatic agents, and type-and-crossed blood products are critical components of surgery on these tumors. Angioembolization should be considered for larger paragangliomas, whether they are clearly jugulare or tympanicum in origin. These tumors should not be biopsied because of their propensity for bleeding.[9,10]

- Blood supply
  - Glomus tympanicum
    - Inferior tympanic artery (a branch of the ascending pharyngeal artery)
  - Glomus jugulare
    - Ascending pharyngeal artery (branch of the external carotid artery)
    - Middle meningeal artery
    - Branches from the petrous internal carotid artery
    - Branches from the vertebral artery
- Effective hemostatic agents
  - Tympanicum
    - Carbon dioxide or argon laser
    - Bipolar cautery
    - Fibrillar
    - High-speed drill with diamond bur (for light use on the cochlear promontory or hypotympanum only)
  - Jugulare
    - Bipolar cautery
    - Angioembolization
    - Oxidized regenerated cellulose
    - Gelatin matrix
    - Microfibrillar collagen

Caution: Vasoconstrictive medications are ineffective for control of bleeding from these tumors, and absorbable gelatin compressed sponge has limited effects on hemostatic control.

SUMMARY

Control of bleeding during otologic and neurotologic surgery is critical for surgical success because of the small size of the surgical field. Before incision, agents used to decrease bleeding should be applied and allowed adequate time for function, particularly in otologic procedures. For otologic or neurotologic surgeries involving paragangliomas or other pathologies with high propensity for bleeding, preoperative angioembolization may be indicated. Agents appropriate for the planned surgery and pathology should be readily available throughout the procedure. For emergent control of bleeding within the external auditory canal, middle ear, temporal bone, and lateral skull base, angioembolization, angiography with stenting, or suture ligation of potential feeding vessels from the external carotid artery may be required.

Post-Test Questions (Correct answers are in italics)

1. Which of the following is *not* porcine derived?
   A. Absorable gelatin hydrostatic matrix
   B. Absorbable gelatin hydrostatic powder
   C. *Fibrin sealant*
   D. None of the above
2. Which vessels can provide the blood supply for glomus jugulare tumors?
   A. Ascending pharyngeal artery
   B. Middle meningeal artery
   C. Feeders from the internal carotid artery
   D. *All of the above*
3. What is the primary blood supply for a glomus tympanicum tumor?
   A. *Ascending pharyngeal artery*
   B. Middle meningeal artery
   C. Feeders from the internal carotid artery
   D. Branches from the vertebral artery
4. What is a possible complication of embolization of the blood supply to a glomus jugulare tumor?
   A. Hydrocephalus
   B. Contralateral hearing loss
   C. Cerebrospinal fluid leak
   D. *Facial nerve paralysis*

REFERENCES

1. Yao HH, Hong MK, Drummond KJ. Haemostasis in neurosurgery: what is the evidence for gelatin-thrombin matrix sealant? J Clin Neurosci 2013;20(3):349–56.
2. Shen Y, Teh BM, Friedland PL, et al. To pack or not to pack? A contemporary review of middle ear packing agents. Laryngoscope 2011;121(5):1040–8.
3. Smith C. Haemostasis in ear surgery. Proc R Soc Med 1971;64(12):1225–6.
4. Perez R, Freeman S, Cohen D, et al. The effect of hydrogen peroxide applied to the middle ear on inner ear function. Laryngoscope 2003;113(11):2042–6.
5. Brodish BN, Woolley AL. Major vascular injuries in children undergoing myringotomy for tube placement. Am J Otolaryngol 1999;20(1):46–50.
6. Ulug T, Basaran B, Minareci O, et al. An unusual complication of stapes surgery: profuse bleeding from the anteriorly located sigmoid sinus. Eur Arch Otorhinolaryngol 2004;261(7):397–9.
7. Spetzler RF, Desai SC, Deshmukh VR, et al. Vascular consideration in neurotologic surgery. In: Brackmann DE, Shelton C, Arriaga MA, editors. Otologic surgery. 3rd edition. Philadelphia: Saunders; 2011.
8. Misaki K, Muramatsu N, Nitta H. Endovascular treatment for traumatic ear bleeding associated with acute epidural hematoma. Neurol Med Chir (Tokyo) 2008;48(5):208–10.
9. Valavanis A. Preoperative embolization of the head and neck: indications, patient selection, goals, and precautions. AJNR Am J Neuroradiol 1986;7(5):943–52.
10. Arriaga MA, Brackmann DE. Surgery for glomus tumors and other lesions of the jugular foramen. In: Brackmann DE, Shelton C, Arriaga MA, editors. Otologic surgery. 3rd edition. Philadelphia: Saunders; 2010.

SUGGESTED READINGS

Arriaga MA, Brackmann DE. Surgery for glomus tumors and other lesions of the jugular foramen. In: Brackmann DE, Shelton C, Arriaga MA, editors. Otologic surgery. 3rd edition. Philadelphia: Saunders; 2010.

This classic article reviews surgery for tumors of the jugular foramen, particularly the glomus jugulare, as well as the vascular issues inherent in these procedures.

Brodish BN, Woolley AL. Major vascular injuries in children undergoing myringotomy for tube placement. Am J Otolaryngol 1999;20(1):46–50.

A must-read for any otolaryngology resident, this article reviews vascular complications in a series of children undergoing myringotomy and tube placement.

Yao HH, Hong MK, Drummond KJ. Haemostasis in neurosurgery: what is the evidence for gelatin-thrombin matrix sealant? J Clin Neurosci 2013;20(3):349–56.

This article provides an excellent review of many of the topical hemostatic agents used in neurotologic and otologic surgical procedures and includes a review of the coagulation cascade.

Hemostasis in Orbital Surgery

Solomon S. Shaftel, MD, PhD[a], Shu-Hong Chang, MD[b], Kris S. Moe, MD[c],*

KEYWORDS

- Orbit • Orbital • Hemostasis • Endoscopic • Cantholysis

KEY LEARNING POINTS

At the end of this article, the reader will:

- Be able to identify the major blood vessels supplying the orbit.
- Be able to describe the key anatomic landmarks of the orbit in relation to major blood vessels and critical structures.
- Know the most common causes of significant orbital hemorrhage and how might they be prevented.
- Know effective options exist for providing hemostasis in the orbit.
- Be able to describe orbital compartment syndrome.
- Be able to describe the acute management of a serious orbital hemorrhage.
- Know the goals of and possible outcomes following cantholysis and canthotomy and its management.

INTRODUCTION

Major Vascular Anatomy of the Orbit

- Internal carotid branches into ophthalmic artery just distal to cavernous sinus
  - Travels through optic canal and is contained within dural sheath along with optic nerve
  - Optic strut lies between superior orbital fissure and optic canal
  - Medially bound by sphenoid sinus wall (occasionally ethmoid sinus or Onodi cells)[1]

Funded by NIH, grant number R21 EB016122-01.
[a] Department of Ophthalmology, Southern California Permanente Medical Group, 4405 Vandever Avenue, San Diego, CA 92120, USA; [b] Division of Orbital and Ophthalmic Plastic Surgery, Department of Ophthalmology, University of Washington, 325 9th Avenue, Seattle, WA 98104, USA; [c] Division of Facial Plastic and Reconstructive Surgery, Departments of Otolaryngology and Neurological Surgery, University of Washington School of Medicine, 1959 Northeast Pacific Street, Seattle, WA 98195, USA
* Corresponding author.
E-mail address: krismoe@uw.edu

Otolaryngol Clin N Am 49 (2016) 763–775
http://dx.doi.org/10.1016/j.otc.2016.02.011
0030-6665/16/$ – see front matter © 2016 Elsevier Inc. All rights reserved.

oto.theclinics.com

The ophthalmic artery is an unusual source of orbital hemorrhage unless the optic nerve is transected as is performed in enucleation or orbital exenteration surgery. In these settings, identification of the optic nerve stump can be facilitated through use of malleable (ribbon) retractors, and hemostasis can be achieved with bipolar cautery of the artery.

- Terminal ophthalmic artery branches are major contributors to serious orbital hemorrhage
  - Supratrochlear artery pierces the septum and exits the orbit ~1.7- to 2.2-cm lateral to midline in the vicinity of the trochlea
  - Supraorbital artery exits the orbit usually in a notch versus foramen
  - Posterior ethmoidal artery lies 6 mm anterior to the optic canal adjacent to the frontoethmoidal suture[2]
  - Middle (accessory) ethmoidal artery is present in as many as one-third of orbits[2,3]
  - Anterior ethmoidal artery is 24 mm from the anterior lacrimal crest
    - Common source of acute orbital hemorrhage during sinus surgery[4]
    - Can retract into the orbit on laceration

Laceration of the ethmoidal arteries can lead to serious orbital hemorrhages during orbital or sinus surgery. During a planned orbital approach to the medial orbital wall, it is both safe and helpful to ligate the anterior ethmoidal artery via a subperiosteal approach before further posterior dissection. The location of this vessel is consistently ~24 mm from the anterior lacrimal crest at the frontoethmoidal suture line. Although this vessel is not always present, knowledge that a middle ethmoidal artery may be encountered can prevent further unwanted hemorrhage. The posterior ethmoidal artery lies in close proximity to the optic canal and optic nerve. Therefore, efforts to ligate this vessel may lead to unwanted damage to the optic nerve and should be attempted only with great care. A useful mnemonic to aid recall of these important anatomic relationships is 24 to 12 to 6: the anterior ethmoidal being 24 mm from the anterior lacrimal crest, posterior ethmoidal located 12 mm posterior to this, and the optic canal positioned 6 mm behind. However, the anatomy, number, and location of these vessels relative to bony landmarks are variable, and these measurements should only be considered rough guidelines.

- The external carotid artery provides most of the inferolateral arterial supply to orbit
  - Dense network of collaterals with the internal carotid
- Zygomaticotemporal and zygomaticofacial arteries enter within lateral and inferolateral portions of lateral orbital wall
- Recurrent meningeal pierces deep lateral wall just anterior to superior orbital fissure
- Infraorbital artery branches enter the orbit along the infraorbital canal

---

These vessels are readily encountered while reflecting the periorbita (periosteum inside the orbit) off of the lateral orbital wall and floor. Pre-emptive ligation with bipolar cautery can save time during dissection because shearing these vessels often results in retraction of the visible stump within the bone. If this occurs, monopolar cautery or bone wax can restore hemostasis. However, monopolar cautery should be used with caution near the orbital roof because this can damage the dura and result in a cerebrospinal fluid leak even in the absence of bone disruption.[5]

- Venous outflow is divided into 2 main pathways
  - Superior ophthalmic vein follows a sinusoidal course from the superomedial orbit into the superior orbital fissure
    - Infrequently encountered because of its close proximity to globe and compressible nature
  - Inferior ophthalmic vein courses through inferior orbital fissure
    - Often encountered and may be sacrificed without lasting functional deficits[1]

Ligation of the superior ophthalmic vein can trigger significant ocular congestion, elevated intraocular pressure, and ultimately, compromise of visual function. Compromise of the inferior ophthalmic vein, however, does not result in significant morbidity. This vein is often transected during manipulation of structures passing through the inferior orbital fissure.

Preoperative Assessment

- Predisposing factors to hemorrhage
  - Hypertension
  - Coagulation disorders
    - Consider checking prothrombin time, partial thromboplastin time, international normalized ratio
  - Anticoagulants
    - Optimally, aspirin and aspirin-containing compounds (Plavix and Aggrenox) should be discontinued 10 to 14 days before surgery
    - Nonsteroidal anti-inflammatory drugs and herbal supplements (eg, fish oil, flaxseed oil, vitamin E, ginkgo, garlic) should be discontinued at least 7 days before surgery
    - Warfarin is generally stopped 5 days before with a bridge to low-molecular-weight heparin (eg, Lovenox) administered subcutaneously if indicated
    - Newer anticoagulants, such as dabigatran (Pradaxa), rivaroxaban (Xarelto), and apixaban (Eliquis), are not easily reversible or assayed and are generally stopped several days before surgery
  - Prior episode of hemorrhage

Optimization of preoperative factors can significantly lessen the risk of orbital hemorrhage. Although it is ideal to stop all anticoagulants before orbital surgery, surgery can still be pursued with concomitant use albeit with greater risk. Aspirin and warfarin discontinuation should only be pursued under the direction of the primary care practitioner or cardiologist because the risk of stopping (eg, cardiac and cerebrovascular) may outweigh the perceived benefit of lessening the risk of hemorrhage. Surgical planning for patients on newer anticoagulants, such as dabigatran, rivaroxaban, and apibaxan, presents significant challenges because these agents are neither easily assayed nor reversed. Antidotes are neither US Food and Drug Administration approved nor fully effective at this time. The most important predictor of orbital hemorrhage is a patient history of a prior bleeding abnormality during surgery.

- Vascular congestion of the orbit
  - Thyroid eye disease (thyroid-associated orbitopathy)
    - Active phase manifests with significant orbital hyperemia
    - Delay surgical intervention until convalescent phase if possible
    - Consider preoperative steroid treatment to reduce vascular congestion
  - Neoplasms
    - Feeder vessels may be identified on imaging
  - Autoimmune disease of the orbit
    - Sarcoidosis, granulomatosis with polyangiitis, polyarteritis nodosa
  - Sinus disease
  - Infections
  - Vascular malformations
    - For example, varices, lymphangioma, arteriovenous malformations
    - Flow characteristics best defined with static (MRI, computed tomography [CT]) and dynamic (angiography) imaging
    - Consider consultation with interventional neuroradiology

The degree of orbital hyperemia can often be characterized on imaging performed with contrast. Consultation with interventional neuroradiology can be helpful in the setting of highly vascular orbital lesions to consider interruption of inflow and outflow pathways before excision. Precise intraluminal delivery of thrombogenic agents can improve the safety profile before excision of orbital vascular tumors.[6]

- Informed consent
  - Must outline risk of orbital hemorrhage
  - Reported rates of orbital hemorrhages
    - Blepharoplasty, 0.05%
    - Sinus surgery, 0.12%
    - Orbital/peribulbar/retrobulbar injections, less than 2%[7]

Although a rare occurrence, the risk of orbital hemorrhage should be outlined in the informed consent process for any eyelid, orbital, and sinus surgery because of the potential for devastating consequences. Patients should be instructed to decrease exertional and provocative activities in the 2 weeks after these surgeries because they increase orbital vascular congestion and can predispose to the development of postoperative orbital hemorrhage. These activities include strenuous exercise, sexual activity, bending the head below chest level, squeezing of facial muscles, lifting greater than 10 pounds, and other Valsalva maneuvers.

Overview of Endoscopic Surgery of the Orbit

- Advantages of endoscopic surgery of the orbit
  - Improved illumination and magnification
  - Ability to involve all attendants to surgery
    - Traditional open approaches only provide optimal view to one surgeon at a time
  - Smaller incisions

- Disadvantages
  - Increased equipment utilization
  - Surgeon and assistants must modify techniques to preserve bimanual surgery capability

- Navigation devices
  - Provide precise anatomic localization
  - Allow for mirror imaging and more accurate orbital reconstruction[8]

Endoscopic surgery of the orbit provides optimal magnification and illumination during orbital surgery to all those in attendance and is ideal for education, training, and involvement of the entire operative team in the surgery. Traditional open approaches often only allow the operating surgeon adequate views, albeit at lower magnification. The use of modern navigation technologies as an adjunct to endoscopy can increase the safety profile of surgery through confirmation of anatomic landmarks with radiologic images. The small expense of navigation devices is greatly outweighed by their benefit.

Causes of Orbital Hemorrhage

- Disruption of major vessels
  - Usually readily apparent during surgery
- Contribution of smaller branches supplying:
  - Orbital fat
  - Periosteum
  - Lacrimal gland
  - Extraocular muscles
- By location:
  - Intraconal
  - Extraconal
  - Subperiosteal

Disruption of smaller blood vessels that supply orbital tissues results in slower development of orbital hemorrhages. These bleeds may not present until after surgery but can still have devastating consequences secondary to development of compartment syndrome and resultant tissue ischemia.

Clinical Signs of Orbital Hemorrhage

- Intraoperative alarm signs
  - Proptosis (bulging) of the globe
  - Tense orbital tissues
  - Increased intraocular pressure
  - Pupillary dilation

Periodic assessment for these signs in orbital and sinus surgery can provide useful information and help to rule out the presence of an orbital hemorrhage. Gentle ballottement of the globe using the tips of the index fingers can help to determine if the orbit is tense. For novice orbital surgeons, performing this maneuver at the start of surgery before incision will provide a baseline for intraoperative assessment of orbital and globe pressure. Precise measurement of intraocular pressure is provided by an automated tonometer, such as a Tono-Pen (Reichert Technologies, Buffalo, NY, USA), which are commonly used by ophthalmic surgeons. Intraocular pressures less than 21 mm Hg are considered normal, and transient pressure readings less than

30 mm Hg rarely cause permanent vision loss. The risk of permanent vision loss increases proportionately as the intraocular pressure increases.

Abnormalities in the size and shape of the pupil may be a sign of excessive pressure on the globe or retrobulbar structures, including the ciliary ganglion. Periodic assessment of pupil size and shape can help detect this and in this way serves as an adjunct measure of intraorbital pressure. Local infiltration of epinephrine-containing local anesthetics can lead to papillary dilation and may interfere with this assessment. Dynamic changes in pupil size noted intraoperatively usually respond to removal of surgical instruments from the orbit and a reduction in intraorbital pressure. A fixed, dilated pupil may be a sign of irreversible damage to the optic nerve and or ciliary ganglion.

Intraoperative Techniques for Hemostasis

- Tools to aid identification of bleeding source:
  - Suction (7- or 8-French cannula)
  - Malleable (ribbon) retractors of various sizes
  - Cottonoids (0.25 inch wide of various lengths)
  - Irrigation
  - Patient positioning
  - Hypotensive anesthesia
  - Deep extubation
  - Antiemetic agents

Identification of the source of hemorrhage is often facilitated through the use of malleable retractors and neurosurgical cottonoids, which provide a barrier to orbital fat from entering the surgical field. Allowing saline to pool in the orbit is a useful technique to determine if hemostasis has been achieved and to detect the point source, which may be seen streaming from within the fluid compartment.

Anesthesia providers can reduce the occurrence and rate of hemorrhage through the use of head-up positioning (reverse Trendelenburg) and lowering of the mean arterial pressure. Although these factors may be overlooked in the search for hemorrhage, they can often be extremely helpful. Deep extubation and antiemetic agents can help reduce coughing and vomiting, which can both lead to increased intracranial pressure. Steroids and serotonin antagonists are particularly effective for postoperative nausea.

Hemostatic Techniques

- Cautery
  - Monopolar
  - Bipolar
- Bone wax

Monopolar (Bovie) cautery is broadly effective but results in greater tissue disruption secondary to the generation of thermal damage to the radial field surrounding the tip. Bipolar cautery lessens surrounding tissue disruption but requires greater access for careful administration secondary to the size of the forceps. Bayonet forceps are very useful within the deep orbit.

Bone wax is extremely effective in sealing hemorrhage from bone-perforating vessels. Effort should be made to remove excess material because it may cause unwanted inflammation.[9]

- Pharmacologic vasoconstriction
  - Oxymetazoline
  - Epinephrine
  - Cocaine

Administration of vasoconstrictors via topical and injectable routes helps to reduce vascular congestion and intraoperative bleeding. They can be administered after bleeding is discovered, but will take several minutes before they reach their maximal effect.

- Procoagulants
  - Hydrogen peroxide
  - Thrombin
  - Gelfoam (absorbable gelatin)
  - Surgicel (oxidized cellulose)
  - Floseal (gelatin matrix and thrombin)
  - Avitene (microfibrillar collagen)
  - Tisseel (fibrinogen and thrombin)

Chemical coagulants and matrix coagulators are particularly helpful in the setting of brisk hemorrhage when a point source is unable to be identified. Hydrogen peroxide is useful for diffuse oozing and leads to vasoconstriction and thrombus formation through aggregation of neutrophils and platelets. Thrombin can be introduced via infused cottonoids or on gelfoam-soaked wedges. Floseal is distributed as a highly viscous paste that easily adheres to different surfaces. The authors have had success with a premade mixture of 5000 units thrombin, 8 mL saline, and surgifoam powder as an alternative to Floseal at reduced cost. Surgicel and Avitene can provide a matrix for clot formation but may add unnecessary volume to the orbit. Administration of hemostatic materials into the orbit should be limited to that which is required for hemostasis because residual material may lead to granuloma formation.[10]

Approaches to the Orbit for Rapid Control of Ethmoidal Hemorrhage

---

- Transcaruncular/postcaruncular
- Medial transcutaneous (Lynch)

Transorbital endoscopic techniques can be extremely useful for the treatment of ongoing orbital hemorrhage. If the hemorrhage is due to sinus surgery, a transorbital approach transfers the procedure to a dry field, where the anterior, middle, and posterior ethmoidal arteries can be easily visualized and ligated. The vector of this approach, coplanar with the vessels, is highly favorable and provides excellent freedom of instrument motion. The ligation can be performed with small vascular clips or bipolar cauterization. When the posterior ethmoidal vessels are involved, visualization of the optic nerve is advisable before ligating the vessels, directly or with surgical navigation.

- Imaging
  - Intraoperative CT
  - Postoperative CT

CT performed without contrast can help to localize the site of blood deposition. Hemorrhages are localized to the intraconal, extraconal, or subperiosteal compartments of the orbit. Intraconal hemorrhages are often focal, but drainage is not advised because of the proximity of critical ocular structures, including extraocular muscles and nerves, ciliary body, and the optic nerve. Extraconal hemorrhages are usually more diffuse and difficult to drain. Subperiosteal hemorrhages often collect in a well-defined compartment and are amenable to drainage with an increased safety profile. The term retrobulbar hemorrhage encompasses all the entities described above (**Fig. 1**).

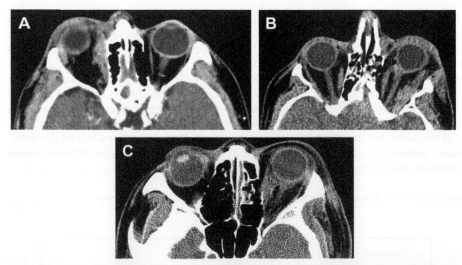

Fig. 1. Axial CT scans demonstrating (*A*) subperiosteal, (*B*) extraconal, and (*C*) intraconal hemorrhages. There is significant tenting of the globe and optic nerve stretch in (*B*).

Postoperative Care

- Signs and symptoms of serious orbital hemorrhage
  - Severe eye pain
  - Proptosis
  - New bleeding from orbit
  - Decreased vision
  - Limitation of eye movement
    - Double vision

After orbital surgery, all patients should be given postoperative instructions that include immediate contact of the surgical team upon development of these findings. Vision should be checked routinely in the postoperative period as part of a postoperative check. Most orbital hemorrhages occur within a few hours of surgery, but can present days after injury especially after provocative measures that increase orbital congestion. Immediate consultation with an ophthalmologist is indicated if these symptoms develop. Whenever possible, the eye should NOT be patched nor a Frost suture placed after surgery because this may obscure symptom development and may increase the potential for orbital compartment syndrome.

Mechanism of Ocular Injury During Orbital Hemorrhages

- Orbital compartment syndrome
  - Development of hemorrhage within the orbit can quickly lead to compartment syndrome and ischemic injury as the eye is compressed
    - As intraocular pressure surpasses perfusion pressure, the blood supply is effectively cut off
  - Retrobulbar hemorrhages also exert increased pressure on the globe, which has limited residual excursion before it is placed on stretch
    - Direct injury to axons and nutrient supply
    - Manifests as globe "tenting" on imaging

Orbital compartment syndrome is an emergency secondary to direct compression of the globe by expansion of orbital volume within the confined orbital space. Globe tenting is seen on imaging as a reduction in the posterior angle of the eye to less than 120°, which may be predictive of impending vision loss. Primate studies have shown that irreversible vision loss occurs approximately 60 to 100 minutes after the onset of ocular tissue ischemia.[7] For this reason, treatment of orbital compartment syndrome should NOT be delayed for any reason including awaiting consultation from ophthalmology or obtaining imaging. It is critical that treatment is carried out in a timely fashion (**Fig. 2**).

Management of Serious Orbital Hemorrhage

- Mainstay of treatment is centered on increasing relative orbital volume

- Canthotomy and cantholysis
  - Most rapid and effective means of reducing intraocular pressure in orbital compartment syndrome
    - Lower canthal tendon release is usually sufficient
    - Most incisions heal well by secondary intention

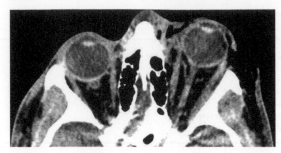

Fig. 2. Axial CT demonstrating significant proptosis, optic nerve stretch, and tenting of the globe.

The ability to perform rapid and effective canthotomy and cantholysis should be in the surgical repertoire of every surgeon that performs surgery in and adjacent to the orbit. Effective performance of this maneuver can frequently reverse vision loss when carried out within the critical time window. Canthotomy alone is ineffective, although often results when the procedure is carried out by inexperienced surgeons.

The canthotomy is performed by incising the skin and orbicularis from the lateral canthal angle laterally for 1 to 2 cm. Pre-emptive clamping of tissues is unnecessary and can be destructive.[1] Next, the eyelid is placed on stretch with forceps directed outward from the orbit. The lower canthal tendon is "strummed" with a ring scissors to facilitate identification and then is incised until the eyelid fully releases from the orbit. Fibers of the orbicularis lateral raphe and lower eyelid retractors can also be released for increased effect.

In the authors' experience, release of the upper canthal tendon provides little additional benefit, causes more bleeding, and has the consequence of completely distorting the lateral canthus requiring subsequent surgical repair. Tonometry can be used before and after the procedure to assess adequate reduction in intraocular pressure. When performed properly, there is limited disfigurement from canthotomy and cantholysis. For this reason, the authors recommend timely performance of this maneuver when suspicion for hemorrhage is high before irreversible vision loss occurs.

When canthotomy and cantholysis fail to reduce intraocular pressure

- Operative management
  - Evacuation
  - Bony orbital decompression
    - Fracture of orbital walls
  - Evacuation of subperiosteal hemorrhage
    - Needle drainage
    - Endoscopic/open approaches
- Medical management of elevated intraocular procedure
  - Intravenous infusion
    - Mannitol
    - Steroids
    - Acetazolamide
  - Eye drops
    - Carbonic anhydrase inhibitors
    - β-Blockers
    - α Agonists
    - Prostaglandin E2 agonists

In cases where canthotomy and cantholysis are ineffective in reducing intraocular pressure or improving visual symptoms, further surgical intervention may be warranted. Emergent CT imaging can be helpful in delineating the location and size of the hemorrhage and presence of direct compression of the optic nerve. Aside from evacuation of the hemorrhage, intraorbital pressure can be reduced further by increasing the orbital volume by fracturing orbital walls. Fracturing orbital walls can be done emergently through use of a rigid device such as a curved hemostat with force directed away from the orbit. The orbital floor is easily fractured into the maxillary sinus and is generally a safe procedure if care is taken to avoid the globe, extraocular muscles, and the infraorbital neurovascular bundle. The lamina papyracea of the medial wall can also be fractured in this manner with careful avoidance of the ethmoidal arteries. Endoscopic bony decompression in the operating room of the medial wall and floor can provide rapid and maximal increases in orbital volume but may result in unwanted delays and resulting damage to ocular structures from tissue ischemia.

Drainage of subperiosteal hemorrhages can be attempted with large-bore (18-gauge) needles when anterior, fresh, and not yet organized. This drainage can be carefully done through a transcutaneous approach in the eyelids or through conjunctiva in the fornices. Surgical approaches are more effective and involve elevation of the periosteum at the orbital rim followed by evacuation with suction. Endoscopic approach to drainage of subperiosteal hemorrhages allows for improved visualization, which can help ensure that all hemorrhage has been evacuated and the point source identified if still bleeding.

Medical management is not first-line therapy but may be effective to maintain intraocular pressure reduction during anticipated postoperative orbital edema after canthotomy and cantholysis. Intravenous mannitol can produce modest decreases in intraocular pressure. Acetazolamide is effective but takes 1 to 2 hours for maximal effect. Steroids can reduce orbital edema but also take time to become effective.

Ophthalmologists frequently use topical medications to effect significant reduction of intraocular pressure. Although these medications, singly or in combination, can treat elevations in intraocular pressure, they are not first-line treatment for acute orbital hemorrhage secondary to their slow onset and modest effects on acute increases in intraocular pressure.

SUMMARY

- Orbital hemorrhage is a rare but serious risk of eye, orbital, and sinus surgery
- Rapid treatment of orbital compartment syndrome can save vision

The anatomic principles and techniques described in this article are effective in preventing and controlling the vast majority of orbital hemorrhages. Endoscopic surgery is particularly well suited to achieving hemostasis in orbital surgery because it provides improved visualization. Although most orbital hemorrhages are self-limited, they can lead to significant functional deficits. Careful attention to danger signs and symptoms will help identify serious orbital hemorrhages. When orbital compartment syndrome is discovered, emergent techniques of restoring normal intraocular pressure should be performed without delay.

Post-Test Questions (Correct answers are in italics)

1. Laceration of which blood vessel can result in a devastating orbital hemorrhage during endoscopic sinus surgery?
   a. Inferior ophthalmic vein
   b. Zygomaticotemporal artery
   c. *Anterior ethmoidal artery*
   d. Recurrent meningeal artery
2. Use of monopolar cautery is relatively contraindicated along which orbital wall?
   a. Floor
   b. *Roof*
   c. Lateral
   d. Medial
3. What is not an advantage of endoscopic orbital surgery versus open approaches?
   a. Higher magnification and brighter illumination of orbital contents
   b. Smaller incisions
   c. *Reduced instrumentation*
   d. Quicker healing and recovery
4. What is the initial acute treatment for orbital compartment syndrome?
   a. Canthotomy
   b. *Canthotomy and cantholysis*
   c. Decrease in systemic blood pressure
   d. Hyperosmotic agents
5. Which of the following is NOT true of image navigation in endoscopic orbital surgery?
   a. Provides precise anatomic correlation with imaging
   b. *Significantly increases costs of surgery*
   c. Allows for precise realignment in orbital reconstruction using mirrored images
   d. Allows for direct visualization of bleeding vessels

SUPPLEMENTARY DATA

Supplementary PDF slides related to this article can be found online at http://www.oto.theclinics.com/.

REFERENCES

1. Rootman J, Stewart B, Goldberg RA. Orbital surgery: a conceptual approach. Philadelphia: Lippincott-Raven; 1995.
2. Takahashi Y, Kakizaki H, Nakano T. Accessory ethmoidal foramina: an anatomical study. Ophthal Plast Reconstr Surg 2011;27:125–7.
3. Wang L, Youseef A, Al Qahtani AA, et al. Endoscopic anatomy of the middle ethmoidal artery. Int Forum Allergy Rhinol 2014;4:164–8.
4. Dallan I, Tschabitscher M, Castelnuovo P, et al. Management of severely bleeding ethmoidal arteries. J Craniofac Surg 2009;20:450–4.

5. Wulc AE, Adams JL, Dryden RM. Cerebrospinal fluid leakage complicating orbital exenteration. Arch Ophthalmol 1989;107:827–30.
6. Couch SM, Garrity JA, Cameron JD, et al. Embolization of orbital varices with N-butyl cyanoacrylate as an aid in surgical excision: results of 4 cases with histopathologic examination. Am J Ophthalmol 2009;148:614–8.e1.
7. Lima V, Burt B, Leibovitch I, et al. Orbital compartment syndrome: the ophthalmic surgical emergency. Surv Ophthalmol 2009;54:441–9.
8. Bly RA, Chang SH, Cudejkova M, et al. Computer-guided orbital reconstruction to improve outcomes. JAMA Facial Plast Surg 2013;15:113–20.
9. Katz SE, Rootman J. Adverse effects of bone wax in surgery of the orbit. Ophthal Plast Reconstr Surg 1996;12:121–6.
10. Ereth MH, Schaff M, Ericson EF, et al. Comparative safety and efficacy of topical hemostatic agents in a rat neurosurgical model. Neurosurgery 2008;63:369–72 [discussion: 372].

SUGGESTED READINGS

Lima V, Burt B, Leibovitch I, et al. Orbital compartment syndrome: the ophthalmic surgical emergency. Surv Ophthalmol 2009;54:441–9.
Excellent overview of presentation, causes, and treatment of orbital compartment syndrome.
Rootman J, Stewart B, Goldberg RA. Orbital surgery: a conceptual approach. Philadelphia: Lippincott-Raven; 1995.
An outstanding textbook with an excellent overview of both orbital anatomy and surgical approaches to the orbit with rich illustrations and photographs.
Wang L, Youseef A, Al Qahtani AA, et al. Endoscopic anatomy of the middle ethmoidal artery. Int Forum Allergy Rhinol 2014;4:164–8.
Nice anatomic and clinical overview of accessory ethmoidal arteries and their clinical significance.

Managing Vascular Tumors—Open Approaches

Cecelia E. Schmalbach, MD[a], Christine Gourin, MD[b],*

KEYWORDS

- Vascular tumors • Head and neck • Carotid artery • Paragangliomas • Embolization

KEY LEARNING POINTS

At the end of this article, the reader will:

- Be able to apply main preoperative assessment principles in the management of vascular head and neck tumors.
- Be able to apply fundamental surgical techniques in the treatment of vascular tumors.
- Be able to discuss the role of preoperative embolization in the management of different head and neck tumors.
- Understand the role of balloon test occlusion in the management of specific tumors.
- Become familiar with the major open approaches to common head and neck tumors.

INTRODUCTION

> **Vascular tumors pose a challenge to surgical extirpation**
>
> - Increased risk of blood loss
> - Incomplete surgery due to poor visualization or bleeding
> - Morbidity
>   - Cranial nerve sacrifice or injury
>   - Cerebrovascular events
>   - Sequelae of blood loss or transfusion

The most common vascular tumors encountered by the otolaryngologist are rare chromaffin cell tumors termed paragangliomas. Within the head and neck region, they commonly arise from the carotid body (**Fig. 1**), vagus nerve (glomus vagale) (**Fig. 2**), and jugular vein (glomus jugulare). Other vascular head and neck tumors include

[a] Department of Otolaryngology, University of Indiana, Indianapolis, IN, USA; [b] Department of Otolaryngology–Head and Neck Surgery, Johns Hopkins University, Baltimore, MD, USA
* Corresponding author.
E-mail address: cgourin1@jhmi.edu

Otolaryngol Clin N Am 49 (2016) 777–790
http://dx.doi.org/10.1016/j.otc.2016.03.001
0030-6665/16/$ – see front matter © 2016 Elsevier Inc. All rights reserved.

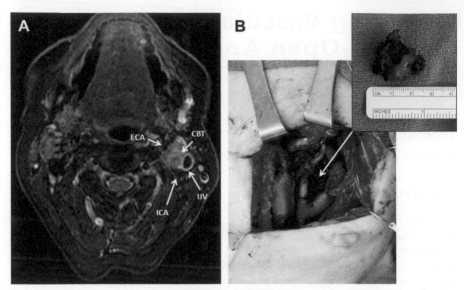

Fig. 1. (*A*) MRI of a left carotid body tumor (CBT). (*B*) Postresection bed demonstrating splaying of the internal and external carotid artery. Inset depicts resected CBT. ECA, external carotid artery; ICA, internal carotid artery; IJV, internal jugular vein.

sinonasal malignancies, because of proximity to or involvement of the pterygoid plexus as well as the rich vascularity of the sinonasal mucosa, juvenile nasopharyngeal angiofibroma, a vascular tumor of male adolescents; unusual vascular tumors such as hemangiopericytoma; and metastatic renal cell cancer, which has a proclivity for an unusually rich blood supply.

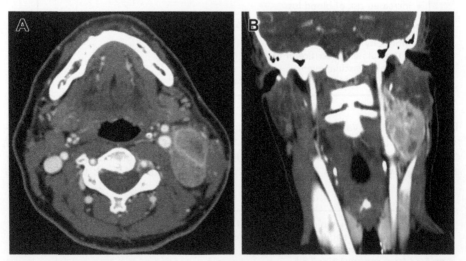

Fig. 2. (*A*) Axial MRI demonstrating a left vagal nerve paraganglioma (glomus vagale). Note the lateral position to the great vessels. (*B*) Coronal MRI of the same tumor. Note the absence of internal and external carotid artery splaying, which is seen in the setting of a carotid body tumor.

Preoperative planning

Adequate imaging is a prerequisite to surgical planning to determine:

- Location of tumor
- Likely diagnosis
- Assess vascularity
- Types of imaging modalities
  - Diagnostic imaging
    - Computed tomography (CT)
    - MRI
    - Computed tomography angiography (CTA)
    - Magnetic resonance angiography (MRA)
    - Angiography

The location and histology of the tumor are key points in considering how to minimize blood loss before surgery begins. CT (**Fig. 3**) or MRI (**Fig. 4**) can be obtained as a first step, and often both are obtained for planning purposes because these are complementary modalities. CT is superior for demonstrating bone involvement, but MRI is superior in demonstrating the soft tissue characteristics of the tumor, delineating tumor from muscle and vascular relationships, and demonstrating classic flow voids (see **Fig. 4**) in paragangliomas.

Angiography (**Fig. 5**) has classically been used in the workup of most vascular lesions. Increasingly, catheter angiography has been replaced by MRA and CTA in the preoperative workup of vascular lesions. However, angiography can be useful when embolization is being considered, and angiography with balloon occlusion testing is necessary if malignancy is suspected and/or if carotid sacrifice or injury is

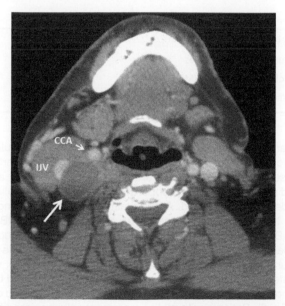

Fig. 3. CT scan of a right glomus vagale (*large arrow*). Note the splaying of the internal jugular vein (IJV) from the common carotid artery (CCA). This patient presented with right vocal cord paralysis and associated hoarseness.

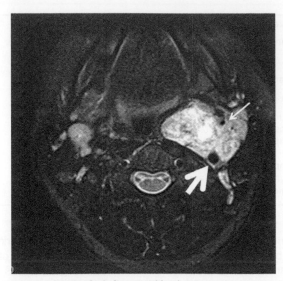

Fig. 4. T2 fat-saturated axial MRI of a left carotid body tumor demonstrating the classic flow voids, which give a salt-and-pepper appearance to the tumor when contrasted imaging is used. The large arrow points to the internal carotid artery; the small arrow points to the external carotid artery. Note how the 2 branches are splayed by the tumor (lyre sign).

anticipated during resection, such as in large carotid body tumors. Embolization has been reported to reduce blood transfusion requirements. However, embolization of paragangliomas remains controversial with some investigators reporting no effect on blood transfusion, an increase in cranial nerve injury, and increased costs.[1]

Additional tests for paraganglioma

- 24-hour urine catecholamines
- Metaiodobenzylguanidine (MIBG) scan
- CT abdomen

When a paraganglioma is suspected, 24-hour urine collection should be performed to detect catecholamine secretion (vanillylmandelic acid, metanephrines). Secreting tumors can cause an intraoperative hypertensive crisis or cardiac arrythmias from manipulation and must be identified preoperatively so α-cardiovascular and β-cardiovascular blockade can be instituted. Approximately 10% of paragangliomas secrete catecholamines. If urine catecholamine levels are elevated, an MIBG scan should be obtained. MIBG scans use a radioisotope similar to norepinephrine and can localize catecholamine uptake and storage, which is important to rule out the primary tumor as the source. Because 10% of paragangliomas are multiple, when catecholamines are elevated, a CT of the abdomen should also be performed to detect an adrenal pheochromocytoma. Paraganglioma metastasis is estimated to occur in 10% to 36% of cases (**Fig. 6**). Patients with malignant paragangliomas are often asymptomatic. The diagnosis is commonly rendered following pathologic evaluation of an enlarged lymph node, which demonstrates chromaffin cells. In such cases, a full

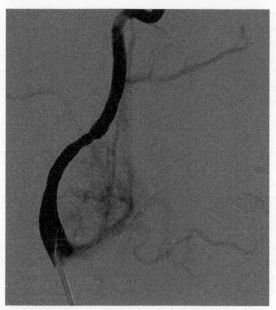

Fig. 5. Angiogram demonstrating a well-vascularized carotid body tumor. Note the hallmark lyre sign in which the internal and external carotid vessels are splayed.

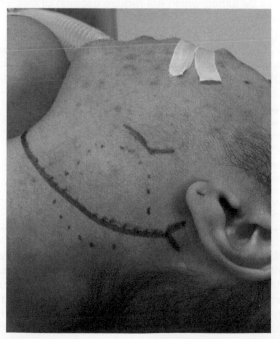

Fig. 6. Transcervical approach to a carotid body tumor. The incision is made at least 2 finger-breadths beneath the mandible to avoid injury to the marginal mandibular nerve.

metastatic workup is warranted to evaluate both regional and distant metastasis. Clinical examination will direct the need for imaging. Both PET and octreotide scintigraphy have proven helpful in this setting.

Treatment options for metastatic disease include surgical resection, targeted therapy with radioactive metaiodobenzylguanidine (^{131}I-MIBG), or chemotherapy. Timely diagnosis and treatment are imperative to avoid myocardial infarction, severe hypertension, stroke, and arrhythmia.

Biopsy

- Should not be performed before imaging

Under most circumstances, a presumptive diagnosis can be made on the basis of the above-named imaging studies. Under no circumstances should biopsy be performed before obtaining the radiologic studies. FNA biopsy can be a useful adjunct when the mass is readily accessible, either transcervically or transorally, and can provide useful information if a diagnosis of malignancy is suspected. However, if imaging studies suggest a vascular lesion, FNA provides little if any useable information and is not indicated. Incisional biopsy should only be considered if the patient is not an operative candidate and FNA is inconclusive, and only if a diagnosis of malignancy or lymphoma is strongly suspected. Transoral open biopsy has been described but carries a risk of hemorrhage and contamination of the pharyngeal mucosa by tumor, which will require excision of that site during subsequent definitive resection.

Embolization

Preoperative embolization may reduce intraoperative blood loss

- Pros:
  - Reduced intraoperative blood loss
  - Reduced need for transfusion
  - Improved visualization

- Cons:
  - May not reduce transfusion requirements
  - Increased cranial nerve injury
  - Obscures subadventitial plane for carotid body tumor removal
  - Increased costs
  - Small risk of stroke associated with procedure

Preoperative embolization may reduce intraoperative blood loss. As a general rule, embolization is advised for vascular tumors that are larger than 3 cm when feeding vessels are identified on angiogram. Branches of the external carotid artery that supply the tumor can be occluded with embolization. The most common feeding vessel for a carotid body tumor is the ascending pharyngeal branch. If the internal carotid artery is involved (usually encasement), balloon occlusion testing can be performed to test the adequacy of the contralateral circulation to determine if carotid sacrifice or bypass is required. It must be noted that in cases of high-grade malignancy, carotid encasement of greater than 270° is considered unresectable, with no improvement in overall survival.[1]

Embolization may reduce intraoperative blood loss and transfusion requirements and facilitates resection of large tumors.[2–4] Embolization of paragangliomas remains controversial with some investigators reporting no effect on blood transfusion, an increase in cranial nerve injury, and increased costs.[5] Glomus vagale tumors rarely have an isolated vascular supply, and resection is usually not associated with significant blood loss. Carotid body paraganglioma are supplied by the adventitia of the carotid and do not usually have an obvious single feeding vessel.[6,7] Several retrospective series have found no significant difference in blood loss with embolization, after controlling for tumor size.[4,6] Risks of embolization include complication rates related to neurologic ischemia or cranial nerve injury of 13% to 18%, which is higher than the rates of 0% to 3% reported for patients who did not undergo embolization.[3,8] Embolization of a carotid body tumor may cause a marked inflammatory response, particularly with newer embolization particles, that can obscure the subadventitial plane in which dissection is performed. The risks and benefits of embolization should be carefully considered in the context of the size of the tumor and the risk of significant blood loss.

BALLOON OCCLUSION TEST

When is balloon occlusion testing indicated?
• Carotid involvement
• High risk of carotid injury

The balloon occlusion test measures the effect of internal carotid artery occlusion on cerebral blood flow (CBF) and the adequacy of the contralateral circulation. It is indicated when imaging studies suggest carotid involvement or when resection of the lesion carries a high risk of intraoperative carotid artery injury. When either situation is suggested, preoperative vascular surgery consultation should be pursued for intraoperative assistance.

Angiography is performed, and the internal carotid artery is occluded using a balloon-tipped catheter for 10 to 15 minutes. In patients who develop neurologic symptoms (approximately 5%), the test is abandoned and no further evaluation is performed: these patients are considered at high risk for stroke and should undergo nonoperative therapy, subtotal resection with carotid preservation, or revascularization before resection.

In patients without neurologic symptoms during balloon occlusion, xenon-enhanced CT scanning is performed to quantitate CBF. CBF is evaluated both before and after balloon occlusion; xenon gas is inhaled, diffuses rapidly into the bloodstream, and causes areas of the brain that are perfused to become radiopaque. Patients with diminished perfusion on xenon-enhanced CT (approximately 25%) are considered at mild to moderate risk of stroke with prolonged carotid occlusion, and interposition grafting of the internal carotid artery is recommended if the artery is to be sacrificed.

There is a 4% incidence of neurologic sequelae from the balloon occlusion test itself, and so the procedure is reserved only for cases in which the carotid is suspected to be involved or at risk. Carotid encasement of greater than 270° in high-grade malignancies is associated with poor overall survival.[1]

SURGICAL STRATEGIES

> **Principles of open surgical approach**
> - Expose tumor from above as well as from below
> - Identify and control major blood vessels
> - Isolate internal carotid artery and its vascular contributions
> - Vascular surgery and neurosurgery consultation where appropriate

Most vascular tumors of the head and neck that are not amenable to an endoscopic approach can be approached through a transcervical approach, which may be combined with mandibulotomy, parotidectomy, or infratemporal fossa approaches, with or without craniotomy for exposure of high lesions. Sinonasal tumors may require maxillectomy or a maxillary swing approach.

Patients must be counseled about the risks of potential carotid sacrifice or injury as well as the possibility of cranial nerve injury and resultant dysfunction. Vagal nerve deficits result in both speech and swallowing impairment, through loss of motor function to the ipsilateral vocal cord as well as loss of sensation to the ipsilateral larynx, both of which predispose to aspiration. The adjacent hypoglossal nerve serves to provide motor function to the tongue, and the glossopharyngeal nerve innervates the palate and constrictor muscles. Multiple cranial nerve deficits should alert the physician to consider gastrostomy tube placement.

Transcervical Approach

The transcervical approach is the preferred method for removal of most vascular tumors involving the poststyloid parapharyngeal space. A transverse incision (see **Fig. 6**) at the level of the hyoid bone, 2 fingerbreadths below the mandible, is performed, and the carotid artery and internal jugular vein are identified (**Fig. 7**). The digastric, stylohyoid, and styloglossus muscles are retracted to allow access to the parapharyngeal space. The submandibular gland can be retracted anteriorly for exposure or removed if necessary. Division of the stylomandibular ligament can increase exposure to the parapharyngeal space by up to 2 cm by facilitating retraction of the mandible; this may not provide adequate exposure for large lesions or those with significant cranial extension.

Transcervical-Transparotid Approach

A transcervical approach may be combined with a transparotid approach for many superiorly located parapharyngeal tumors to protect the facial nerve while enhancing exposure to the parapharyngeal space. By extending the cervical incision into a preauricular incision, the facial nerve can be identified and protected and the styloid process removed in addition to the stylomandibular ligament to enhance exposure. This approach is usually reserved for tumors involving the deep lobe of the parotid gland.[9] Vascular tumors in this area requiring more exposure superiorly require mandibulotomy.

Mandibulotomy

The transcervical approach can be combined with mandibulotomy, or mandibular swing, which greatly facilitates exposure. A midline mandibulotomy is preferred, for 2 reasons: to limit injury to the inferior alveolar nerve, which is disrupted with a lateral mandibulotomy and causes permanent anesthesia to the lower lip; and because of the potential for osteoradionecrosis if postoperative radiation is required. The exception

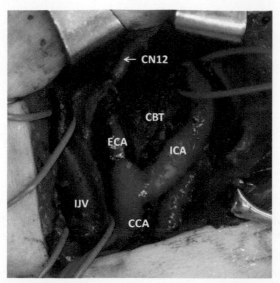

Fig. 7. Left carotid body tumor (CBT) with identification of key vascular structures above and below the tumor to allow safe and expeditious control of major bleeding. CCA, common carotid artery; CN12, hypoglossal nerve; ECA, external carotid artery; ICA, internal carotid artery; IJV, internal jugular vein.

would be for tumor involvement of the mandible, in which case segmental mandibulectomy is performed. Mandibulotomy is often required for vascular tumors that extend into the parapharyngeal space above the level of the mandible, tumors located in the superior parapharyngeal space, and tumors involving the skull base.

A midline lip-splitting incision (**Fig. 8**) is used, and a mucosal incision is then made along the ipsilateral floor of mouth, leaving sufficient mucosa for closure laterally and extending the incision back to the level of the anterior tonsil pillar and soft palate. Deep to these structures is the superior extent of the parapharyngeal space, great vessels, and cranial nerve. This approach essentially opens the superior parapharyngeal space "like a book" and facilitates visualization up to the level of the skull base; however, tracheostomy is required because of postoperative mucosal edema (**Fig. 9**).

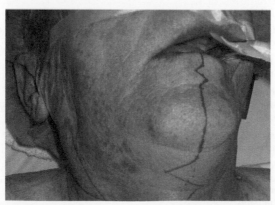

Fig. 8. Midline split incision. A stair-step technique can be used to ensure precise reapproximation of the vermillion boarder.

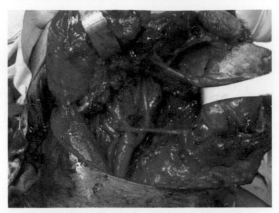

Fig. 9. A mandibulotomy approach opens up the parapharyngeal space "like a book" with excellent exposure of the great vessels above the digastric tendon.

Infratemporal Fossa Approach

A preauricular infratemporal fossa approach as described by Fisch can be used for malignant tumors involving the skull base or jugular foramen.[10] This approach can be combined with frontotemporal craniotomy for removal of tumors with significant intracranial extension (**Fig. 10**A). A parotidectomy incision with cervical extension as described above is extended superiorly into a hemicoronal scalp incision (**Fig. 10**B). The temporalis muscle is elevated to expose the glenoid fossa, which is removed laterally. The temporomandibular joint can be displaced inferiorly, or the mandible condyle can be transected for improved exposure. Orbitozygomatic osteotomies are performed, and the infratemporal skull base and distal carotid are exposed. The facial nerve and vascular structures in the neck are identified through the cervical and preauricular approaches (**Fig. 10**C).

MANAGEMENT OF THE CAROTID ARTERY

When the carotid artery is at risk during surgery, several decisions need to be made preoperatively

- Is disease resectable?
  - Carotid encasement greater than 270° or skull base erosion are considered unresectable for high-grade malignancy
- Consider the goals of surgery
  - Weigh morbidity of treatment against morbidity of the disease
- What is the best surgical approach?
  - Adequate visualization of the tumor is key to avoiding intraoperative complications
- Carotid sacrifice or bypass?
  - Vascular and/or neurosurgical consultation preoperatively
- Prepare for blood loss
  - Communication with anesthesiologist preoperatively
  - Preoperative optimization of medical status
  - Blood banking
  - Use cell saver

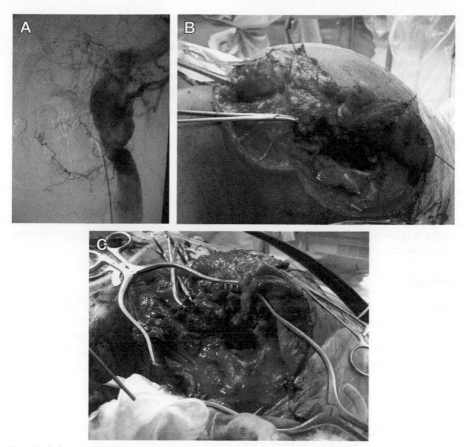

Fig. 10. (*A*) Angiogram showing large glomus vagale. (*B*) A parotidectomy incision with cervical extension is extended superiorly into a hemicoronal scalp incision. (*C*) The transcervical/transparotid approach is combined with a lateral skull-base approach to reach tumors with significant skull base extension.

STAGING SURGERY

Staging of surgery should be considered in the case of large tumors that may require a combined approach such as craniotomy for complete removal. In the case of tumors involving the carotid artery, staging may allow carotid bypass before more definitive resection. Staging removal is also a good strategy if excessive blood loss or length of surgery would be anticipated for complete removal. The goals of surgery should be carefully discussed with patients. The risks of morbidity from resection of vascular tumors of the head and neck are primarily those of blood loss, neurological ischemia, and cranial neuropathies, which may be multiple. Leaving some residual disease behind can be considered for patients who are poor candidates for complete extirpative surgery, if tumor size is causing symptoms.

Nonoperative Management

Nonoperative management should be considered for patients who are poor surgical candidates because of comorbid disease, selected elderly patients, patients who fail balloon occlusion, unresectable lesions, and for those patients with benign slow-growing tumors in whom resection would carry a significant risk of sacrifice of multiple cranial nerves. The risks and benefits of surgery must be weighed in every case. The incidence of neurovascular complications, including cranial nerve injury and cerebrovascular injury, is increased in patients with paragangliomas and malignancies. Alternatives to surgical therapy consist of observation or radiation therapy.

POSTOPERATIVE CARE

Patients undergoing open resection of large vascular lesions of the head and neck should be observed for at least 24 hours in the intensive care unit. Bleeding, neurologic injury, and aspiration from cranial neuropathies require close monitoring in the postoperative period for detection and intervention. Speech and swallowing consultation is highly recommended, especially in the management of glomus vagale tumors and glomus jugulare when cranial nerves are sacrificed. Transmandibular approaches require tracheostomy because significant upper airway edema can result from the procedure, causing obstruction.

SUMMARY

Vascular tumors of the head and neck can be successfully approached through open approaches but require careful preoperative planning, including embolization when appropriate, consideration of the carotid artery, preoperative consultation with vascular surgery, neurosurgery, and anesthesiology to plan an approach to minimize complications and blood loss, and selection of the best approach for adequate exposure.

Post-Test Questions (Correct answers are in italics)

1. What is the correct initial step in the workup of a vascular tumor?
   a. 24-hour urine catecholamines
   b. Fine needle aspiration
   c. *Imaging*
   d. Embolization
2. A transcervical approach is best suited for vascular tumors involving the:
   a. *Poststyloid parapharyngeal space*
   b. Skull base
   c. Prestyloid parapharyngeal space
   d. Jugular foramen
3. Balloon occlusion testing identifies:
   a. Carotid body tumors
   b. Carotid involvement
   c. Neurologic deficits
   d. *Cerebral blood flow*
4. Preoperative embolization may reduce:
   a. Cranial nerve injury
   b. *Intraoperative blood loss*
   c. Costs
   d. Extent of surgery

SUPPLEMENTARY DATA

Supplementary PDF slides related to this article can be found online at http://www. oto.theclinics.com/.

REFERENCES

1. Manzoor NF, Russell JO, Bricker A, et al. Impact of surgical resection on survival in patients with advanced head and neck cancer involving the carotid artery. JAMA Otolaryngol Head Neck Surg 2013;139:1219–25.
2. Persky MS, Setton A, Niimi Y, et al. Combined endovascular and surgical treatment of head and neck paragangliomas–a team approach. Head Neck 2002; 24:423–31.
3. Li J, Wang S, Zee C, et al. Preoperative angiography and transarterial embolization in the management of carotid body tumor: a single-center, 10-year experience. Neurosurgery 2010;67:941–8.
4. Kasper GC, Welling RE, Wladis AR, et al. A multidisciplinary approach to carotid paragangliomas. Vasc Endovascular Surg 2007;40:467–74.
5. Chan JY, Li RJ, Gourin CG. Short-term outcomes and cost of care of treatment of head and neck paragangliomas. Laryngoscope 2013;123:1645–51.
6. Kruger AJ, Walker PJ, Foster WJ, et al. Important observations made managing carotid body tumors during a 25-year experience. J Vasc Surg 2010;52:1518–23.
7. Zeitler DM, Glick J, Har-El G. Preoperative embolization in carotid body tumor surgery: is it required? Ann Otol Rhinol Laryngol 2010;119:279–83.
8. Litle VR, Reilly LM, Ramos TK. Preoperative embolization of carotid body tumors: when is it appropriate? Ann Vasc Surg 1996;10:464–8.
9. Bradley PJ, Bradley PT, Olsen KD. Update on the management of parapharyngeal tumors. Curr Opin Otolaryngol Head Neck Surg 2011;104:92–8.
10. Sanna M, Shin SH, Piazza P, et al. Infratemporal fossa approach type A with transcondylar-transtubercular extension for Fisch type C2 to C4 tympanojugular paragangliomas. Head Neck 2014;36:1581–8.

SUGGESTED READINGS

Bradley PJ, Bradley PT, Olsen KD. Update on the management of parapharyngeal tumors. Curr Opin Otolaryngol Head Neck Surg 2011;104:92–8.
Chan JY, Li RJ, Gourin CG. Short-term outcomes and cost of care of treatment of head and neck paragangliomas. Laryngoscope 2013;123:1645–51.
Kasper GC, Welling RE, Wladis AR, et al. A multidisciplinary approach to carotid paragangliomas. Vasc Endovascular Surg 2007;40:467–74.
Kruger AJ, Walker PJ, Foster WJ, et al. Important observations made managing carotid body tumors during a 25-year experience. J Vasc Surg 2010;52:1518–23.
Li J, Wang S, Zee C, et al. Preoperative angiography and transarterial embolization in the management of carotid body tumor: a single-center, 10-year experience. Neurosurgery 2010;67:941–8.
Litle VR, Reilly LM, Ramos TK. Preoperative embolization of carotid body tumors: when is it appropriate? Ann Vasc Surg 1996;10:464–8.
Manzoor NF, Russell JO, Bricker A, et al. Impact of surgical resection on survival in patients with advanced head and neck cancer involving the carotid artery. JAMA Otolaryngol Head Neck Surg 2013;139:1219–25.
Persky MS, Setton A, Niimi Y, et al. Combined endovascular and surgical treatment of head and neck paragangliomas–a team approach. Head Neck 2002;24:423–31.

Sanna M, Shin SH, Piazza P, et al. Infratemporal fossa approach type A with transcondylar-transtubercular extension for Fisch type C2 to C4 tympanojugular paragangliomas. Head Neck 2014;36:1581–8.

Zeitler DM, Glick J, Har-El G. Preoperative embolization in carotid body tumor surgery: is it required? Ann Otol Rhinol Laryngol 2010;119:279–83.

Endoscopic Management of Vascular Sinonasal Tumors, Including Angiofibroma

 CrossMark

Carl H. Snyderman, MD, MBA[a],*, Harshita Pant, BMBS[b]

KEYWORDS

- Angiofibroma • Coblation • Embolization • Harmonic scalpel • Internal carotid artery
- Juvenile nasopharyngeal angiofibroma • Staging system • Vascularity

KEY LEARNING POINTS

At the end of this article, the reader will:

- Know which techniques can be used to devascularize a sinonasal tumor.
- Know the major source of morbidity when removing vascular tumors such as angiofibromas.
- Be able to describe a staging system for angiofibromas that incorporates residual vascularity of the tumor as a prognostic factor.
- Know the most common source of blood supply from the internal carotid artery for an angiofibroma.
- Know the key anatomic landmarks for locating the petrous segment of the internal carotid artery.
- Know which blood-sparing strategies can be used to minimize the need for blood transfusion.

▶ Video content accompanies this article at http://www.oto.theclinics.com

---

Conflicts of Interest: The authors have no conflict of interest to disclose.
[a] Department of Otolaryngology, Center for Cranial Base Surgery, University of Pittsburgh Medical Center, University of Pittsburgh School of Medicine, 200 Lothrop Street, EEI Suite 500, Pittsburgh, PA 15213, USA; [b] Department of Otolaryngology, Head and Neck Surgery, University of Adelaide School of Medicine, Eleanor Harrald Building, Frome Road, Adelaide, South Australia 5005, Australia
* Corresponding author. Department of Otolaryngology, University of Pittsburgh School of Medicine, 200 Lothrop Street, EEI Suite 500, Pittsburgh, PA 15213.
E-mail address: snydermanch@upmc.edu

INTRODUCTION

> **Juvenile nasopharyngeal angiofibroma**
>
> - Rare, benign, vascular tumor
> - Male adolescents
> - Origin: nasopharynx in region of pterygoid canal
> - Symptoms: nasal obstruction, recurrent unilateral epistaxis
>   - Facial swelling
>   - Orbit: proptosis, diplopia, visual loss
>   - Facial hypesthesia (V2)
> - Primary treatment is surgery

Juvenile nasopharyngeal angiofibroma (JNA) is a rare, benign tumor that is characteristically found in male adolescents. It arises in the lateral nasopharynx and can spread in multiple directions: nasal cavity, oropharynx, paranasal sinuses, orbit (via inferior orbital fissure), and infratemporal fossa (via pterygomaxillary fissure). Intracranial extension occurs through skull base foramina and erosion of bone. Early symptoms include nasal obstruction and recurrent unilateral epistaxis. Large tumors can displace normal structures, resulting in facial swelling, proptosis, diplopia, visual loss, and facial hypesthesia. The primary treatment is surgical excision. The greatest challenge of surgery is bleeding caused by the hypervascular nature of JNA.

WHY IS BLEEDING A PROBLEM?

> - Increased risk of injury caused by poor visualization
> - Incomplete surgery caused by poor visualization or volume of blood loss
> - Medical morbidity:
>   - Postoperative nausea and fatigue
>   - Hypoxia (from blood loss and nasal packing)
>   - Transfusion of blood products
> - Increased medical cost

Surgical bleeding is to be expected with the management of large and vascular tumors such as JNA. Other tumors that are characterized by increased vascularity are meningioma, sinonasal malignancy, hemangiopericytoma, and metastatic renal cell carcinoma. Bleeding with poor visualization is a primary risk factor for complications such as cranial nerve injury, cerebrospinal fluid leak, and vascular injury. Poor visualization and excessive blood loss also limit the ability to completely remove the tumor; staging of surgery may be necessary. Additional morbidities include postoperative nausea from swallowed blood, postoperative anemia, and the risks of blood transfusion. Deaths still occur from unmanaged blood loss. Excessive blood loss increases the costs of health care because of greater use of resources, treatment of complications, and prolonged hospitalization.

Small JNAs receive their blood supply from the external carotid artery (ECA) and can be effectively devascularized by preoperative embolization or surgical ligation of the internal maxillary artery. Intraoperative endoscopic ligation of the ethmoid and sphenopalatine arteries can often be performed by working around the periphery of the tumor or through an external approach.

Larger JNAs receive a blood supply from multiple sources, including the internal carotid artery (ICA). For such tumors, the best treatment strategy is controversial and depends on the capabilities and resources of the surgical team. With proper planning, even giant JNAs can be effectively managed using minimally invasive surgical approaches.

GOALS OF TREATMENT

- Complete removal of tumor
  - Access to routes of extension
  - Vascular control
- Minimize morbidity
  - Blood loss and transfusion
  - Cranial nerve injury
  - Disruption of growth centers/cosmesis
  - Brain manipulation
  - Soft tissue injury/pain
- Avoid radiation therapy
  - Long-term side effects

In addition to complete removal, the goals of treatment are to minimize morbidity and avoid the use of radiation therapy. Intraoperative bleeding is the major source of morbidity and contributes to incomplete tumor resection and complications caused by poor visualization. Concerns about bleeding or incomplete surgery may result in inappropriate use of radiation therapy.

STAGING OF ANGIOFIBROMAS

Potential prognostic factors
- Age, weight
- Prior treatment
- Tumor size, volume
- Sites of tumor involvement
- Skull base involvement
- Intracranial extension
- ICA contribution
- Residual vascularity

Potential prognostic factors for the treatment of JNAs include the size, location, and extent of the tumor. Multiple staging systems have been proposed over the years for prognostic classification of JNA (**Table 1**). Key staging criteria include the tumor extent and presence of skull base involvement and intracranial extension. The greatest challenge of these surgeries is not the size or extent of the tumor but intraoperative hemorrhage that cannot be controlled by embolization or ligation of branches of the

Table 1
Staging systems for JNA

Stage	Onerci et al,[1] 2006	Radkowski et al,[2] 1996	Andrews et al,[3] 1989	Chandler et al,[4] 1984	Sessions et al,[5] 1981
I	Nose, NP, ethmoid and sphenoid sinuses, or minimal extension into PMF	a. Limited to nose or NP b. As in (a) with extension into ≥1 sinus	Limited to NP Bone destruction negligible or limited to SPF	Limited to NP	a. Limited to nose and NP b. Extension into ≥1 sinus
II	Maxillary sinus, full occupation of PMF, extension to anterior cranial fossa, limited extension into ITF	a. Minimal extension through SPF and into medial PMF b. Full occupation of PMF, displacing posterior wall of maxilla forward, orbit erosion, displacement of maxillary artery branches c. ITF, cheek, posterior to pterygoid plates	Invading PPF or maxillary, ethmoid, or sphenoid sinus with bone destruction	Extension into nasal cavity or sphenoid sinus	a. Minimal extension into PMF b. Full occupation of PMF with or without erosion of orbit c. ITF with or without cheek extension
III	Deep extension into cancellous bone at pterygoid base or body and GW sphenoid; significant lateral extension into ITF or pterygoid plates; orbital, cavernous sinus obliteration	Erosion of skull base a. Minimal intracranial extension b. Extensive intracranial extension ± cavernous sinus	Invading ITF or orbital region a. No intracranial involvement b. Extradural (parasellar) involvement	Tumor into antrum, ethmoid sinus, PMF, ITF, orbit, and/or cheek	Intracranial extension
IV	Intracranial extension between pituitary gland and ICA, tumor localization lateral to ICA, middle fossa extension, and extensive intracranial extension	—	Intracranial, intradural tumor a. With b. Without cavernous sinus, pituitary or optic chiasm infiltration	Intracranial extension	—

Abbreviations: GW, greater wing; ITF, infratemporal fossa; NP, Nasopharynx; PMF, pterygomaxillary fossa; PPF, pterygopalatine fossa; SPF, sphenopalatine foramen.

From Snyderman CH, Pant H, Carrau RL, et al. A new endoscopic staging system for angiofibromas. Arch Otolaryngol Head Neck Surg 2010;136(6):589; with permission.

ECA. In particular, these staging systems do not account for the vascularity of the tumor (following embolization) and the route of intracranial extension (medial or lateral to ICA and cavernous sinus).

The University of Pittsburgh Medical Center (UPMC) staging system (**Table 2**), proposed in 2010, separates JNA tumors into 3 groups based on the vascularity and extent of the tumor. Tumors in stages I and II receive their entire blood supply from branches of the ECA and are readily excised (following embolization) using endoscopic techniques with little morbidity. Stage III tumors are intermediate risk and are characterized by skull base erosion or lateral extension but without residual vascularity. Stage IV and V tumors are challenging to treat because of significant blood supply from the ICA. Routes of intracranial extension may be from the sphenoid sinus medial to the cavernous sinus or lateral to the ICA through the orbital fissures to the middle cranial fossa (**Fig. 1**).

The most important discriminating factor is the presence of significant residual vascularity following embolization. Assessment of residual vascularity is subjective and is defined as significant tumor blush. In contrast with the other staging systems, the UPMC staging system provides a strong correlation between tumor stage and intraoperative blood loss (**Fig. 2**).

The UPMC staging system also provides superior correlation with the need for staged surgeries and the presence of residual or recurrent disease.

TREATMENT OF ANGIOFIBROMAS

Preoperative embolization

- ECA
  - Unilateral or bilateral
- ICA
  - Contribution
  - Balloon occlusion with proximal embolization
    - Risk of stroke

Table 2
UPMC staging system

Stage	UPMC Staging Criteria
I	Nasal cavity, medial pterygopalatine fossa No residual vascularity
II	Paranasal sinuses, lateral pterygopalatine fossa No residual vascularity
III	Skull base, orbit, infratemporal fossa No residual vascularity
IV	Skull base, orbit, infratemporal fossa Residual vascularity
V	Intracranial extension: medial; lateral Residual vascularity

From Snyderman CH, Pant H, Carrau RL, et al. A new endoscopic staging system for angiofibromas. Arch Otolaryngol Head Neck Surg 2010;136(6):590; with permission.

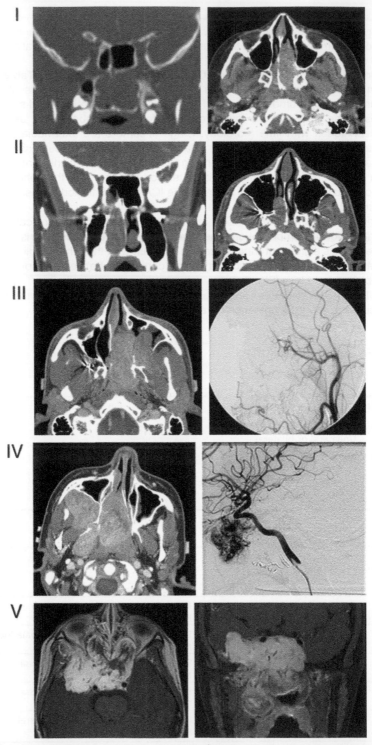

Fig. 1. Examples of UPMC stages I to V. (*From* Snyderman CH, Pant H, Carrau RL, et al. A new endoscopic staging system for angiofibromas. Arch Otolaryngol Head Neck Surg 2010;136(6):590; with permission.)

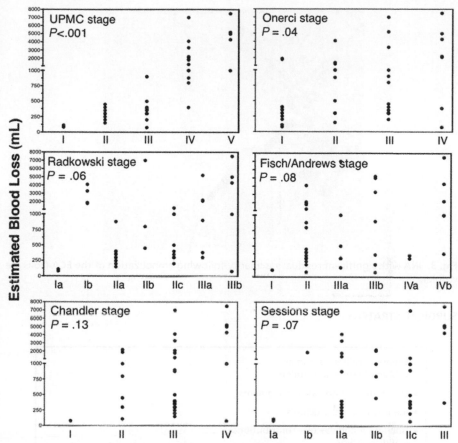

Fig. 2. UPMC staging system. (*From* Snyderman CH, Pant H, Carrau RL, et al. A new endoscopic staging system for angiofibromas. Arch Otolaryngol Head Neck Surg 2010;136(6):592; with permission.)

Preoperative embolization is performed for all but the smallest of tumors. Embolization is usually restricted to branches of the ECA (internal maxillary artery, ascending pharyngeal artery) and may be bilateral for larger tumors that cross the midline. Following embolization of the ECA, residual vascularity from branches of the ICA may be observed and can be profound. Embolization of these branches (with temporary distal occlusion of the ICA) can be considered in select cases but carries significant risk of stroke caused by release of embolized particles. If there is complete encasement of the ICA, balloon test occlusion of the ICA may be performed to assess the adequacy of collateral circulation and the feasibility of carotid sacrifice if necessary.

The vidian artery (second genu of the petrous ICA) is the most common source of blood supply from the ICA. Other contributing vessels typically arise from the cavernous segment of the ICA (**Fig. 3**).

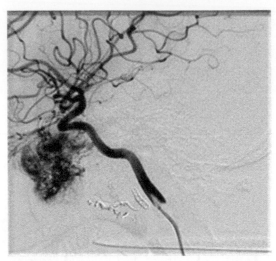

Fig. 3. JNA with significant residual vascularity following embolization of the ECA (coils are visible).

SURGICAL STRATEGY

- Expose periphery of tumor
  - Multiple surgical corridors
- Divide tumor into vascular segments
- Identify midline structures
- Isolate ICA and vascular contributions
  - Vidian artery
- One bleeder at a time
- Staging of surgery
  - Blood loss, coagulopathy
  - Avoid mixing of blood and cerebrospinal fluid

For all JNAs, the surgical strategy consists of dissection around the periphery of the tumor to establish the limits of the tumor, identifying key anatomic landmarks, and minimizing manipulation of the tumor until necessary. Multiple surgical corridors are used, as needed, to gain access to the margins of the tumor: transnasal, transmaxillary, and infratemporal. Most tumors can be excised endoscopically using a combination of endonasal and anterior transmaxillary approaches (Video 1).

For large tumors, it is helpful to divide the tumor into segments corresponding with vascular territories. For example, a large bilateral tumor may have 3 vascular segments corresponding with the ECA on each side and the ICA on 1 side. Each vascular segment is removed sequentially (1 bleed at a time) to limit blood loss and allow staging of the surgery if necessary. Extracranial segments are removed first with identification of skull base landmarks. The vidian artery is the most prominent blood supply from the ICA and is usually approached medially after tumor has been dissected from the walls of the sphenoid sinus and the course of the ICA has been delineated. The vidian nerve travels with the vidian artery through the pterygoid canal at the inferolateral aspect of the sphenoid sinus. Complete removal of tumor requires drilling of the bone of the pterygoid canal to the plane of the ICA (**Fig. 4**).[6] The vidian nerve is a useful landmark for the plane of the petrous ICA.

Intracranial extensions of tumor are removed last after the tumor has been devascularized and orienting landmarks are more apparent (Video 2). If there is a dural opening, it is important to avoid mixing of cerebrospinal fluid and blood because this can result in cerebral vasospasm and postoperative intracranial hypertension. The decision to stage the surgery depends on multiple factors. Excessive blood loss with associated coagulopathy should be corrected before performing intracranial dissection.

SURGICAL TOOLS

- Bipolar electrocautery
- Ultrasonic cautery
  - Harmonic scalpel (Ethicon, Cincinnati, OH)
- Radiofrequency energy
  - Aquamantys (Medtronic Advanced Energy, Minneapolis, MN)
  - Coblation (Smith & Nephew, London, United Kingdom)

Large tumors need to be divided into smaller fragments in order to deliver them and to improve visualization of key anatomic structures. The Harmonic scalpel is a useful device for transection of large angiofibromas (Video 3). It uses ultrasonic energy to

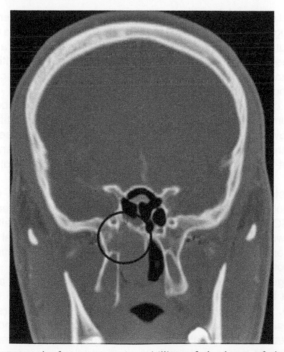

Fig. 4. Complete removal of tumor requires drilling of the bone of the pterygoid base (*circle*) along the course of the vidian nerve.

coagulate the tissue as it cuts. There is less thermal damage to the surrounding tissues compared with standard monopolar electrocautery. The large size of the instrument may require an anterior maxillotomy (sublabial approach) in addition to an endonasal route.

Another technique that has been used effectively for dissection of vascular tumors is coblation.[7,8] Coblation uses radiofrequency energy to disrupt the tissues without generating significant heat. The greatest experience has been with tonsillectomy procedures. Although the experience with coblation for the treatment of angiofibromas is limited, it may offer advantages for endoscopic surgery.

MANAGEMENT OF INTERNAL CAROTID ARTERY

Clinical decisions

- Is the tumor operable?
- Embolization
- What is the best surgical approach?
- Management of ICA
- Blood transfusion/sparing
- Staged operations
- Treatment of residual tumor

There are several clinical decisions to be made as part of the treatment of angiofibromas. For large angiofibromas with skull base erosion, a key decision is management of the ICA. Even tumors that partially envelop the ICA usually have a good plane of dissection. Increased difficulty of dissection is noted in patients with prior surgery/embolization or radiation therapy. In such cases, there is an increased risk of intraoperative injury and leaving residual tumor.

A 14-year-old boy had a transpalatal excision of a JNA 7 years before presentation. Tumor recurrence was missed because of extensive metal artifact from dental braces on a follow-up MRI scan. He was subsequently misdiagnosed with dyslexia because of severe visual loss in both eyes. The MRI scan shows an extensive JNA with encasement of both ICAs and intracranial extension (left middle cranial fossa) (**Fig. 5**).

Visual field testing revealed severe scotomas of both eyes (**Fig. 6**A, B). Angiography after embolization showed extensive tumor blush from feeders from the ICA bilaterally (**Fig. 6**C). Because of tumor encasement of both ICAs, balloon test occlusion of the ICA was performed to assess the adequacy of collateral intracranial circulation in case one of the ICAs was injured and needed to be sacrificed. Symmetric perfusion was noted (**Fig. 6**D).

Staging of surgery was performed because of the extent of tumor and risk of injury to both ICAs. At the first stage, removal of half of the extracranial tumor was performed (**Fig. 7**A). At the second stage, the remainder of the extracranial tumor was removed (see **Fig. 7**B). At a third and final stage, the intracranial tumor was successfully removed (see **Fig. 7**C). Final results are shown with a hypodense area (meningocele) at the site of tumor excision in the left middle cranial fossa (marked with an asterisk).

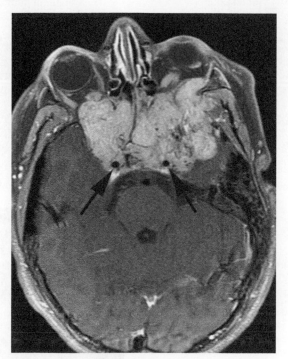

Fig. 5. MRI scan showing an extensive JNA with encasement of both ICAs (*arrows*) and intracranial extension (left middle cranial fossa).

INTERNAL CAROTID ARTERY

- Location of feeding vessels
  - Vidian artery
  - Cavernous sinus
- Endovascular
  - Preoperative embolization?
  - Preoperative sacrifice?
  - Intraoperative balloon occlusion?
- Identification of landmarks
- Dealing with ICA injury

Bleeding from the ICA can be minimized by careful cauterization of feeding vessels, most commonly from the vidian artery and small branches from the cavernous ICA. Although preoperative embolization of branches of the ICA is feasible using temporary distal balloon occlusion, there is a significant risk of a stroke from loss of embolization material into the intracranial circulation. If the risk of ICA injury is increased (tumor encasement, prior surgery/embolization, prior radiation therapy) and the patient has adequate collateral circulation, preoperative sacrifice of the ICA may be considered but has not been necessary in our experience. Intraoperative temporary occlusion of the ICA may also be considered to decrease bleeding from ICA branches while tumor is dissected.

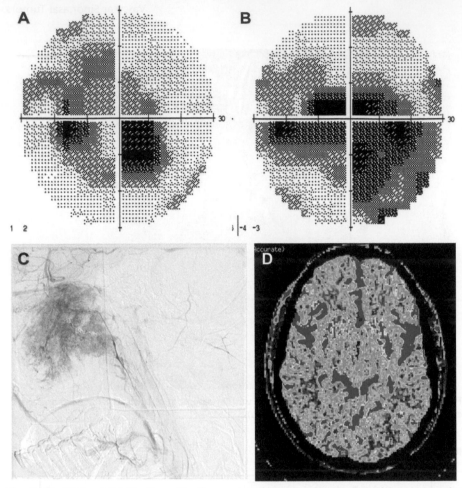

Fig. 6. (*A, B*) Visual field testing of both eyes reveals severe visual defects. (*C*) Angiography after embolization demonstrates marked residual vascularity from the ICA. (*D*) Balloon test occlusion of the ICA demonstrates good collateral circulation.

A graduated surgical experience with strong knowledge of anatomic relationships of the ICA is most important for avoiding catastrophe. Key landmarks include the bony features of the sphenoid sinus and the vidian nerve and canal.[9] Although prevention of injury to the ICA is the best strategy, the surgical team should be prepared for a carotid injury and have treatment protocols in place for such events.

BLOOD-SPARING STRATEGIES

Blood-sparing protocol

• Acute normovolemic hemodilution
  ○ Blood substitutes
  ○ Autotransfusion (maintain connection to patient)

• Tranexamic acid
• Cell-saver system
• Perioperative erythropoietin, iron, and folate
• Hemostatic surgical technique

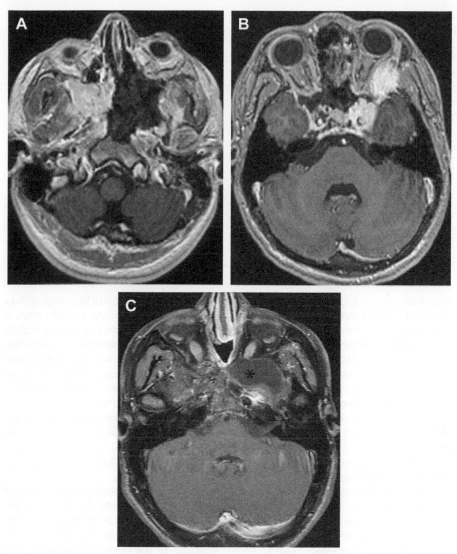

Fig. 7. (*A*) First stage: removal of half of the extracranial tumor. (*B*) Second stage: removal of the remainder of the extracranial tumor. (*C*) Final results are shown with a hypodense area (meningocele) at the site of tumor excision in the left middle cranial fossa (*asterisk*). (*From* Snyderman CH, Pant H, Carrau RL, et al. A new endoscopic staging system for angiofibromas. Arch Otolaryngol Head Neck Surg 2010;136(6):593; with permission.)

In surgeries in which excessive blood loss is anticipated, there are several strategies for minimizing blood loss. These strategies are especially important in pediatric patients with a low blood volume and patients who are unable or unwilling to receive transfusion of blood products. Acute normovolemic hemodilution includes the administration of blood substitutes as well as autotransfusion of the patient's blood that is withdrawn at the beginning of the surgery and reinfused following blood loss. Tranexamic acid (oral, intravenous, and topical) has been used during endoscopic sinus surgery to promote coagulation. Use of the cell saver to salvage blood for reinfusion is not practical in most cases with potential bacterial contamination but might be considered for some aspects of tumor dissection. Postoperative recovery from anemia resulting from operative blood loss can be hastened by the postoperative administration of erythropoietin, iron, and folic acid. In addition, hemostatic surgical technique can minimize the risk of bleeding in the perioperative period.

STAGING OF SURGERY

- Multiple vascular territories
- Excessive blood loss
- Intracranial extension
- Duration of surgery

Staging of surgery should be considered when the ability to complete the surgery may be limited by excessive blood loss or a prolonged surgery. Pediatric patients have a smaller blood volume and can tolerate less blood loss before staging of surgery should be considered. The amount of tolerable blood loss should be established through discussion with the anesthesiologist before surgery. Staging can minimize the risk of coagulopathy from excessive blood loss and the morbidity of excessive fluid and blood replacement. A second-stage surgery can be performed in several days, after body fluids have equilibrated and postoperative anemia has been treated.

Fig. 8 shows an example of a large JNA that was judged inoperable and failed radiation therapy at an outside institution. There is extensive skull base erosion with involvement of both ICAs and intracranial extension (**Fig. 8**A, B). Staging of surgery was planned because of vascular contribution from the ICAs and expected tumor scarring from radiation therapy.

Endoscopic surgical access was augmented with an anteromedial maxillotomy and medial maxillectomy (**Fig. 8**C). The middle fossa component was the last vascular segment removed (**Fig. 8**D). Four surgeries were required to achieve a complete resection because of extensive tumor fibrosis, intraoperative blood loss, and the need for recovery between stages. Tumor invasion of the dura was noted at the time of surgery.

Residual or recurrent tumor in proximity to the ICA can be observed for growth before making a decision about additional therapy. In approximately 50% of cases, no additional growth is observed and involution eventually occurs. If growth is observed, endoscopic surgery or radiosurgery may be considered. In this case, there was tumor invasion of the cavernous sinus and complete tumor excision was not achieved. A small residual (shown at 6 months following surgery) has remained stable without the need for additional therapy (**Fig. 8**E).

SUMMARY

Highly vascular sinonasal tumors such as angiofibromas can be successfully managed through a combination of strategies, including proper preoperative planning, devascularization of the tumor's blood supply, segmentation of surgical dissection,

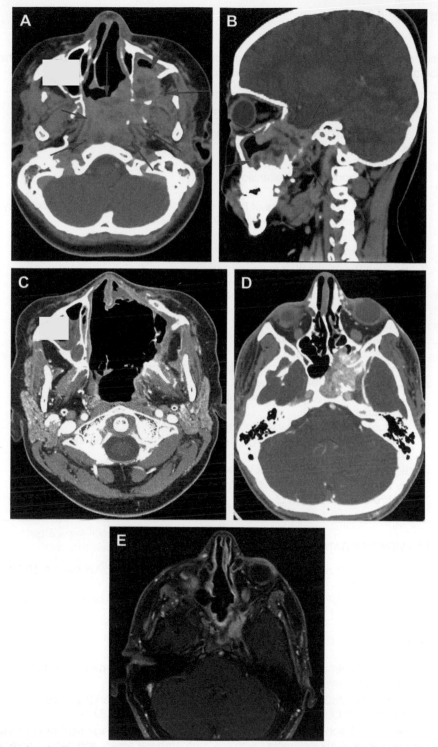

Fig. 8. (*A, B*) Large JNA (*arrows*) that was judged inoperable and failed radiation therapy at an outside institution. (*C*) Staged surgeries including an anteromedial maxillotomy and medial maxillectomy were necessary to achieve resection. (*D*) The middle fossa component was the last vascular segment removed. (*E*) A small residual of tumor in the left cavernous sinus remains without further growth.

staging of surgeries, and blood-sparing techniques. New surgical tools facilitate hemostasis during surgery of vascular tumors.

Post-Test Questions (Correct answers are in italics)

1. What factor differentiates UPMC stage IV JNA from UPMC stage III JNA?
   a. Skull base erosion
   b. Orbital involvement
   c. Infratemporal fossa extension
   d. *Residual vascularity*
2. What is the primary source of blood supply for JNA with residual vascularity following embolization of the internal maxillary artery?
   a. Anterior ethmoid artery
   b. *Vidian artery*
   c. Posterior septal artery
   d. Middle meningeal artery
3. A key landmark for locating the petrous segment of the ICA is:
   a. Foramen rotundum
   b. Lateral optic-carotid recess
   c. *Pterygoid (vidian) canal*
   d. Descending palatine nerve
4. Which of the following is not a blood-sparing strategy:
   a. *Preoperative radiation therapy*
   b. Acute normovolemic hemodilution
   c. Tranexamic acid
   d. Postoperative administration of erythropoietin
5. Valid reasons for staging surgery include all of the following except:
   a. Tumor has multiple vascular territories
   b. Excessive blood loss in a pediatric patient
   c. *Extensive skull base erosion*
   d. Prolonged duration of surgery

SUPPLEMENTARY DATA

Supplementary data related to this article can be found at http://dx.doi.org/10.1016/j.otc.2016.02.009.

Supplementary PDF slides related to this article can be found online at http://www.oto.theclinics.com/.

REFERENCES

1. Onerci M, Ogretmenoglu O, Yucel T. Juvenile nasopharyngeal angiofibroma: a revised staging system. Rhinology 2006;44(1):39–45.
2. Radkowski D, McGill T, Healy GB, et al. Angiofibroma: changes in staging and treatment. Arch Otolaryngol Head Neck Surg 1996;122(2):122–9.
3. Andrews JC, Fisch U, Valavanis A, et al. The surgical management of extensive nasopharyngeal angiofibromas with the infratemporal fossa approach. Laryngoscope 1989;99(4):429–37.
4. Chandler JR, Goulding R, Moskowitz L, et al. Nasopharyngeal angiofibromas: staging and management. Ann Otol Rhinol Laryngol 1984;93(4 Pt 1):322–9.

5. Sessions RB, Bryan RN, Naclerio RM, et al. Radiographic staging of juvenile angio-fibroma. Head Neck Surg 1981;3(4):279–83.
6. Thakar A, Hota A, Bhalla AS, et al. Overt and occult vidian canal involvement in juvenile angiofibroma and its possible impact on recurrence. Head Neck 2015. [Epub ahead of print].
7. Ruiz JW, Saint-Victor S, Tessema B, et al. Coblation assisted endoscopic juvenile nasopharyngeal angiofibroma resection. Int J Pediatr Otorhinolaryngol 2012;76(3): 439–42.
8. Ye L, Zhou X, Li J, et al. Coblation-assisted endonasal endoscopic resection of ju-venile nasopharyngeal angiofibroma. J Laryngol Otol 2011;125(9):940–4.
9. Vescan AD, Snyderman CH, Carrau RL, et al. Vidian canal: analysis and relation-ship to the internal carotid artery. Laryngoscope 2007;117(8):1338–42.

SUGGESTED READINGS

Alshaikh NA, Eleftheriadou A. Juvenile nasopharyngeal angiofibroma staging: An overview. Ear Nose Throat J 2015;94(6):E12–22.

This is a comprehensive review of all staging systems for angiofibromas, high-lighting the advantages and limitations of each system. Although the UPMC stag-ing system was judged to be the most comprehensive regarding prognostic factors, it needs to be further validated by other centers.

Ashour R, Aziz-Sultan A. Preoperative tumor embolization. Neurosurg Clin North Am 2014;25(3):607–17.

This review provides a comprehensive summary of embolization materials and techniques for the management of a variety of vascular tumors, including angio-fibromas. Embolization with Onyx, either by transarterial or direct injection, pro-vided excellent results.

Boghani Z, Husain Q, Kanumori VV, et al. Juvenile nasopharyngeal angiofibroma: a systematic review and comparison of endoscopic, endoscopic-assisted, and open resection in 1047 cases. Laryngoscope 2013;123:859–69.

This is a systematic review of treatment outcomes for JNA comparing endo-scopic, endoscopic-assisted, and open surgical approaches. In this study, endo-scopic resection had decreased blood loss and lower recurrence rate compared with open resection. However, after adjusting for tumor grade (Radkowski/Ses-sions tumor stage), there was no difference in recurrence rates.

Snyderman CH, Pant H, Carrau RL, et al. A new endoscopic staging system for an-giofibromas. Arch Otolaryngol Head Neck Surg 2010;136(6):588–94.

This article proposes a new staging system for JNA that incorporates residual vascularity as a prognostic factor for surgery. The UPMC staging system was su-perior to other staging systems for predicting intraoperative blood loss, residual tumor, and risk of recurrence.

Management of Major Vascular Injury: Open

Samuel A. Tisherman, MD

KEYWORDS

- Hemorrhage • Carotid artery • Vascular surgery • Cancer

KEY LEARNING POINTS

At the end of this article, the reader will:

- Understand the risk factors for vascular injury.
- Be able to identify and classify vascular injuries.
- Know the options for emergency management of vascular injuries.
- Know the options for definitive management of vascular injuries.

INTRODUCTION

> **Why is vascular injury a problem?**
>
> - Major blood vessels are in proximity to other vital structures in the neck and base of skull.
> - Infections and tumors of the head and neck can invade vascular structures.
> - Vascular injuries can lead to massive hemorrhage.
> - Vascular injuries can lead to cerebral ischemia or stroke.
> - Emergency and definitive management can be challenging.

Intraoperative injury to the carotid artery can rapidly lead to exsanguinating hemorrhage. Depending on the location of the injury, vascular control may be straightforward or extremely challenging. Exposure of the carotid artery at the base of the neck or the base of the skull may require a coordinated effort between 2 or 3 surgical subspecialty services. Potential for neurologic injury (ie, stroke) may affect management strategies.

The author has no disclosures related to the content of this article.
Department of Surgery, RA Cowley Shock Trauma Center, University of Maryland School of Medicine, 22 South Greene Street, Baltimore, MD 21201, USA
E-mail address: stisherman@umm.edu

Otolaryngol Clin N Am 49 (2016) 809–817
http://dx.doi.org/10.1016/j.otc.2016.02.004
0030-6665/16/$ – see front matter © 2016 Elsevier Inc. All rights reserved.

Endovascular approaches, if available and feasible, have revolutionized the management of these situations. Open procedures, however, may be necessary or preferable in some circumstances. This article focuses on the open surgical approaches for control of hemorrhage intraoperatively and postoperatively. Open operative management of the carotid blowout is discussed briefly with more in-depth discussion in other articles.

Risk factors for vascular injury

- Tumor in close proximity to carotid artery
- Previous radiation
- Presence of infection
- Previous operations
- Level of surgeon's experience

Intraoperative injury to major vascular structures can be avoided with appropriate preoperative evaluation of the patient and meticulous operative technique. Tumors near vital structures may be amenable to neoadjuvant therapy to shrink the tumor and facilitate the resection. This potential benefit should be weighed against the downside of the tissue changes caused by radiation, however. Previous operations and infections may also add fibrosis that makes the dissection more difficult.

INITIAL RESUSCITATION FROM VASCULAR INJURY

Overview

- Airway management
- Breathing
- Circulation

The management of a life-threatening situation is initially focused on airway, breathing, and circulation. If a patient does not already have an endotracheal tube or surgical airway in place, the airway should be secured in most of these situations. Once airway access is assured, the adequacy of ventilation should be assessed. Bleeding from the oral cavity can enter the airway via the larynx. Bleeding from the neck can enter the airway via a surgical stoma. Significant amounts of blood in the lungs can cause severe hypoxemia. The airway should be aggressively suctioned. Fiberoptic bronchoscopy may be needed to adequately clear the airway.

Management of circulatory compromise from hemorrhage involves simultaneous fluid resuscitation and procedures to achieve hemostasis.

Fluid resuscitation

- Adequate venous access
- Activate massive transfusion protocol
- Transfuse packed red blood cells
- Hemostatic resuscitation

Fluid resuscitation from intraoperative or postoperative hemorrhage should follow the principles of resuscitation from traumatic hemorrhagic shock. Venous access needs to be obtained with at least 2 large-bore catheters. The blood bank should be alerted because there may be a need for large amounts of blood products quickly. Many hospitals have established transfusion protocols in preparation for vascular emergencies. If a patient is hypotensive, that patient has most likely lost at least 30% to 40% of blood volume. Blood products should be administered as soon as possible, using O-negative blood if necessary. If a patient is hypotensive, the goal of fluid resuscitation should be to prevent cardiac arrest but not necessarily to achieve normotension unless cerebral blood flow may be comprised at this time. This permissive hypotension may decrease hemorrhage temporarily but may, in some cases, increase the risk of stroke.

Once bleeding has been controlled, restoring adequate vital organ perfusion as rapidly as possible should be the priority. Recent trauma literature suggests that a hemostatic resuscitation approach, in which fresh frozen plasma and platelets are transfused along with the red cells to prevent dilutional coagulopathy, may be beneficial.[1] The optimal ratio for these products is not clear. All fluids should be warmed during infusion to help prevent hypothermia. The antifibrinolytic agent, tranexamic acid, may also decrease blood loss.

Emergency approach to hemorrhage

- Vascular surgery principles
  - Obtain proximal vascular control
  - Obtain distal vascular control
  - Restore flow as soon as possible
  - Consider temporary vascular shunt to restore cerebral perfusion
  - Assess the injury location and severity
  - Options for definitive management
    - Ligation
    - Repair
    - Bypass
- Zones of the neck (trauma perspective)
  - Zone I: sternal notch to cricoid
  - Zone II: cricoid to angle of mandible
  - Zone III: above the angle of the mandible

If possible, digital pressure directly on the site of injury is helpful while resuscitating the patient and preparing for definitive management. This may not be possible in some situations; focused packing can at least help decrease hemorrhage until adequate exposure is obtained. The most important next step in achieving hemostasis is to obtain vascular control proximal to the site of injury. Vessel loops are placed around the vessel to facilitate the placement of a clamp across the vessel. Exposure of the vessel proximal and distal to the injury may require expeditious dissection and may involve extending the operative field into other body cavities.

Trauma surgeons have defined 3 zones in the neck based on the specific challenges involved in accessing and controlling blood vessels in these zones. In nontrauma situations, these zones remain conceptually helpful for planning a course of action during a crisis.[2]

For injuries in zone I, a sternotomy may be required to obtain proximal control. Immediate assistance from cardiothoracic or trauma surgeons is invaluable. Control of either the innominate artery or the proximal common carotid artery (CCA) is needed.

Vascular control for injuries in zone II is typically more straightforward during a neck dissection. The carotid sheath proximal and distal to the site of injury should be opened to allow direct control of the vessel.

Obtaining control of injuries in zone III, like those in zone I, can be challenging. For injuries to the carotid artery during procedures on the base of the skull, control of the carotid artery in the neck may be necessary. This can be accomplished expeditiously via an incision along the anterior border of the sternocleidomastoid. Once the platysma is divided, the carotid sheath is identified by lateral retraction of the sternocleidomastoid. The carotid sheath is incised and the carotid artery separated from the internal jugular vein and vagus nerve. More distal dissection of the artery can be facilitated by division of the digastric muscle. This exposure allows for separate control of the internal carotid artery (ICA) and external carotid artery (ECA). Care should be taken to avoid injury to the ansa cervicalis and the superior laryngeal, vagus, and hypoglossal nerves. More distal access to the carotid may necessitate subluxation of the mandible or mandibular osteotomy.

A Fogarty catheter can also be advanced distally via the CCA. Balloon inflation can temporarily control more distal hemorrhage. After hemostasis is achieved with this technique, the options include distal dissection from the neck with repair or ligation of the vessel, arteriographic embolization and stenting, or at least 48-hour balloon occlusion if there are no signs of cerebral ischemia. After 48 hours to 72 hours, the balloon is deflated and the patient observed closely for recurrent hemorrhage. A crossover angiogram should be performed to rule out bleeding or pseudoaneurysm formation distal to the original injury. If cerebral ischemia occurs, one option is a cervical ICA to the petrous ICA bypass. Working with a neurosurgeon is essential when managing injuries in this area.

A more direct approach to bleeding at the base of the skill is placement of bone wax directly into the carotid canal.

MONITORING

Surgical procedures on the carotid artery can cause a stroke by:
• Intraoperative ischemia
• Emboli of plaque or air
• Thrombosis
• Conversion of a previous ischemic stroke to a hemorrhagic stroke with reperfusion

While managing active hemorrhage from the carotid artery, there may be no way to avoid the risk of temporary occlusion of the vessel. Unfortunately, the concomitant systemic hypotension only exacerbates the cerebral ischemia.

Tolerance to temporary occlusion of the carotid artery is variable, depending on a patient's anatomy, that is, blood flow within the circle of Willis, duration of occlusion, and systemic blood pressure. For patients who demonstrate high risk of significant cerebral ischemia or who are already demonstrating ischemia, intraoperative temporary vascular shunt can be life-saving.[3] Preoperative CT brain perfusion mapping may identify patients who do not tolerate temporary occlusion well and should have a vascular shunt placed during the procedure. Typically, elective operations on the carotid are conducted under general anesthesia with electroencephalographic monitoring or awake with regional anesthesia. If ischemia is suggested by electroencephalogram (decreased amplitude or slowing of the rhythm) or clinical examination during 3 minutes of test clamping, a vascular shunt can be placed. Measurement of the back pressure in the carotid artery and shunting if the pressure is less than 25 mm Hg is another option. Some investigators also advocate the use of a shunt in patients who have suffered a previous stroke and others advocate shunting all patients. Such monitoring is not typically possible in the emergency situation. At most, the surgeon may be able to measure back pressure in the carotid artery.

Vascular shunts can maintain cerebral blood flow while the surgeon operates on the carotid artery. Shunts, however, are not without risk. The flow through the shunt is not monitored, so the shunt may not actually accomplish what it was meant to do. Also, the shunt itself can injure the intima, increasing the risk of thrombosis. Air and plaque debris are embolized through the shunt. Furthermore, the presence of the shunt can complicate a surgeon's ability to conduct the operation as meticulously as possible.

DAMAGE CONTROL

- Control hemorrhage
- Minimize contamination
- Minimize operative time
- Restore homeostasis in the intensive care unit
- Delayed definitive management

Since the mid-1990s, trauma surgeons have used the term, *damage control surgery*, to describe an operative approach that does not include definitive management of all injuries but focuses only on specific, life-saving procedures. By doing this, a patient who is already in extremis is spared the physiologic cost of an additional operative insult, allowing more rapid restoration of homeostasis.

Specifically, the highest priority with the damage control approach is hemostasis. For arteries, this may involve ligation, shunting, or repair. Most veins are ligated without significant morbidity. Packing of the wound can control small vessel bleeding and most venous bleeding.

Once hemostasis is achieved, the patient is taken to the ICU, where fluid resuscitation is continued and coagulopathy and hypothermia corrected.

SHUNTING

If a shunt is to be used, it is placed expeditiously after the CCA, ICA, and ECA are clamped, and a vertical arteriotomy is performed. The distal tip is advanced into the ICA first. The proximal end is then advanced into the CCA. There are several types of shunts available. They differ in whether or not they remain totally within the vessel or are looped outside the vessel during the procedure.[3]

The shunt is removed when the suture line for closure of the arteriotomy (often with a patch angioplasty) is near complete. Clamps are replaced on the ICA and CCA. The artery is flushed copiously with heparinized saline solution to remove any material that could embolize. The ICA clamp is released to allow back bleeding. It is reclamped while the CCA and ECA clamps are removed to allow debris to be flushed into the ECA distribution. The ICA clamp is then removed as the suture line is completed.

For patients in extremis requiring other emergent procedures or ongoing resuscitation, it is possible to leave a shunt in place for up to 24 hours.

DEFINITIVE MANAGEMENT

Trauma surgeons have significant experience with the management of injuries to the carotid artery. This experience may help with decision making in nontraumatic injuries as well. In trauma patients with a carotid artery injury, clinical examination is critical to operative decision making. If patients have a completed stroke preoperatively, reperfusion carries significant risk of hemorrhagic conversion and little hope of neurologic improvement. Ligation is usually the procedure of choice.[2]

For minor lacerations of the vessel, direct arteriorrhaphy should be undertaken. Simple closure can be accomplished with interrupted monofilament suture if the lumen of the vessel is not compromised. If it is, a patch angioplasty with autogenous vein, bovine pericardium, or prosthetic may be needed. It is important to achieve coaptation of the intima to minimize the risk of microemboli from the repair site.

For more severe injuries, a bypass may be required. This can be accomplished with an autogenous or prosthetic vein graft. Polytetrafluoroethylene is often appropriate for CCA injuries, whereas autogenous vein is a better choice for the ICA due to the size of the vessel and better patency rates. For injuries near the carotid bulb, an ECA to ICA bypass is also an option. The proximal ICA and distal ECA are ligated and the proximal ECA is anastomosed to the distal ICA.

Injury to the ICA at the base of the skull can present significant challenges. If the injury is an avulsion of a small branch, bipolar electrocautery may suffice for achieving hemostasis.[4] For larger injuries, direct suture repair is preferred. If this is not possible, crushed muscle patches have been used with success. If necessary, the ICA is sacrificed using aneurysm clips or packing. Unless test occlusion of the carotid preoperatively demonstrated adequate collateral circulation, ligation of the ICA carries significant risk of stroke. A bypass from the ICA to the middle cerebral artery may be a consideration.

INJURY TO SMALL VESSELS

Operative injury to small arteries usually does not cause significant hemorrhage. On the other hand, ligation of small arteries that supply critical brain structures may lead to significant neurologic deficits. This may occur when dissecting tumors that are near these structures, such as the brainstem or anterior cranial fossa. Care should be taken when retracting these tumors.

INTERNAL CAROTID ARTERY INJURIES DURING ENDONASAL SURGERY

The proximity of the ICA to the sphenoid sinus puts the vessel at risk for injury during endonasal or transsphenoidal procedures. Risk factors include vascular anatomy, previous operations, acromegaly, radiation therapy, and bromocriptine therapy.[5] Preoperative imaging can help define the proximity of the vessel to the planned operative field.

When a vascular injury occurs during endoscopic procedures, maintaining visualization of the operative field becomes challenging. Strategic placement of suction devices and assistance from a second surgeon can help tremendously. The next step is frequently the placement of nasal packing. The resultant hypotension from hemorrhage may help with hemostasis. Achieving normotension before achieving hemostasis, may not be the best strategy. If available, absorbable or biocompatible agents should be used so that removal is unnecessary. Overpacking should be avoided because the resultant occlusion or stenosis may increase the risk of stroke or death. Direct suture repair or placement of a surgical clip may be successful. Endovascular approaches, if available, are the next step. Further information on this topic is discussed elsewhere in this issue (see Jovin T, Aghaebrahim A: Endovascular Management of Diseases in Relation to Otolaryngology, in this issue).

Delayed hemorrhage can also occur from a pseudoaneurysm of the ICA. Packing may help, but endovascular stent placement is usually the procedure of choice. Rarely, an extracranial to intracranial graft is indicated.

POSTOPERATIVE HEMORRHAGE

After extensive operative dissections, postoperative bleeding is not uncommon.[6] If the bleeding seems to be from a subcutaneous vessel at the wound edges, direct pressure, sutures, or infiltration with an anesthetic and epinephrine can control the bleeding. A slowly enlarging hematoma is likely of venous origin. Milking of the drains may suffice to release the hematoma and promote hemostasis by reapproximation of the tissues. If the bleeding is causing recurrent ballooning of the skin flaps after milking the drains or active bleeding through the skin closure, re-exploration to rule out a more significant vascular injury is indicated.

CAROTID ARTERY BLOWOUT

Types of carotid blowout syndromes[6]

- Threatened blowout because of exposure of the carotid
- Impending blowout with minor, sentinel bleeding episodes
- Active hemorrhage

Patients who suffer a carotid blowout have often undergone radiation therapy, have nodal disease, or have undergone a neck dissection. A salivary fistula is a major contributing factor as are wound infection and soft tissue necrosis. The rupture typically occurs in the CCA. Patients may first present with the so-called sentinel bleed or may present with immediately life-threatening massive hemorrhage.

Bleeding may be external or internal (into the hypopharynx or mouth). If possible, direct pressure with a finger on the site of hemorrhage is the best temporizing maneuver. Large, bulky dressings are not effective and only tend to cover up the amount of bleeding. Passing a Fogarty catheter through the site of rupture and inflating the balloon may help temporize, allowing the surgeon to obtain vascular control. Aggressive fluid and blood product administration, along with airway protection, are the key principles for initial resuscitation.

Endovascular approaches to control bleeding with embolization or stent placement are preferable to open approaches because there is less morbidity, such as damage to nearby nerves and veins or stroke, and mortality.[7] A stent may be preferable to embolization in patients who fail a balloon occlusion test of the carotid, have an incomplete circle of Willis, or have significant carotid disease on the contralateral side. If a patient is unstable or this approach fails, an open procedure is needed. Vessel ligation is the next best life-saving choice. Repairing the vessel is usually impossible in this situation.

After either an endovascular procedure or ligation, anticoagulation postoperatively may be appropriate to prevent clot propagation. Patients may also require flap coverage of the wound.

SUMMARY

Emergency management of vascular injuries during operations in the neck or base of skull involves airway management, fluid resuscitation, and hemostasis. Handling injuries within the skull base, high in the neck, or just above the thoracic inlet can pose significant challenges. Ultimately, the decisions regarding definitive management should include the timing of the recognition of the injury (intraoperative, postoperatgive, or carotid blowout), any delay in recognition, neurologic examination (if available), information regarding collateral circulation, wound infection, previous radiation therapy, and overall prognosis. Coordination between subspecialty surgical teams is critical.

Post-Test Questions (Correct answers are in italics)

1. For a patient who is bleeding from the carotid artery intraoperatively, the best initial management of the bleeding is
   a. Placing vessel loops around the artery distal to the injury
   b. Directly repairing the injury
   c. *Applying digital pressure to the bleeding site*
   d. Placing vessel loops around the artery proximal to the injury.
2. Which procedure is most helpful for attaining proximal vascular control in a patient who has suffered an injury to the CCA just above the clavicle?
   a. *Median sternotomy*
   b. Left thoracotomy
   c. Supraclavicular incision
   d. Mandibular osteotomy
3. Using trauma terminology, an injury to the ICA at the base of the skull is in zone
   a. I
   b. II
   c. *III*
   d. IV
4. The best test for determining if a patient will develop a stroke after ligation of the ICA is
   a. Ligating the artery and examining the patient postoperatively
   b. Monitoring somatosensory evoked potentials during test occlusion of the artery
   c. *Monitoring continuous electroencephalography intraoperatively*
   d. Monitoring pupil responsivity intraoperatively

SUPPLEMENTARY DATA

Supplementary PDF slides related to this article can be found online at http://www.oto.theclinics.com/.

REFERENCES

1. Holcomb JB, Tilley BC, Baraniuk S, et al. Transfusion of Plasma, Platelets, and Red Blood Cells in a 1:1:1 vs a 1:1:2 Ratio and Mortality in Patients With Severe Trauma. The PROPPR Randomized Clinical Trial. JAMA 2015;313(5):471–82.
2. Knipp BS, Gillespie DL. Vascular trauma. In: Moore WS, editor. Vascular and endovascular surgery. A comprehensive review. 8th edition. Philadelphia: Elsevier Saunders; 2013. p. 721–53.
3. Moore WS. Extracranial cerebrovascular disease. In: Moore WS, editor. Vascular and endovascular surgery. A comprehensive review. 8th edition. Philadelphia: Elsevier Saunders; 2013. p. 328–68.

4. Pinheiro-Neto CD, Snyderman CH, Gardner PA. Cranial base surgery. In: Johnson J, Rosen C, editors. Bailey's head and neck surgery-otolaryngology, 2 volume set. 5th edition. Philadelphia: Lippincott Williams & Wilkins; 2014.
5. Valentine R, Wormald PJ. Carotid artery injury after endonasal surgery. Otolaryngol Clin North Am 2011;44(5):1059–79.
6. Medina JE, Vasan NR. Neck dissection. In: Johnson J, Rosen C, editors. Bailey's head and neck surgery-otolaryngology, 2 volume set. 5th edition. Philadelphia: Lippincott Williams & Wilkins; 2014.
7. Rimmer J, Giddings CE, Vaz F, et al. Management of vascular complications of head and neck cancer. J Laryngol Otol 2012;126(2):111–5.

SUGGESTED READINGS

Valentine R, Wormald PJ. Carotid artery injury after endonasal surgery. Otolaryngol Clin North Am 2011;44(5):1059–79.

This paper describes the risk factors for carotid artery injury during endonasal injury and how to minimize the risk. Once an injury occurs, they describe approaches for achieving hemostasis and definitive management.

Rimmer J, Giddings CE, Vaz F, et al. Management of vascular complications of head and neck cancer. J Laryngol Otol 2012;126(2):111–5.

Through a series of cases, this paper describes the evaluation and management of several vascular complications of head and neck cancer.

Management of Major Vascular Injury During Endoscopic Endonasal Skull Base Surgery

Paul A. Gardner, MD[a],*, Carl H. Snyderman, MD, MBA[a,b],
Juan C. Fernandez-Miranda, MD[a], Brian T. Jankowitz, MD[a]

KEYWORDS

- Endoscopic skull base surgery • Internal carotid artery • Pseudoaneurysm
- Vascular injury

KEY LEARNING POINTS

At the end of this article, the reader will:

- Understand how major vasculature can be evaluated preoperatively.
- Understand how ischemia can be evaluated intraoperatively.
- Know which tumor types are at greatest risk for internal carotid artery (ICA) injury during endoscopic endonasal skull base surgery (ESBS).
- Know what techniques can be used to preserve a vessel injury during ESBS.
- Be able to determine if bleeding from the ICA or circle of Willis can be controlled during ESBS.
- Know how and when arteries can be evaluated following injury.
- Be able to identify the endovascular adjuncts that are currently available following vascular injury.

INTRODUCTION

The endoscopic endonasal approach to the ventral skull base has gained popularity over the past decade. Through collaboration between otolaryngologists and neurosurgeons, these approaches have provided increasingly expanded access to the skull base, in modules that extend from the crista galli to the odontoid process and laterally

Disclosure Statement: The authors have no conflict of interest to disclose.
[a] Department of Neurological Surgery, University of Pittsburgh School of Medicine, 200 Lothrop Street, PUH B-400, Pittsburgh, PA 15213, USA; [b] Department of Otolaryngology, University of Pittsburgh School of Medicine, 200 Lothrop Street, EEI 500, Pittsburgh, PA 15213, USA
* Corresponding author.
E-mail address: gardpa@upmc.edu

Otolaryngol Clin N Am 49 (2016) 819–828
http://dx.doi.org/10.1016/j.otc.2016.03.003
0030-6665/16/$ – see front matter © 2016 Elsevier Inc. All rights reserved.

oto.theclinics.com

to the cavernous sinus, middle fossa, and orbit. Great advances have been made in instrumentation and reconstruction to allow the progression of these approaches.

During any surgery involving the skull base, surgeons must have anatomic knowledge of the internal carotid artery (ICA) with respect to the operative field and have strategies for dealing with inadvertent injury to this and other major vessels of the circle of Willis. There remains significant concern about the ability to manage such injuries when working with an endoscope through limited openings such as "keyhole" craniotomies or through the paranasal sinuses.

INJURY AVOIDANCE

> - The best strategy for dealing with major vessels is to avoid injury.
> - Understand the anatomic landmarks and course of the arteries and recognize how an individual tumor may have affected the anatomic location of the vessel.
> - For the ICA, there are well-established landmarks to its various segments from an endonasal perspective.

Segment of internal carotid artery and anatomic landmark	
Segment of ICA	Anatomic Landmark
Paraclinoid	Medial opticocarotid recess[1]
Anterior genu	Medial pterygoid plate/wedge[2]
Horizontal petrous	Vidian nerve[2]
Ascending/parapharyngeal	Eustachian tube[3]

> All tumors of the skull base have the potential to
>
> - Encapsulate
> - Invade
> - Displace the ICA

Cavernous and petroclival meningiomas can encircle the cavernous or petrous ICA and basilar artery, with narrowing of the vessel or invasion of the adventitia (**Fig. 1**). Pituitary adenomas can invade the cavernous sinus and encircle the ICA, but do not tend to invade the adventitia. Chondroid tumors, such as chordomas and chondrosarcomas, can significantly displace the ICA or basilar artery. Rarely, they can weaken or invade the adventitia (**Fig. 2**). Chondroid tumors were the most common tumor type injured during endonasal skull base surgery (ESBS) in the authors' series of more than 2000 patients.[4] Juvenile nasal angiofibromas (JNAs) frequently derive blood supply from the cavernous ICA via branches such as the vidian artery (**Fig. 3**) but are rarely adherent to the ICA. Nasopharyngeal and other paranasal sinus carcinomas can invade soft tissue or bone up to or surrounding the ICA. Rarely, this can lead to rupture of the vessel, especially following radiation therapy.

Technologies that can be used intraoperatively to localize the ICA and prevent its injury include the following:

- Doppler ultrasound
- Navigation or image guidance
- Computed tomographic (CT) angiography, which is best for evaluating major vasculature

---

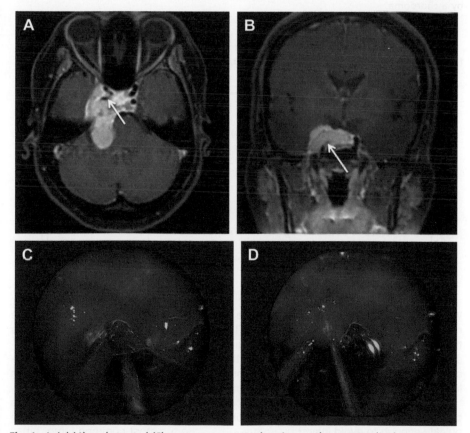

Fig. 1. Axial (*A*) and coronal (*B*) postcontrast MRI showing a sphenopetroclival meningioma with encasement, displacement, and narrowing of the right ICA (*arrows*). (*C*) Intraoperative injury of the right ICA during resection of the petroclival meningioma. This was controlled with an aneurysm clip without sequelae (*D*). Doppler is used to confirm flow in the preserved ICA after clipping.

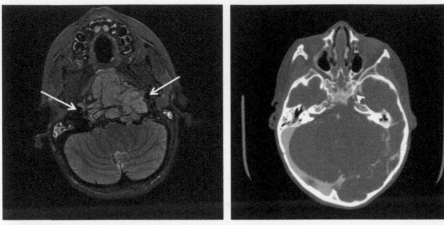

Fig. 2. Preoperative T2 MRI and CT angiogram showing involvement of bilateral parapharyngeal ICAs (*arrows*) and displacement and narrowing of the left petrous ICA (*arrowhead*) by a chordoma.

MANAGEMENT STRATEGIES FOR CONTROLLING ARTERIAL INJURY

1. Sacrifice
   a. Approximately 80% patients will initially tolerate ICA sacrifice
   b. Role of balloon test occlusion (BTO) and neurophysiological monitoring

2. Bypass
   a. Prophylactic
   b. Emergent

3. Vessel preservation techniques
   a. Bipolar electrocautery
   b. Aneurysm clips
   c. Muscle or other packing
   d. Suture

When considering sacrifice, preoperative ICA testing with BTO or intraoperative neurophysiologic monitoring is helpful. BTO is recommended for recurrent tumors that may invade the artery wall (ie, meningiomas, chordomas). The addition of perfusion study during the BTO can risk-stratify those patients who clinically tolerate occlusion. Most patients (80%–87%) will initially tolerate ICA sacrifice, based on intraoperative carotid endarterectomy shunting studies.[5,6]

Bypass surgery is best used prophylactically when the patient has failed BTO or has borderline perfusion. Emergent bypass following injury often cannot be performed quickly enough to avoid infarct.

Vessel preservation techniques are designed to control bleeding while maintaining flow within the ICA. These strategies include sealing of the edges with bipolar electrocautery, placement of aneurysm clips, direct suture repair, and nonocclusive packing. Endonasal suturing is generally not feasible for most ICA injuries because of the inherent limitations posed by the location of vessel, access, and nature of injury.

Any arterial injury, regardless of approach, should be managed by

- Localizing and controlling the site of bleeding (often with a cottonoid and suction)
- Gaining proximal and distal control
- Increasing exposure to better identify the injury

Muscle can be harvested from abdominal rectus, sternocleidomastoid, or temporalis muscle. Crushing the muscle graft releases calcium that may promote the initial fibrin plug and improve arterial wall healing.[7]

Advantages of team surgery

- Dynamic endoscopy allows close visualization of site of bleeding while maintaining a view, even if the endoscope is contaminated repeatedly with blood.
- Maintaining calm during a major, stressful complication.
- Troubleshooting and problem-solving.

Working as a team is essential for controlling a major endonasal vascular injury.

NEUROPHYSIOLOGIC MONITORING AND ITS ROLE DURING VASCULAR INJURY

Somatosensory evoked potentials and electroencephalography monitoring can provide surrogate information for BTO in the setting of an intraoperative injury. Surrogate information includes the following:

- A general idea on the distribution of hemispheric ischemia
- A guide for intraoperative and immediate postoperative management.
- Determination about whether the vessel can be sacrificed without stroke-related morbidity or whether it must be preserved.

The tests can be performed with the vessel controlled or occluded under hypotensive conditions to evaluate a perfusion deficit. However, active bleeding can lead to a transient decrement in evoked potentials which does not clearly predict impact of sacrifice; therefore, testing for necessity of preservation should be done after bleeding is controlled.

ENDOVASCULAR EVALUATION AND MANAGEMENT OF MAJOR VASCULAR INJURY

An immediate postoperative digital subtracted angiogram (DSA) should be performed before waking the patient.

Further vascular evaluation should be performed at least a week after injury to ensure that no pseudoaneurysm has formed, even if the initial DSA is normal. CT

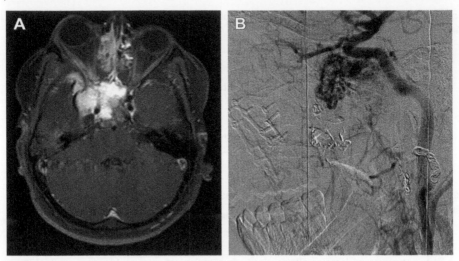

Fig. 3. (*A*) Preoperative, postcontrast axial MRI showing encasement of the right ICA by a JNA. (*B*) ICA injection following tumor embolization showing significant residual vascularity from the involved ICA.

angiography can be used for future evaluation, although DSA remains the gold standard.

Pseudoaneurysm formation is common and follow-up imaging for up to 6 months postoperatively should include vascular imaging (CT angiography, MR angiography, DSA).

Reasons for endovascular salvage
• Active extravasation
• Pseudoaneurysm
• ICA stenosis from packing

Endovascular treatment options vary depending on the injury and patient anatomy/physiology. For patients with active extravasation on a postoperative angiogram, immediate treatment is mandated. Options include pseudoaneurysm treatment with coils or a liquid embolic, ICA occlusion (if patient has visible collaterals and passes a balloon test occlusion with neurophysiologic monitoring or awake evaluation with provocative hypotension), OR flow diverson/covered stenting. Finally, critical stenosis (>50% or resulting in delayed distal flow) can be treated with observation, balloon angioplasty, or stenting.

INTERNAL CAROTID ARTERY INJURY MANAGEMENT ALGORITHM

The algorithm in **Fig. 4** is based on the authors' experience with ICA injury during ESBS.[4]

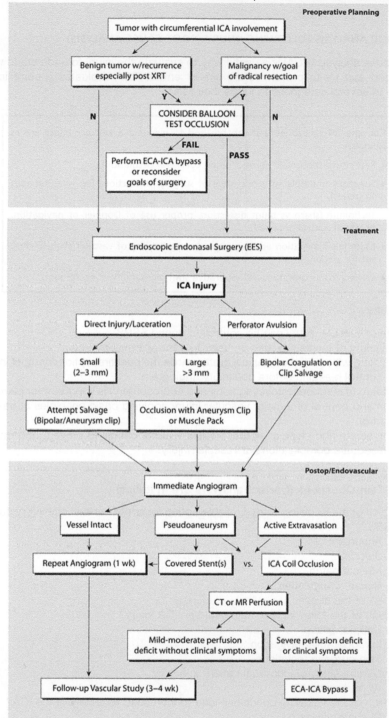

Fig. 4. ICA injury management algorithm. ECA, external carotid artery; ICA, internal carotid artery; XRT, radiation therapy. (*From* Gardner PA, Tormenti MJ, Pant H, et al. Carotid artery injury during endoscopic endonasal skull base surgery: incidence and outcomes. Neurosurgery 2013;73(2 Suppl Operative):ons267; with permission.)

POST-HOC ANALYSIS FOLLOWING INJURY (ROOT CAUSE ANALYSIS)

Root cause analysis (RCA) is a useful way to evaluate the injury to understand why it happened and try to prevent future similar errors. RCA evaluates a complication looking at several categories to judge their role.

Examples of categories that can be used to evaluate a vascular injury are as follows:

- Patient (tortuous ICA, fibrotic tumor, collateral circulation)
- Surgeons (multiple surgeons, goal of surgery, distractions [eg, simultaneous surgeries])
- Technique (sharp vs blunt dissection, proper use of Doppler or navigation, proximal control obtained)
- Materials (navigation accuracy, Doppler, availability of vascular clamps, clips, suture, packing)
- Process (communication with operative staff, availability of equipment)

SUMMARY

- Major vascular injury can be controlled during ESBS.
- A variety of techniques can be used to control a major injury.
- Packing with a crushed muscle graft may be the best first option for most injuries to control bleeding before postinjury angiogram.
- A team of surgeons (otolaryngology and neurosurgery) is important for identification and control of a major vascular injury applying basic principles of vascular control.
- Immediate and close angiographic follow-up is critical to prevent and manage subsequent complications of vascular injury.

Post-Test Questions (Correct answers are in italics)

1. Which of the following is not a reliable option for control of vascular injury during ESBS?
   a. Aneurysm clip
   b. *Suturing*
   c. Muscle patch
   d. Bipolar coagulation
   e. All of the above
2. Which of the following can help avoid an ICA injury?
   a. Doppler probe
   b. Intraoperative navigation
   c. Two-surgeon technique
   d. Careful study of individual patient anatomy
   e. *All of the above*
3. Which of the following conditions lead to increased tortuosity of the ICA?
   a. Cushing disease
   b. Esthesioneuroblastoma
   c. Juvenile nasal angiofibroma
   d. *Acromegaly*

4. Which of the following are possible sequelae of ICA injury?
   a. Stenosis
   b. Distal embolus
   c. Nasoseptal flap infarct
   d. Pseudoaneurysm
   e. *a, b, and d*
5. Which of the following is a critical anatomic relationship for ICA identification?
   a. The lateral OCR is pneumatization of the optic strut.
   b. *The vidian nerve crosses the horizontal petrous ICA.*
   c. The vidian nerve and maxillary nerve converge on Meckel cave.
   d. The sphenopalatine artery can be found behind the crista ethmoidalis.

SUPPLEMENTARY DATA

Supplementary PDF slides related to this article can be found online at http://www.
oto.theclinics.com/.

REFERENCES

1. Fernandez-Miranda JC, Prevedello DM, Madhok R, et al. Sphenoid septations and their relationship with internal carotid arteries: anatomical and radiological study. Laryngoscope 2009;119(10):1893–6.
2. Vescan AD, Snyderman CH, Carrau RL, et al. Vidian canal: analysis and relationship to the internal carotid artery. Laryngoscope 2007;117(8):1338–42.
3. Ozturk K, Snyderman CH, Gardner PA, et al. The anatomical relationship between the Eustachian tube and petrous internal carotid artery. Laryngoscope 2012; 122(12):2658–62.
4. Gardner PA, Tormenti MJ, Pant H, et al. Carotid artery injury during endoscopic endonasal skull base surgery: incidence and outcomes. Neurosurgery 2013;73(2 Suppl Operative):ons261–9.
5. Modica PA, Tempelhoff R, Rich KM, et al. Computerized electroencephalographic monitoring and selective shunting: influence on intraoperative administration of phenylephrine and myocardial infarction after general anesthesia for carotid endarterectomy. Neurosurgery 1992;30(6):842–6.
6. Plestis KA, Loubser P, Mizrahi EM, et al. Continuous electroencephalographic monitoring and selective shunting reduces neurologic morbidity rates in carotid endarterectomy. J Vasc Surg 1997;25(4):620–8.
7. Padhye V, Valentine R, Paramasivan S, et al. Early and late complications of endoscopic hemostatic techniques following different carotid artery injury characteristics. Int Forum Allergy Rhinol 2014;4(8):651–7.

SUGGESTED READINGS

AlQahtani A, Castelnuovo P, Nicolai P, et al. Injury of the internal carotid artery during endoscopic skull base surgery: prevention and management protocol. Otolaryngol Clin North Am 2016;49(1):237–52.
   The authors describe their approach to the prevention and management of ICA injuries during ESBS.

Chin OY, Ghosh R, Fang CH, et al. Internal carotid artery injury in endoscopic endonasal surgery: a systematic review. Laryngoscope 2016;126(3):582–90.

This is a systematic review of ICA injuries during endoscopic endonasal surgery, including sinus surgery and skull base surgery. Twenty-five articles with 50 cases were included in this review. The most commonly injured ICA segment was the cavernous (34 cases) segment. Injuries occurred more commonly on the left (1.3:1). Initial hemostasis was achieved with packing in 35 cases, endoscopic clip sacrifice in 4 cases, bipolar coagulation with the intent to seal defect in 3 cases, and bipolar coagulation with the intent to sacrifice the ICA in 1 case.

Gardner PA, Tormenti MJ, Pant H, et al. Carotid artery injury during endoscopic endonasal skull base surgery: incidence and outcomes. Neurosurgery 2013;73(2 Suppl Operative):ons261–9.

This article describes the authors' collective experience with ICA injuries during ESBS. Most injuries involved the left paraclival ICA. Risk factors include a diagnosis of chondroid neoplasm. A treatment strategy with algorithm is presented for the management of small and large vascular injuries.

Padhye V, Valentine R, Paramasivan S, et al. Early and late complications of endoscopic hemostatic techniques following different carotid artery injury characteristics. Int Forum Allergy Rhinol 2014;4(8):651–7.

This study compares the efficacy of the muscle patch, bipolar diathermy, and aneurysm clip on hemostasis, pseudoaneurysm formation, and long-term vessel patency for different injury types in a sheep model of carotid bleeding. Standardized linear, punch, and stellate injuries were made. Randomization of sheep to receive 1 of 3 hemostatic techniques was performed (muscle, bipolar, clip). This study shows that the crushed muscle patch and aneurysm clip can be viable options in the management of ICA injury with short-term and long-term benefits. Complications associated with these techniques were comparable if not reduced when compared with the published literature.

Management of Carotid Blowout from Radiation Necrosis

John Gleysteen, MD[a], Daniel Clayburgh, MD, PhD[a],
James Cohen, MD, PhD[b],*

KEYWORDS

- Carotid blowout • Endovascular • Radiation complication

KEY LEARNING POINTS

At the end of this article, the reader will:

- Understand the main risk factors for the development of carotid blowout syndrome.
- Understand how carotid blowout syndrome can be prevented.
- Recognize the difference between threatened and impending carotid blowout syndrome.
- Appreciate the role of computed tomography in the management of carotid blowout syndrome.
- Understand the role of angiography in the management of carotid blowout syndrome.
- Define the role of surgery in the management of carotid blowout syndrome.

Carotid blowout syndrome (CBS) remains one of the most serious and dramatic complications of head and neck surgery. Prevention of the syndrome is paramount and is primarily accomplished by prophylactic coverage of the major vasculature with well-vascularized tissue, especially in an irradiated field. Modern reconstructive techniques have therefore significantly decreased its occurrence and the development of endovascular techniques has significantly altered its management, with an associated decrease in short-term morbidity and mortality.[1–3] However, the long-term mortality of patients experiencing this complication remains essentially unchanged because it usually occurs in the setting of recurrent and/or uncontrolled tumors in the head and neck region.[4]

Disclosures: The authors have no financial or nonfinancial relationships to disclose.
[a] Department of Otolaryngology/Head and Neck Surgery, Portland VA Medical Center, Oregon Health Sciences University, Portland, OR, USA; [b] ENT, Department of Otolaryngology/Head and Neck Surgery, Portland VA Medical Center, Oregon Health Sciences University, P3-OC, 3710 Southwest US Veteran's Hospital Road, Portland, OR 97239, USA
* Corresponding author.
E-mail address: James.Cohen2@va.gov

Otolaryngol Clin N Am 49 (2016) 829–839
http://dx.doi.org/10.1016/j.otc.2016.02.001
0030-6665/16/$ – see front matter Published by Elsevier Inc.

oto.theclinics.com

This article outlines a practical and rational approach to this problem, incorporating modern diagnostic and therapeutic techniques that can be applied to any patient in whom this possible complication is considered.

The most effective management of CBS is preventing it from developing in the first place. Although some cases are inevitable, recognition of the long-term risk of CBS at the time of patients' primary or salvage surgery may steer surgeons toward the use of various reconstructive techniques that may prevent CBS from developing. As mentioned previously, the incidence of CBS has been decreasing with the development of more modern surgical techniques. The shift from true radical neck dissection to selective neck dissection with preservation of the internal jugular vein (IJV) and/or the sternocleidomastoid muscle (SCM) over the past few decades has resulted in fewer patients with the carotid artery covered only by the skin and platysma muscle.[1,5] When a radical neck dissection is needed and both the IJV and SCM are sacrificed, placement of a pectoralis flap or a fasciocutaneous free flap into the neck may provide coverage of the carotid with healthy vascularized tissue and prevent the development of CBS.[6] Similarly, it has been shown that use of either a pectoralis overlay flap or an interposed fasciocutaneous free flap for pharyngeal closure after salvage laryngectomy is superior to primary closure in reducing fistula formation,[7] which is a key risk factor for the development of CBS. Thus, every effort should be made at the time of surgery to provide well-vascularized tissue coverage of the carotid artery, particularly in previously irradiated patients. Despite this, there is a subset of patients who inevitably develop CBS (**Table 1**).

Patients facing this potential complication generally present in one of 3 different categories. Perhaps most common are patients who have an exposed carotid artery in the neck, from prior surgery, wound breakdown, or tumor, but no history of bleeding. This condition has been termed threatened carotid blowout. The second group, termed impending carotid blowout, are patients with the same physical findings as group 1 but who have also experienced a self-limited bleeding event (sentinel bleed) thought to have arisen from the carotid artery system. The third group is the patients who present with active carotid bleed or carotid rupture. With this group, diagnosis is straightforward and clinicians proceed directly to active management (discussed later). In the threatened and impending groups, decision making can be more difficult because the likelihood that carotid bleeding will occur or has occurred and the degree to which further diagnostic and therapeutic strategies are needed must be determined.

Factors associated with CBS
• Prior radiotherapy
• Prior radical neck dissection
• Mucocutaneous fistula
• Flap necrosis
• Wound infection
• Poor nutrition or compromised wound healing
• Recurrent tumor

Carotid blowout is almost exclusively associated with patients who have undergone prior radiation therapy, although prior neck dissection, mucocutaneous

Table 1
Classification of CBS

Category	Definition
Threatened carotid blowout	Exposed carotid artery, no evidence of bleeding
Impending carotid blowout	Exposed carotid artery with self-limited sentinel bleed
Active carotid blowout	Massive hemorrhage from exposed carotid artery

fistula, flap necrosis, wound infection, poor nutrition/unhealthy supporting tissue, and recurrent tumor are also strongly associated.[1,4] Therefore, when evaluating a patient with suspected CBS, the presence or absence of these risk factors must be evaluated. The amount of prior radiation (risk is proportional to dose), the radiation ports (was the carotid artery in the port?), and the period of time since irradiation (risk is higher with a longer period of time after irradiation because tissue devascularization increases with time) should be determined.[8,9] If there has been a prior neck dissection, knowledge of whether the carotid sheath was opened (risk increased[5]), whether the IJV was taken (if present, the IJV is a possible source of bleeding[10,11]), and whether there was close proximity of the tumor to the carotid wall helps determine risk and what vessels are most likely involved. If the patient has had prior removal of an upper aerodigestive tract malignancy, knowledge of the primary site and whether there was/is a postoperative mucocutaneous fistula or wound breakdown is important. History of a prior tracheotomy raises the possibility that a tracheoinnominate fistula exists. If recurrent tumor is present, its location is important in determining the possible site of bleeding and the tumor prognosis is important as a context for future decision making about the aggressiveness of management (**Table 2**).

It can be challenging to determine whether or not a sentinel bleed has occurred. Patients often report small amounts of blood in their saliva/tracheal secretions or wound drainage and these may or may not be significant. Questioning the patient as to the chronology and amount of bleeding, whether it was pulsatile, and whether the bleeding was in their mouth, airway, or both is important in determining the likelihood that a bleed from the head and neck vasculature has occurred. It must be differentiated from other sources such as wound granulation tissue, ulcerated tumor, tracheal mucosa, or gastrointestinal mucosa that could be responsible for the bleeding. If a

Table 2
Initial assessment of suspected CBS

History	Physical Examination
Chronology of bleeding?	Vital signs/hemodynamic stability?
Amount of bleeding?	Presence and location of fistula?
Blood in saliva/tracheal secretions/neck wound?	External wound breakdown?
Presence of fistula?	Carotid exposure?
Previous neck dissection? Vessels preserved?	Tumor recurrence?
Previous radiation? Dose and elapsed time?	Status of tracheal mucosa/blood in the airway?
Presence of tracheostomy?	Blood or clot present in neck wound?
Previous microvascular reconstruction?	—
Oncologic prognosis and comorbidities?	—

tracheotomy is present, the clinician should try to ascertain whether bleeding has come through or around the tube. In addition, if a microvascular free flap reconstruction has been performed, it is important to know the vessel that was used in the anastomosis and whether it is viable, because this may influence subsequent decisions to sacrifice or stent vasculature.

Physical examination is directed toward ascertaining hemodynamic stability, the status of the patient's airway, the presence of tumor, the presence of a mucocutaneous fistula and its proximity to the carotid vasculature, and any wound breakdown. The presence or absence of blood in the neck wound, oral cavity, pharynx, or airway should be noted to determine the possible site of the bleeding. If significant clot is present in the neck it should not be disrupted before subsequent investigations. If a tracheostomy exists, the presence of blood in the airway and the status of the tracheal mucosa are important. Particular attention should be paid to the anterior tracheal mucosa at the site of the innominate artery. Flexible endoscopy through the nose, tracheostomy, and/or fistula should be performed as indicated.

Key points guiding evaluation and management of CBS

- Is the patient at high risk for carotid blowout based on the history and examination?
- Has a sentinel bleed occurred?
  - If so, which vessel is most likely involved?
  - Can this vessel be sacrificed?
- Is the patient's airway secure or easily secured?
- What is the patient's overall prognosis from the cancer and comorbidities?

Preliminary investigations should include hemoglobin level and hematocrit to determine the extent of blood loss, blood urea nitrogen and serum creatinine levels to determine the risk of contrast administration with subsequent radiologic studies, and a type and cross for blood products if active bleeding has occurred. With this information, clinicians should be able to answer several critical questions and determine the need for, and nature of, subsequent management.

Low-risk patients with carotid exposure only may be initially observed with local wound care while planning for potential procedures to provide coverage for the exposed vessel. High-risk patients with a compelling history for a sentinel bleed need subsequent investigation after medical stabilization. This investigation should include establishing large-bore intravenous access, fluid resuscitation, securing of the airway, and a type and cross for a sufficient amount of blood products should rebleeding occur. These steps should not be bypassed regardless of the perceived risk of impending or active bleeding, which can nearly always be controlled with pressure while these crucial steps occur. Experience has shown that short-term overall morbidity/mortality is related to hemodynamic instability during the course of patient work-up and management rather than the overall amount of bleeding[11,12]; thus, rapid stabilization with temporary control of the bleeding is critical before moving on to definitive management of the hemorrhage (**Figs. 1** and **2**).

In stabilized and nonbleeding patients, the author's preferred next step is a computed tomography (CT) scan with contrast of the neck. The primary focus of this imaging study is to determine the proximity between any fistulous tract or tumor and the neck vasculature, which could indicate a bleeding source. The air contained

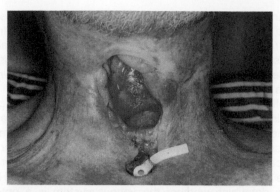

Fig. 1. External appearance of a patient with a large pharyngocutaneous fistula and history of a sentinel bleed.

within the wound/fistula helps to outline this relationship. This information is sometimes necessary in making the final determination about a patient being high or low risk for CBS (and thus the need for angiography) when the history and physical examination are indeterminate. If there is significant soft tissue between the air shadow of a fistula or wound and the vessels, this may suggest the patient is at low risk for CBS. It

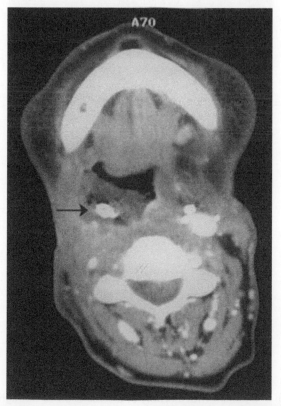

Fig. 2. Computed tomography (CT) scan of the same patient showing the right common carotid artery (*arrow*) surrounded by air and debris in the fistulous tract.

can also determine which vessels (carotid, IJV, or other named vessels) are still present and may be involved in bleeding. This information may be extremely helpful in directing angiography to the appropriate site. Even though the addition of a CT scan with contrast adds to the overall contrast load that patients must receive in their management, the information gained and the potential for streamlining the angiography sequences is worth the added risk to the patients (**Fig. 3**).

In high-risk patients, angiography is the next step from both a diagnostic and therapeutic standpoint. Diagnostically, the angiogram can show the status of the major vasculature in the neck (innominate artery and vein, carotid systems, jugular veins, and completeness of the circle of Willis) and determine whether either contrast extravasation or significant aneurysmal dilatation and vessel irregularity is present to suggest a recent or active bleed. The venous phase should always be studied in addition to the arterial phase to determine whether the venous system is a potential source of bleeding. Because of the contrast load, patients should be fully fluid resuscitated, if possible, before beginning.

Decision making after the diagnostic phase of the angiogram can often be complex. The angiography team and the head and neck team should communicate in advance as to the index of suspicion for CBS, what vessels are thought to be at risk, and

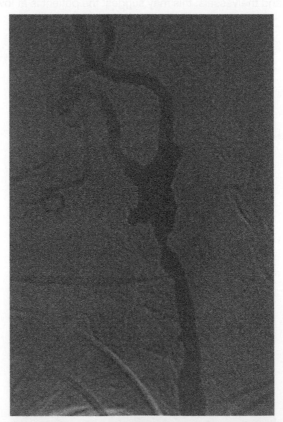

Fig. 3. Angiogram of a patient with a history of a sentinel bleed through a pharyngocutaneous fistula after composite resection. Note the pseudoaneurysmal dilatation of the carotid bifurcation and irregularity of the common carotid artery lumen.

whether sacrifice (embolization) or reconstruction (stenting) of the vessels is preferred. The decision between embolization and stenting may be driven by many factors, including the adequacy of cross circulation, overall prognosis and patient functional status, and the presence of microvascular reconstructive flaps dependent on those vessels. In patients in whom the risk of CBS is thought to be low, a negative diagnostic angiogram may be all that is necessary. Alternatively, high-risk patients with a compelling history for a sentinel bleed and CT scan showing a fistula in proximity to the carotid artery may need to undergo embolization or stenting of a major vessel that is thought to be at high risk, even if extravasation or vessel irregularity and pseudoaneurysm are not seen, in an effort to prevent subsequent rebleeding (**Fig. 4**).

There has been a trend toward reconstruction (stenting) rather than sacrifice (embolization/balloon occlusion) of the carotid artery system because of concerns of immediate or delayed cerebral ischemia associated with embolization.[1,13,14] Although it initially seemed that reconstructive stent grafts had unfavorable durable hemostasis and long-term outcomes,[11,15] a more recent study found no significant differences in the technical and hemostatic outcomes of reconstructive and deconstructive endovascular management.[2] However, it is important to remember that endovascular stenting may temporarily prevent bleeding but does not ultimately solve the problem that led to the bleeding in the first place. Following stenting, efforts should be made to provide tissue coverage of the vessel with well-vascularized tissue to exclude it from the outside environment. Clinicians could also consider extra-anatomic bypass of the involved vessel outside the irradiated field (ie, subclavian to internal carotid artery

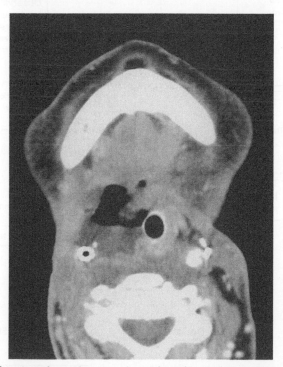

Fig. 4. CT scan of patient from **Figs. 1** and **2** with endovascular stenting of right common carotid artery as a prelude to extra-anatomic bypass from the right subclavian to internal carotid artery and subsequent balloon occlusion and coverage of the stent with a pectoralis major flap reconstruction.

bypass) followed by embolization of the involved/stented segment. However, this extensive reconstructive process may not be possible in all patients. For example, in patients with recurrent tumor, adequate cross circulation as determined by balloon occlusion, and a poor prognosis, initial embolization may be wiser. Reconstruction or stenting of vessels in a contaminated field must be viewed as a temporary solution to acute bleeding or a high-risk situation until a more permanent solution can be found. Without subsequent reconstruction and vessel coverage, rebleeding is virtually guaranteed.

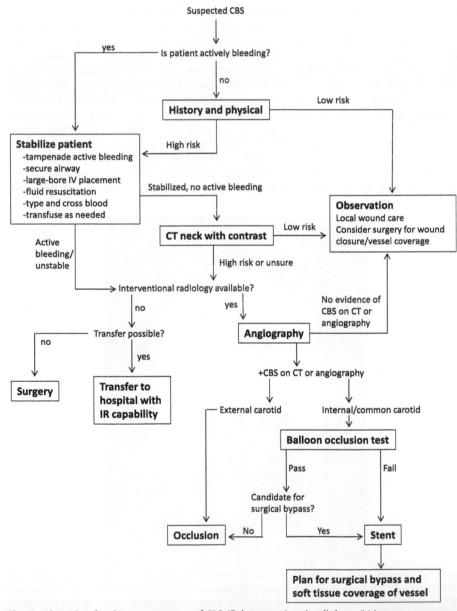

Fig. 5. Algorithm for the management of CBS. IR, interventional radiology; IV, intravenous access.

Surgery for vessel ligation has no significant role to play in the management of CBS in the modern era in which diagnostic and therapeutic angiography are available. These operations are technically difficult, with morbidity and mortality much higher than can now be accomplished with angiography.[1] With emergency surgery, hypotension and cardiac events/cerebrovascular accident often complicate the anesthetic management. Neck exploration frequently initiates rebleeding with subsequent difficulty in nerve identification and preservation, complicated by a struggle to obtain proximal and distal control of the involved vessel while maintaining pressure on a fragile vessel. Surgery for vessel ligation should be reserved for the rare situations in which acute bleeding cannot be stopped and angiography is not available. It is preferable, in the authors' opinion, to stabilize and transfer the patient to an angiography center with ongoing external pressure on the neck to tamponade bleeding rather than undertake an attempt at vessel ligation. Surgery for CBS should be reserved for vessel coverage (including coverage of embolized vessels to prevent subsequent extrusion), salivary diversion with flaps, wound debridement after vessel management, or extra-anatomic bypass after vessel stenting.

A summary algorithm for management of CBS is shown in **Fig. 5**.

SUMMARY

Although the incidence of carotid blowout has decreased with the advent of better reconstructive techniques it remains a real risk after major head and neck surgery, especially in an irradiated field. A systematic multidisciplinary approach incorporating appropriate history and physical examination, adequate resuscitation, diagnostic CT, and diagnostic and therapeutic angiography can manage most of these patients in a safe and effective management. Surgery has a limited role to play in acute management and is primarily reserved for subsequent wound management.

Post-Test Questions (Correct answers are in italics)

1. Which of the following factors is not associated with an increased risk of CBS?
   a. Pharyngocutaneous fistula
   b. Wound breakdown
   c. Prior radiation therapy
   d. *Preservation of the sternocleidomastoid muscle*
   e. Poor nutrition
2. The first priority in the management of patients with threatened CBS is:
   a. Ensuring hemodynamic stability
   b. *Ensuring a secure airway*
   c. CT scan to determine the site of bleeding
   d. Angiogram to determine the site of bleeding
   e. Flexible fiberoptic laryngoscopy to determine the site of bleeding
3. Compared with angiography, CT scan can add what additional important information in the assessment and management of patients with CBS?
   a. Determine which vessel is the site of active bleeding
   b. Determine the status of the circle of Willis
   c. *Determine the proximity of a mucocutaneous fistula or open wound to the carotid artery*
   d. Determine the presence of a pseudoaneurysm
   e. Assess the degree of atherosclerosis in the carotid artery

4. Assuming adequate interventional radiology support, the primary role of surgery in the acute management of CBS is:
   a. Carotid artery ligation
   b. Carotid artery bypass
   c. Closure of a mucocutaneous fistula
   d. *Vascularized tissue coverage of the involved carotid artery*
   e. Neck exploration to ascertain whether recurrent tumor is present

SUPPLEMENTARY DATA

Supplementary PDF slides related to this article can be found online at http://www.oto.theclinics.com/.

REFERENCES

1. Chaloupka JC, Putman CM, Citardi MJ, et al. Endovascular therapy for the carotid blowout syndrome in head and neck surgical patients: diagnostic and managerial considerations. AJNR Am J Neuroradiol 1996;17:843–52.

2. Chang F-C, Lirng JF, Luo CB, et al. Patients with head and neck cancers and associated postirradiated carotid blowout syndrome: endovascular therapeutic methods and outcomes. J Vasc Surg 2008;47:936–45.

3. Chang F-C, Luo CB, Lirng JF, et al. Evaluation of the outcomes of endovascular management for patients with head and neck cancers and associated carotid blowout syndrome of the external carotid artery. Clin Radiol 2013;68:e561–9.

4. Powitzky R, Vasan N, Krempl G, et al. Carotid blowout in patients with head and neck cancer. Ann Otol Rhinol Laryngol 2010;119:476–84.

5. Maran AG, Amin M, Wilson JA. Radical neck dissection: a 19-year experience. J Laryngol Otol 1989;103:760–4.

6. Cohen J, Rad I. Contemporary management of carotid blowout. Curr Opin Otolaryngol Head Neck Surg 2004;12:110–5.

7. Patel UA, Moore BA, Wax M, et al. Impact of pharyngeal closure technique on fistula after salvage laryngectomy. JAMA Otolaryngol Head Neck Surg 2013;139: 1156–62.

8. Murros KE, Toole JF. The effect of radiation on carotid arteries. A review article. Arch Neurol 1989;46:449–55.

9. Dorresteijn LDA, Kappelle AC, Scholz NM, et al. Increased carotid wall thickening after radiotherapy on the neck. Eur J Cancer 2005;41:1026–30.

10. Timon CV, Brown D, Gullane P. Internal jugular vein blowout complicating head and neck surgery. J Laryngol Otol 1994;108:423–5.

11. Citardi MJ, Chaloupka JC, Son YH, et al. Management of carotid artery rupture by monitored endovascular therapeutic occlusion (1988-1994). Laryngoscope 1995; 105:1086–92.

12. Porto DP, Adams GL, Foster C. Emergency management of carotid artery rupture. Am J Otol 1986;7:213–7.

13. Chaloupka JC, Roth TC, Putman CM, et al. Recurrent carotid blowout syndrome: diagnostic and therapeutic challenges in a newly recognized subgroup of patients. AJNR Am J Neuroradiol 1999;20:1069–77.

14. Lesley WS, Chaloupka JC, Weigele JB, et al. Preliminary experience with endovascular reconstruction for the management of carotid blowout syndrome. AJNR Am J Neuroradiol 2003;24:975–81.
15. Warren FM, Cohen JI, Nesbit GM, et al. Management of carotid 'blowout' with endovascular stent grafts. Laryngoscope 2002;112:428–33.

SUGGESTED READINGS

Chang F-C, Lirng JF, Luo CB, et al. Patients with head and neck cancers and associated postirradiated carotid blowout syndrome: endovascular therapeutic methods and outcomes. J Vasc Surg 2008;47:936–45.
   This study evaluates the outcomes of reconstructive and deconstructive endovascular management of carotid blowout syndrome involving the main trunk of the carotid artery. It provides a summary of different therapeutic techniques and lists indications and merits for each. They found that clinical severity correlated well with angiographic severity. They also discuss complications and offer thoughtful suggestions on how to reduce them.
Powitzky R, Vasan N, Krempl G, et al. Carotid blowout in patients with head and neck cancer. Ann Otol Rhinol Laryngol 2010;119:476–84.
   This article not only reviews the carotid blowout cases at their own institution, but also provides a meta-analysis of all studies documenting carotid blowout cases within the past 15 years. Using a total of 140 cases, they are able to identify significant risk factors, bleeding location, and outcome data including morbidity and mortality. They also include an algorithm for management.

Endovascular Management of Diseases in Relation to Otolaryngology

Tudor Jovin, MD*, Amin Aghaebrahim, MD

KEYWORDS

- Endovascular treatment • Embolization • Tinnitus • Epitaxis • Pseudoaneurysm
- Coiling • Onyx

KEY LEARNING POINTS

At the end of this article, the reader will:

- Understand the role of endovascular treatments in common otolaryngologic conditions.
- Be familiar with endovascular techniques used for these diseases.

Procedures to discuss
Venous stenting (pseudotumor cerebri, tinnitus)
Embolization (tumors, epistaxis, dural arteriovenous fistula)
Balloon test occlusion (vessel sacrifice, tinnitus)
Arterial stenting (carotid stenosis postradiation, carotid blow out)
Coiling (traumatic pseudoaneurysm)

PULSATILE TINNITUS

The differential diagnosis of pulsatile tinnitus includes the following[1] (**Fig. 1**):

- Middle ear conductive hearing loss
  - Middle ear effusion
  - Chronic otitis: Tympanic Membrane or ossicular abnormalities
  - Otosclerosis
- Neoplasm
  - Glomus tympanicum or jugulare
  - Middle ear adenoma

University of Pittsburgh Medical Center, 200 Lothrop Street, PUH C-424, Pittsburgh, PA 15213, USA
* Corresponding author.
E-mail address: jovitg@upmc.edu

Otolaryngol Clin N Am 49 (2016) 841–862
http://dx.doi.org/10.1016/j.otc.2016.03.005
0030-6665/16/$ – see front matter © 2016 Elsevier Inc. All rights reserved.

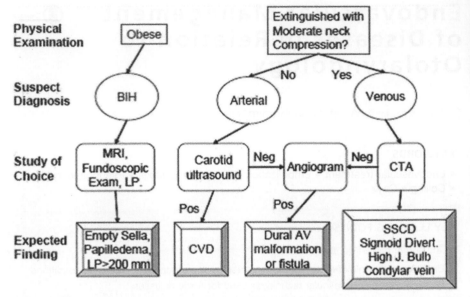

Fig. 1. Diagnostic work-up. AV, arteriovenous; BIH, Benign intracranial hypertension. CTA, CT angiogram; CVD, cardiovascular disease; LP, lumbar puncture; SSCD, superior semicircular canal dehiscence. (*From* Mattox D, Hudgins P. Algorithm for evaluation of pulsatile tinnitus. Acta Otolaryngol 2008;128(4):430; with permission.)

- ○ Geniculate ganglion hemangioma
- • Arterial
  - ○ Atherosclerotic disease
    - ■ Carotid (ipsilateral or contralateral)
    - ■ Subclavian
  - ○ Dural arteriovenous fistulas
  - ○ Carotid-cavernous fistula
  - ○ Fibromuscular dysplasia of carotid artery
  - ○ Carotid artery dissection
  - ○ Aberrant internal carotid artery
  - ○ Hyperdynamic states (anemia, thyrotoxicosis, pregnancy)
  - ○ Hypertension
  - ○ Internal auditory canal vascular loops
- • Venous
  - ○ Benign intracranial hypertension
  - ○ Sigmoid or jugular diverticulum
  - ○ High jugular bulb
  - ○ Transverse or sigmoid stenosis
  - ○ Condylar vein abnormalities

Sinus Venous Stenosis

Case example

A 23-year-old previously healthy woman presents with 3 months of pulsatile tinnitus in the right ear with normal examination (**Figs. 2–5**). The patient had immediate resolution of her pulsatile tinnitus after stent placement. She was started on aspirin and clopidogrel. At 3-month follow-up, the patient remained symptom-free.

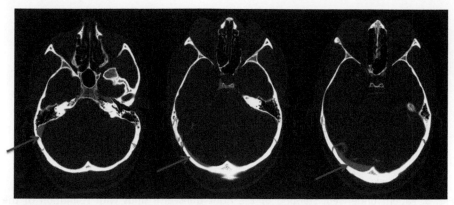

Fig. 2. Computed tomography (CT) venogram: *arrows* point to stenosis of the right transverse sinus.

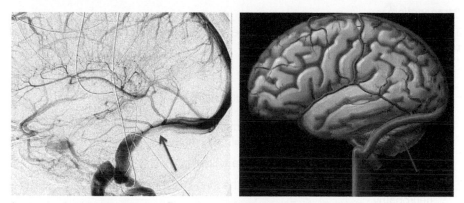

Fig. 3. Cerebral angiogram: confirms right transverse sinus stenosis (*arrows*).

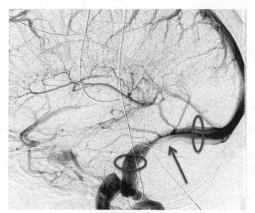

31/25 (27) mm Hg

20/16 (17) mm Hg

Fig. 4. Venous pressure showed 10 mm Hg gradient across the stenosis (*arrow*). *Circles* highlight the proximal and distal part of the transverse sinus.

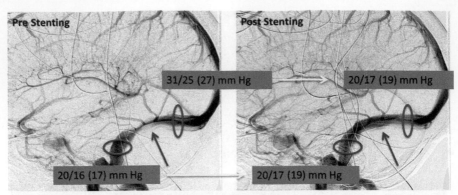

Fig. 5. Patient underwent stenting of the right transverse sinus with resolution of the gradient. *Circles* highlight the proximal and distal part of the transverse sinus. Transverse sinus stenosis (*left arrow*), resolution of the stenosis (*right arrow*).

Paragangliomas

These are highly vascular neuroendocrine tumors arising from chemoreceptors of paraganglia.[2,3]

- Types
  - Carotid body
  - Temporal bone: glomus tympanicum, glomus jugulare, jugular fossa
  - Glomus vagale
- Associated with familial paraganglioma, neurofibromatosis type 1, von Hippel-Lindau disease, Carney triad, and multiple endocrine neoplasia type 2 (**Table 1**)

Symptoms of paraganglioma include the following[4]:

- Temporal bone paragangliomas: hearing loss, pulsatile tinnitus, cranial neuropathy
- Carotid body tumor: slow growing, painless neck mass
- 5% of cases have signs/symptoms of catecholamine hypersecretion

Case example
A 63-year-old woman developed pulsatile tinnitus for the last 2 months with a normal examination (**Figs. 6** and **7**).

Table 1	
Classification of glomus jugularis tumors of the temporal bone as proposed by Fishch	
Type	**Description**
A	Tumors restricted to middle ear (glomus tympanicum tumors)
B	Tumors restricted to tympanomastoid site
C	Tumors involving the infralabyrinth portion toward the petrous apex
D1	Tumor with intracranial invasion (<2 cm)
D2	Tumor with intracranial invasion (>2 cm)

From Fisch U. Infratemporal fossa approach for glomus tumors of the temporal bone. Ann Otol Rhinol Laryngol 1982;92:474–9; with permission.

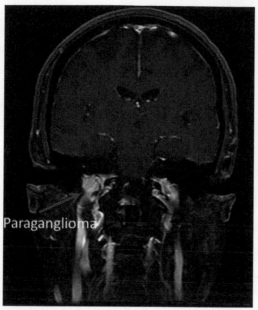

Fig. 6. MRI head: 2-cm right jugular bulb mass consistent with paraganglioma (*arrow*).

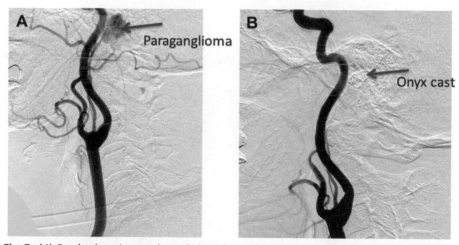

Fig. 7. (*A*) Cerebral angiogram lateral view showed tumor blush (*arrow*). (*B*) Cerebral angiogram postembolization with onyx.

Dural Arteriovenous Fistula

Dural arteriovenous fistula refers to direct shunting of arterial blood into the wall of a dural venous sinus or a cortical vein. Clinical presentation is as follows[5]:

- Pulsatile tinnitus
- Cranial nerve deficits

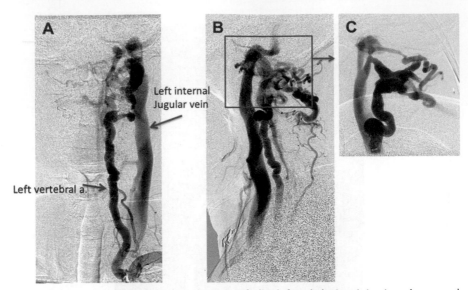

Fig. 8. (*A*) Anteroposterior (AP) projection of the left subclavian injection shows early drainage of the internal jugular vein from the left vertebral artery. (*B*) Lateral projection. (*C*) Zoomed-in view of the left vertebral artery showing the fistula and their connections.

- Visual symptoms and headache
- Focal neurologic deficit caused by venous hypertension, which leads to edema in the surrounding parenchyma
- Intraparenchymal hemorrhage

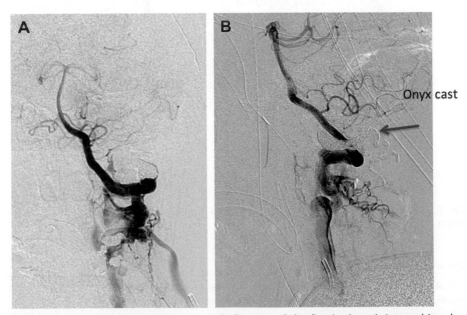

Fig. 9. Patient underwent transvenous embolization of the fistula though internal jugular vein with significant reduction of flow across the fistula. (*A*) AP and (*B*) lateral projection and improvement of her symptoms. *Arrow* points to the onyx cast postembolization.

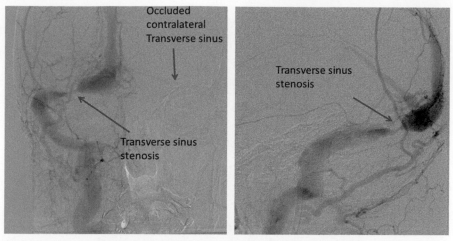

Fig. 10. Cerebral angiogram showed right transverse sinus stenosis with occluded contralateral transverse sinus.

The prognosis for dural arteriovenous fistula depends on venous outflow. Symptomatic dural arteriovenous fistulas have hemorrhage or nonhemorrhagic complications of at least 15% to 19% per year. Asymptomatic dural arteriovenous fistulas with cortical reflux have a much lower rate of complications (<2% per year).[6]

Case example

A 67-year-old woman presents with pulsatile tinnitus for the last 3 months. She is initially diagnosed with mastoiditis, but continued to be symptomatic despite antibiotic

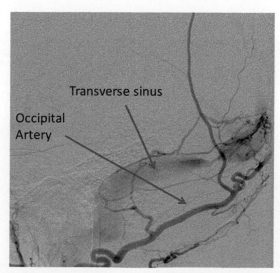

Fig. 11. External carotid artery injection showed direct occipital artery fistula to the right transverse sinus.

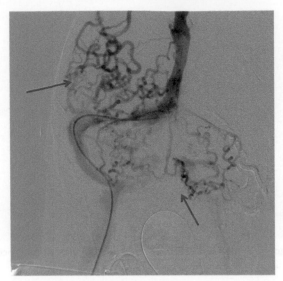

Fig. 12. Transvenous injection showed retrograde filling of cortical veins (*arrows*) suggesting reversal of flow.

therapy. She had normal examination. Cerebral angiogram showed a direct left vertebral artery to internal jugular vein fistula located at C1 level with retrograde filling of the left sigmoid and transverse sinus but no cortical venous reflux (cognard type IIa) (**Figs. 8** and **9**).

Case example
A 70-year-old woman presents with headache, ataxia, and pulsatile tinnitus (**Figs. 10–14**).

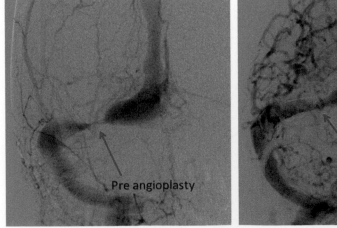

Fig. 13. Patient underwent transarterial embolization through the occipital artery in addition to right transverse sinus angioplasty with resolution of the fistula.

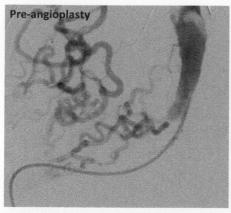
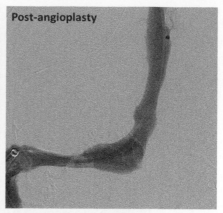

Fig. 14. Postangioplasty injection showed no retrograde filling of cortical veins.

Juvenile Nasopharyngeal Angiofibroma

The characteristics of juvenile nasopharyngeal angiofibroma are as follows:

- Benign tumor that is markedly vascular
- Occurs primarily in adolescent boys, arises in the lateral nasopharynx, and is hormonally sensitive
- Can cause severe epistaxis
- Blood supply is mostly derived from internal maxillary artery[7]

Case Example

A 15-year-old boy presents with nasal congestion and witnessed apnea and snoring (**Figs. 15–17**).

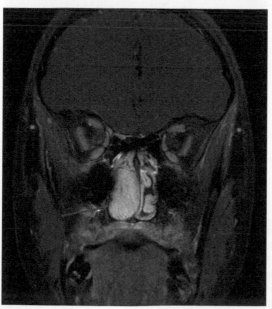

Fig. 15. MRI head showed a right-sided juvenile nasopharyngeal angiofibroma (*arrow*).

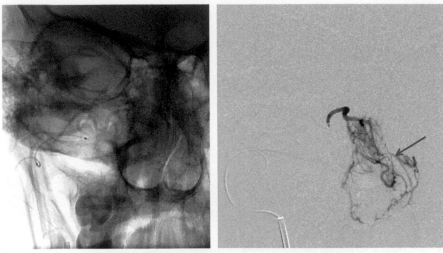

Fig. 16. Cerebral angiogram showed tumor blush (*arrow*) from distal internal maxillary injection.

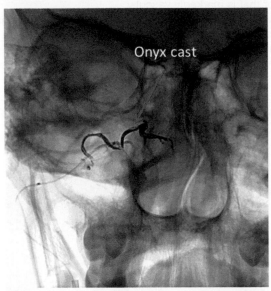

Fig. 17. Patient underwent selective tumor embolization via onyx before surgical resection.

Epistaxis

Ninety percent of epistaxis occurs from the anterior nasal septum (Kiesselbach plexus), and posterior epistaxis occurs in the rest of the cases. Anterior nasal septum blood supply are from the external carotid artery through the superior labial branch of the facial artery and the terminal branches of the sphenopalatine artery and from the internal carotid artery through the anterior and posterior ethmoidal arteries. The blood supply to the posterior nasal septum are from the external carotid artery through the sphenopalatine branch of the internal maxillary artery.[8]

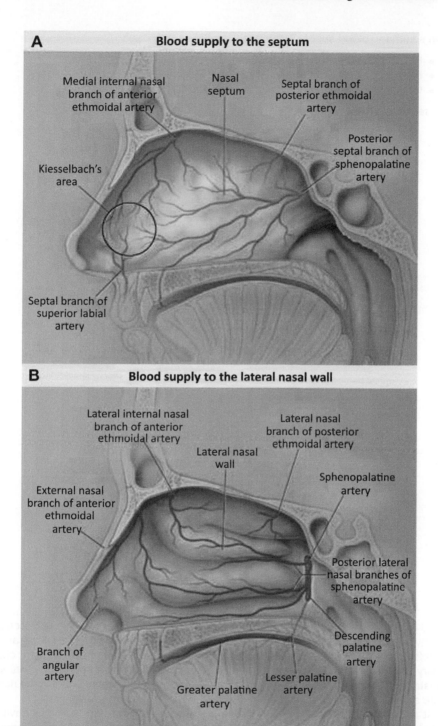

Fig. 18. Blood supply to the nasal septum (*A*) and lateral nasal wall (*B*). (*From* Schlosser RJ. Clinical practice. Epistaxis. N Engl J Med 2009;360(8):785; with permission.)

In summary, blood supply of the nasal cavities are through

- Facial artery (superior labial branch)
- Internal maxillary artery (inferior orbital branch and Sphenopalatine artery)
- Ophthalmic artery (ethmoidal arteries) (**Fig. 18**)

Causes of epistaxis

The following are causes of epistaxis:

- Digital trauma
- Illicit drugs
- Septal perforation
- Rhinosinusitis
- Neoplasms
- Coagulopathies
- Hypertension
- Trauma/surgery
- Pseudoaneurysm

Treatment options include the following:

- Direct pressure applied to the nostril
- Chemical agents
- Electrocautery
- Topical hemostatic vasoconstriction agents
- Cryotherapy
- Anterior nasal packing
- Endovascular embolization
- Surgical ligation

Some points of endovascular embolization are as follows:

- Usually consists of super selective catheterization with particle embolization
- Typically involves distal internal maxillary artery, which ideally includes the infraorbital and sphenopalatine arteries
- Facial artery ipsilateral to the side of nasal bleeding to collateralized flow to the nasal mucosal of the lateral nasal wall via its angular branch
- Close attention to important collaterals, such as ophthalmic artery to avoid complications[9]

Case Example

An 84-year-old man underwent sinus surgery for a right-sided soft tissue infection overlying the right maxillary sinus. Bilateral packing was removed on postoperative Day 2 after surgery without issue. The patient was on aspirin and clopidogrel for coronary stents and on postoperative day 10 developed bleeding through both nares. Epistat was placed in the left nare and an anterior rapid rhino was inserted in the right nare at an outside facility.

At an ear-nose-throat evaluation the packing was removed and the nasal cavity/oropharynx was irrigated with saline. Afrin/lidocaine pledgets were inserted. Endoscopy revealed posterior pharynx bleeding (**Fig. 19**). The patient underwent combination of coil and onyx embolization of his bilateral internal maxillary arteries and middle meningeal artery with resolution of the epistaxis.

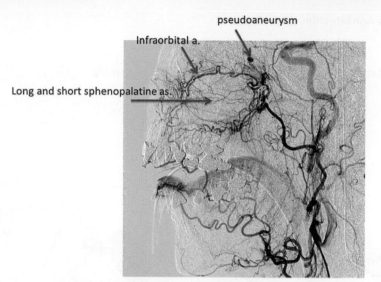

Fig. 19. Cerebral angiogram revealed right middle meningeal artery pseudoaneurysm.

Idiopathic Intracranial Hypertension (Pseudotumor Cerebri)

Symptoms of idiopathic intracranial hypertension are caused by elevated intracranial pressure (headache, papilledema, vision loss, and tinnitus) with normal cerebrospinal fluid composition and no other cause of intracranial hypertension evidence on neuro-imaging.[10] Twenty-five percent of individuals are at risk of severe, permanent vision loss. Treatment options are weight loss, acetazolamide or topiramate, and cerebrospinal fluid shunting procedure for patients with progressive visual loss or medication failure. Alternatively, cerebral sinus stenting is another option for selected patients.

Case Example

A 27-year-old woman presents with headache and blurred vision. On examination she had papilledema and her opening pressure was 50 mm Hg (**Figs. 20–22**).

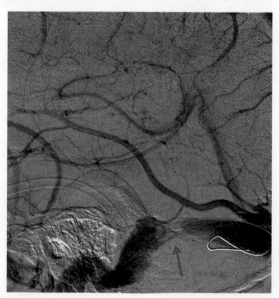

Fig. 20. Cerebral angiogram showed significant right transverse sinus stenosis with hypo-plastic contralateral transverse sinus (*arrow*).

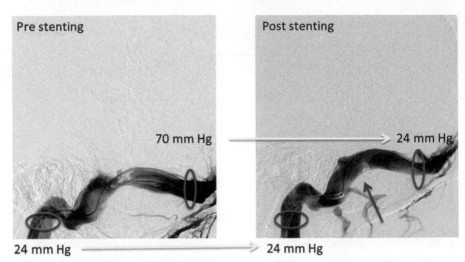

Fig. 21. Venous exploration showed 46 mm Hg gradient across the stenosis. The patient underwent successful stent revascularization with normalization of the gradient (*arrow points to the stent*). Proximal circle (*left*) sigmoid sinus, distal circle (*right*) distal part of the transverse sinus.

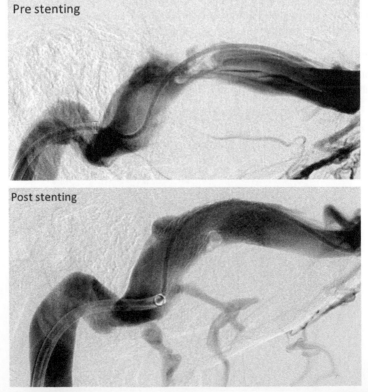

Fig. 22. Zoomed-in view of the transverse sinus stenosis pre and post stent placement. Following the procedure, the patient's headache resolved and her papilledema improved.

Pseudoaneurysm

These are uncommon vascular lesions that may occur following blunt trauma, radiation necrosis, mycotic infection, iatrogenic insult, or neoplastic invasion of the vessel

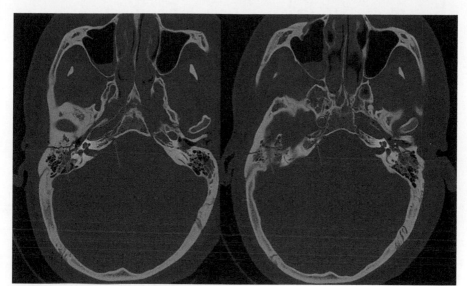

Fig. 23. CT head shows proximity of the skull base fracture (*arrows*) to the carotid artery (*circle*).

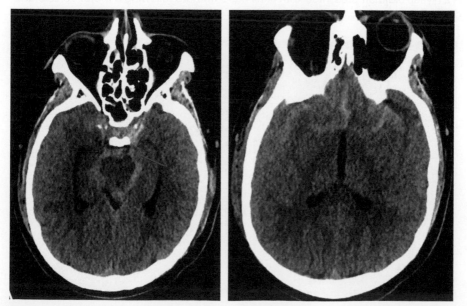

Fig. 24. Head CT showed subarachnoid hemorrhage (*arrows*).

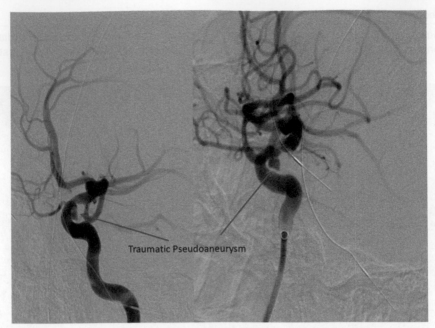

Fig. 25. Patient underwent cerebral angiogram, which showed traumatic pseudoaneurysm in the posterior carotid wall.

wall.[9] If untreated, they may enlarge, causing progressive occlusion of the parent vessel; they may cause symptoms related to local mass; or they may rupture.

Case Example

A 21-year-old man presented with skull base fracture following a motor vehicle accident (**Figs. 23–26**).

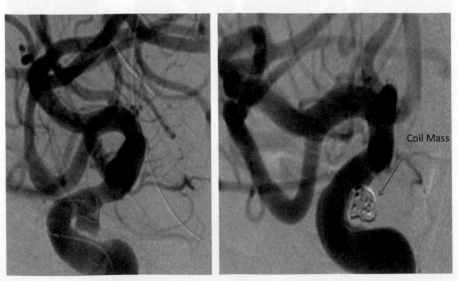

Fig. 26. Patient underwent coil embolization of the aneurysm.

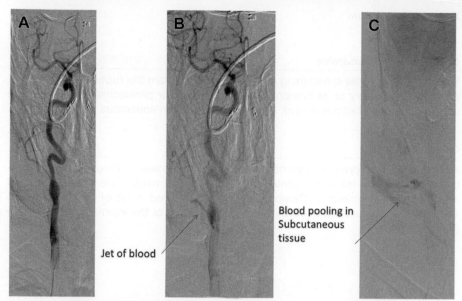

Fig. 27. (A) Right common carotid injection. (B) Delayed run shows jet of blood. (C) Delayed run shows pooling of the blood.

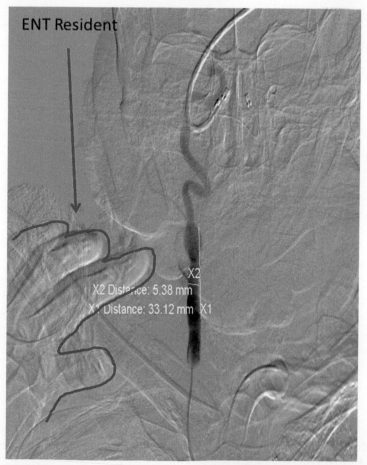

Fig. 28. At that point, direct pressure was applied with the help of the ear-nose-throat (ENT) resident.

Carotid Blowout Syndrome

This an emergent, life-threatening condition resulting from the rupture of the exteracranial carotid artery or its branches with oral, nasal, or peritracheal bleeding.[9] It is usually caused by head and neck neoplasm, most often squamous cell carcinoma.

Case Example

A 68-year-old man presents with neck hematoma, decreased hemoglobin, and hemodynamic changes. He had recently undergone radical neck dissection because of squamous cell carcinoma. Cerebral angiogram showed a jet of blood filling the extravascular space from the proximal cervical portion of the internal cerebral artery (**Figs. 27–30**).

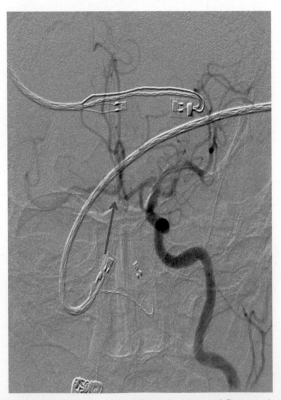

Fig. 29. Contralateral carotid injection showed good collateral flow to the right hemisphere through anterior communicating artery (*arrow*).

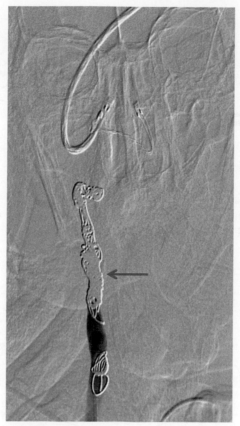

Fig. 30. Patient underwent successful coil (*arrow*) sacrifice of the right internal carotid artery with resolution of the hematoma.

Carotid Artery Stenting

Case Example

A 39-year-old woman underwent endonasal resection of a pituitary adenoma. The procedure was complicated by carotid injury with laceration of the distal cavernous segment of the right internal carotid artery, which was packed. Following this, significant changes in neurophysiologic monitoring were noted that were blood pressure dependent, suggesting hypoperfusion of the right hemisphere. Patient was then taken emergently for a cerebral angiogram (**Figs. 31–33**).

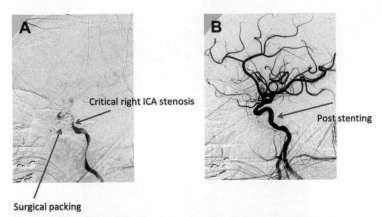

Fig. 31. (*A*) Cerebral angiogram showed critical cavernous segment of the carotid artery stenosis. (*B*) Patient underwent stent and angioplasty of the lesion.

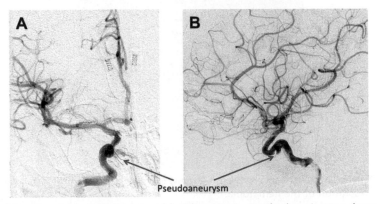

Fig. 32. A few days later patient presented with epistaxis. Cerebral angiogram showed pseudoaneurysm in the site of prior treated carotid artery.

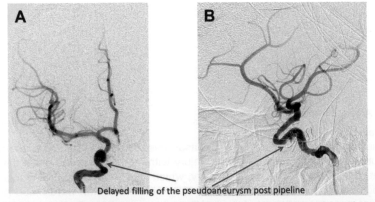

Fig. 33. Patients underwent telescoping flow diverter stent (Pipeline) with resolution of the patient's epistaxis. (*A*) Anterioposterior. (*B*) Lateral projection.

Post-Test Questions (Correct answers are in italics)

1. Which are the following is the most common symptoms associated with dural AV fistula?
   a. Nose bleed
   b. *Pulsatile tinnitus*
   c. Stroke
   d. Cranial nerve deficit
2. Which of the following is one of the arteries that typically is used for endovascular embolization of an epitaxis?
   a. Lingual
   b. *Sphenopalatine*
   c. Artery of Percheron
   d. Anterior ethmoidal artery
   e. None of the above
3. What percentage of patients with idiopathic intracranial hypertension are at risk of severe permanent vision loss?
   a. *25%*
   b. 15%
   c. 50%
   d. 10%

SUPPLEMENTARY DATA

Supplementary PDF slides related to this article can be found online at http://www.oto.theclinics.com/.

REFERENCES

1. Mattox D, Hudgins P. Algorithm for evaluation of pulsatile tinnitus. Acta Otolaryngol 2008;128(4):427–31.
2. DeLellis RA, Lloyd RV, Heitz PU, et al, editors. Pathology and genetics of tumours of the endocrine organs. WHO classification of tumours. Lyon (France): IARC Press; 2004.
3. Fisch U. Infratemporal fossa approach for glomus tumors of the temporal bone. Ann Otol Rhinol Laryngol 1982;92:474–9.
4. Erickson D, Kudva YC, Ebersold MJ, et al. Benign paragangliomas: clinical presentation and treatment outcomes in 236 patients. J Clin Endocrinol Metab 2001; 86(11):5210.
5. Lasjaunias P, Chiu M, ter Brugge K, et al. Dural arteriovenous shunts: a new classification of craniospinal epidural venous anatomical bases and clinical correlations. Stroke 2008;39(10):2783–94.
6. Satomi J, van Dijk JM, Terbrugge KG, et al. Benign cranial dural arteriovenous fistulas: outcome of conservative management based on natural history of the lesion. J Neurosurg 2002;97(4):767–70.
7. Gullane PJ, Davidson J, O'Dwyer T, et al. Juvenile angiofibroma: a review of the literature and a case series report. Laryngoscope 1992;102(8):928.
8. Schlosser RJ. Clinical practice. Epistaxis. N Engl J Med 2009;360(8):784.
9. Gonzalez F, Albuquerque F, McDougall C. New York: Neurointerventional techniques. 2015.

10. Wall M, Kupersmith MJ, Kieburtz KD, et al. NORDIC Idiopathic Intracranial Hypertension Study Group. The idiopathic intracranial hypertension treatment trial: clinical profile at baseline. JAMA Neurol 2014;71(6):693–701.

SUGGESTED READINGS

Pearse Morris P. Practical Neuroangiography (Third Edition). Philadelphia: Lippincott Williams & Wilkins; 2013.

Spetzler RF, Kalani YS, Nakaji P, editors. Neurovascular Surgery. New York: Thieme Medical Publishers Inc; 2015.

Gonzalez LF, Albuquerque FC, McDougall C. Neurointerventional Techniques: Tricks of the Trade. New York: Thieme Medical Publishers Inc; 2014.

Education and Training in Hemostasis

Perspectives of the Early Practitioner and Expert Practitioner

Rebecca Harvey, MD, Kelly Michele Malloy, MD*

KEYWORDS

- Simulation in otolaryngology • Epistaxis • Neck hematoma • Surgical education
- Task trainers

KEY LEARNING POINTS

At the end of this article, early practitioners will:

- Be able to identify the common presentations of hemorrhage in otolaryngology.
- Understand how knowledge of relevant anatomy helps to form the basis for effective management.
- Be able to identify the most common sources of bleeding in otolaryngology emergencies and how can they be controlled.

At the end of this article, expert practitioners/educators will:

- Understand how management of head and neck hemorrhage can be taught and practiced.
- Understand how early practitioner skill and confidence can be developed in the management of hemorrhage in otolaryngology.
- Know which educational tools are available to train early practitioners in control of hemorrhage techniques.

No conflicts of interest or financial disclosures to make.
Department of Otolaryngology - Head and Neck Surgery, University of Michigan, 1904 Taubman Center, 1500 E. Medical Center Drive, Ann Arbor, MI 48109, USA
* Corresponding author.
E-mail address: Kellymal@med.umich.edu

Otolaryngol Clin N Am 49 (2016) 863–876
http://dx.doi.org/10.1016/j.otc.2016.02.006
0030-6665/16/$ – see front matter © 2016 Elsevier Inc. All rights reserved.

oto.theclinics.com

INTRODUCTION

> **How do we learn to manage hemorrhage in the head and neck as early practitioners?**
>
> • Traditional model was experiential: "see one, do one, teach one."
> • Today's early learners often have initial experience as the first responder while the junior resident on call.
> • Modern limitations on time in training and concerns surrounding patient safety have produced practice gaps for the early practitioner.
>   ○ Learners may not encounter a bleeding event or emergency early in their practice when perhaps more supported by an expert teacher.
>   ○ The learner's initial management may be suboptimal if unfamiliar with hemostatic procedures and equipment, thus posing potential concerns regarding patient safety.

Given the current challenges of expeditiously bringing the early, inexperienced learner to a basic level of safe practice and competence, new educational models have been developed to facilitate this process. Although traditional didactics such as lectures and the Socratic method of teaching rounds remain valuable, surgical simulation has entered the expert practitioner's educational armamentarium. Surgical simulation has emerged as effective tool to help build learner confidence and early skill acquisition.[1] Here, we briefly describe 2 otolaryngology hemorrhagic emergencies that can be taught and practiced in a simulated environment. Simulation must be used in the context of a thoughtful curriculum. A robust discussion of curriculum development and the process of prebriefing and debriefing is outside the scope of this article; however, these processes remain vital to the successful implementation of surgical simulation.

EPISTAXIS

> **What are the education gaps for an early practitioner?**
>
> • Knowledge of the common sources of bleeding from the nose and causative factors (hypertension, antiplatelet/anticoagulation, dry oxygen delivery nasal cannula O_2, winter weather).
> • Use of equipment to stop epistaxis (headlight, suction, nasal speculum, bayonet forceps, various nasal packing, and hemostatic products).
> • Postpacking management knowledge (management of causative factors, antibiotic coverage, admission to intensive care for posterior packing, plan for packing removal).

A CURRICULUM IN EPISTAXIS MANAGEMENT

Epistaxis is the most common otolaryngologic emergency, reported to occur in up to 60% of the general population.[2] Effective management poses challenges to the earlier learner who must integrate principles in resuscitation and airway management, nasal anatomy, and sophisticated knowledge of the equipment and methods in epistaxis control (**Figs. 1** and **2, Table 1**).[3,4]

Curriculum design

- Uses a task-specific skills trainer.
- Requires an epistaxis simulator.
  - Easily designed and adapted model using Laerdal Airway Trainer (Laerdal Medical Corporation Wappingers Falls, New York).[3]
  - May also consider cadaver based simulators as described by Chin and colleagues.[4]
  - Hands-on practice with simulator with real-time feedback from expert practitioners/educators
- Skill competency and confidence can be assessed using a task specific check list and global rating scale.
- The goal is to improve skill and confidence in placement of anterior and posterior nasal packs and identify those patients who may require escalation of care.

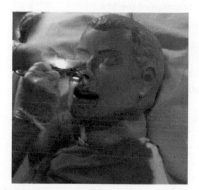

Fig. 1. Epistaxis task trainer.

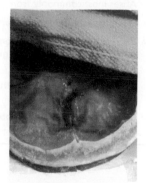

Fig. 2. Cadaver based epistaxis trainer.

Table 1
Summary of anterior and posterior epistaxis

	Anterior Epistaxis	Posterior Epistaxis
Incidence	More common (90%)	Less common (10%)
Source	Anterior to the plane of pyriform aperture	Posterior to the plane of pyriform aperture
Blood flows	Out from the front of nose	Back into the throat
Age	Children or young adults	>40 y
Localization	Easy	Difficult
Common site	Keisselbach's plexus	Woodruff's plexus
Common cause	Local trauma	Spontaneous, skull base of facial trauma
Severity	Less severe	Severe
Treatment	Usually controlled by local pressure or anterior pack	Requires hospitalization and posterior nasal pack is often required

OUTLINE OF LEARNER CURRICULUM

> **Anatomy**
>
> - Epistaxis is typically described as anterior or posterior based on the source of the bleeding vessel(s).
>
> - Anatomic distinction provides important basis for management.
>
> - Anterior epistaxis:
>   - 90% of all nosebleeds.
>   - Most commonly, Kiesselbach's plexus and the anterior septum.
>   - Formed by anastomosis of the septal branch of the anterior ethmoidal artery, the lateral nasal branch of the sphenopalatine artery (SPA), or the septal branch of the superior labial artery.
>   - Bleeding from anterior nostril is usually of lower volume.
>
> - Posterior Epistaxis
>   - Arises most commonly from posterolateral branches of the SPA.
>   - Bleed into the posterior pharynx; may be high volume, brisk.
>   - Knowledge about the anatomic position of the SPA is very important owing to the need for possible surgical ligation in the case of refractory posterior bleeding.
>   - Enters the nose through the sphenopalatine foramen at the posterior end of the middle turbinate.
>   - If bleeding is from a high posterior source, anterior and posterior ethmoid arteries must be considered.

RISK FACTORS AND IMPORTANT COMPONENTS OF HISTORY

> - Anticoagulation.
>
> - Hereditary hemorrhagic telangiectasia.
>
> - Blood dyscrasias, platelet disorders, von Willebrand disease, and hemophilia.
>
> - Aneurysms of the head and neck vasculature secondary to prior regional surgery.
>
> - Nasal neoplasms.
>   - Most common associated with epistaxis: juvenile nasopharyngeal angiofibroma, sinonasal melanoma, squamous cell carcinoma, adenoid cystic carcinoma, and inverted papilloma.
>
> - Chronic alcohol abuse.
>
> - Intranasal steroid use.

EQUIPMENT AND SUPPLIES

An epistaxis tray can be created using common supplies and a few specialized instruments

- Nasal decongestant spray, such as oxymetazoline
- Local anesthetic, such as 2% lidocaine
- Headlight
- Bayonet forceps
- Nasal speculum
- Frazier tip suction
- Lubricating jelly, bacitracin, mupirocin or other antistaphylococcal ointment
- Anterior nasal packs: Merocel (Medtronic Minneapolis, MN), Rapid Rhino (Shippert Medical Technologies Centennial, Colorado) (4.5 cm pediatric, 5.5 cm adult)
- Posterior nasal packs: Rapid Rhino (7.5 cm), Epistat (Medtronic Xomed Minneapolis, MN), urinary balloon catheter
- Additional materials: silver nitrate cautery sticks, thrombogenic agents: Fibrillar, Surgiflo, thrombin spray, transexamic acid.

A stepwise approach should be followed in the treatment of epistaxis. Nonsurgical treatments should initially be pursued including topical treatment, cauterization, thrombogenic therapies, and nasal packs. These treatments will generally stop bleeding in 90% of patients. If the bleed is refractory to these treatments, surgical intervention should be pursued.

EVALUATE HEMODYNAMIC AND AIRWAY STATUS
Initial Management

- Check pulse and blood pressure.
- Asses airway: secure airway with elective intubation if patient unable to protect airway owing to excessive bleeding.
- Ensure intravenous access and volume resuscitation as indicated.
- Treat hypertension.
- Initial laboratory tests: Full blood examination, coagulation panel.

Prepare Patient for Procedure

- Use universal precautions.
- Have patient attached to necessary monitors.
- Patient positioning: sitting position, head and neck in neutral position or sniffing position, avoid extension of the neck.
- Procedure explained to patient in detail.

Pretreatment

- Adequate anesthesia achieved with combination of anesthetic and vasoconstrictive agent:
  - 2% lidocaine, lidocaine with epinephrine, 4% cocaine, or
  - Oxymeazoline adds important vasoconstrictive benefit.
- Digital pressure applied to anterior nasal sidewalls by patient or health care provider for at least 5 minutes.

Look for a Source of Bleeding

- Ask patient to blow all clots from nose, suction remaining clots.
- Insert nasal speculum vertically with 1 hand resting on dorsum of the nose.
- Examine the anterior nasal septum, evaluate inferior to superior, anterior to posterior.
- Examine posterior pharynx for bleeding and clot.
  - A clot in the posterior pharynx serves as high aspiration risk.
- Not uncommonly, a primary bleeding source cannot be identified.
  - Have higher suspicion for posterior source.
- Brisk bleeding often requires immediate management with definitive packing.
  - Imperative to move quickly, not waste time searching for exact source.

HEMOSTASIS FOR ANTERIOR BLEEDS

- May consider nasal tampon such as Merocel (Medtronic Minneapolis, MN) pack or nasal balloon such as Rapid Rhino (Shippert Medical Technologies Centennial, CO).
- Each inserted using same general technique.
- Merocel nasal tampon coated in antibiotic ointment before insertion.
  - Afrin (Schering-Plough HealthCare Products Kenilworth, NJ) or saline may then be injected into nasal cavity for expansion of tampon.
- Rapid Rhino must be soaked in sterile water for 30 seconds.
  - Do not apply lubricants or topical antibiotics, which impair the carboxymethylcellulose fibers (act to promote thrombosis).
  - Balloon inflated with air after insertion; amount will vary with nasal cavity size.
- Insert pack along the floor of the nasal cavity underneath the inferior turbinate until the proximal ring lies within the nares.

Brisk bleeding despite proper packing strongly suggests a posterior source. If bleeding persists despite initial packing, the contralateral naris may be packed, providing a counterforce to promote tamponade.

POSTERIOR EPISTAXIS

- Requires placement of posterior nasal pack to occlude the choanal arch.
- Options:
  - Posterior Rapid Rhino Pack (7.5 cm).
    - Inserted via similar mechanism to other Rapid Rhino packs.
    - Dual balloon system, anterior and posterior balloons.
    - Additional commercial nasal balloon packs are available for both anterior and posterior epistaxis management and are inserted using similar technique.
  - Urinary balloon catheter (10- to 14-Fr can be used).

Placement of a urinary balloon catheter involves passage of the catheter coated with antibiotic ointment through the nares and into posterior pharynx. A tonsil clamp is used to grab the catheter transorally and pull it through the mouth. A gauze pad is tied to the catheter with suture and passed back into the posterior nasopharynx and lodged against the choana. Alternatively, insert a urinary balloon catheter through the nares and advance until the tip of the catheter can be visualized in the back of the pharynx. The balloon is then filled with 10 mL of sterile water and pulled back into the nasopharnx. Anterior nose may then also be packed around the catheter using a variety of techniques including hemostatic agents or ribbon gauze to prevent anterior passage of blood.

POTENTIAL COMPLICATIONS OF PACKING

- Toxic shock syndrome.
- Sinusitis.
- Nasal septal and alar pressure necrosis.
- Abscess.
- Neuorgenic syncope.
- Persistent bleeding despite intervention.

POSTPROCEDURE CARE AND FOLLOW-UP

- Antibiotics must be prescribed with packing.
  - Cover *Staphylococcus* species: cephalexin, amoxicillin, ampicillin, trimethoprim-sulfamethoxazole.
  - Prevent sinusitis and toxic shock.
- Packing should be removed in 3 to 5 days.
- Ensure follow-up for pack removal and evaluation by an otolaryngologist.
- Educate patient on epistaxis prevention.
- Persistent bleeding is indication for escalation of therapy.

CONSIDERATIONS FOR HOSPITAL ADMISSION

- Particularly important in posterior bleeds.
  - More likely to rebleed or require escalation of management.
- Airway compromise may develop in patients with underlying obesity or sleep apnea.
- Posterior packs may lead to nasopulmonary reflex—hypoxia, hypoventilation, and arrhythmia.
- Bilateral or posterior packs may require telemetry monitoring and possibly intensive care monitoring.

INDICATIONS FOR SURGERY/EMBOLIZATION

- Continued bleeding despite packing.
- Patient requires transfusion.
- Nasal anomaly precludes packing.
- Failed medical management after 48 to 72 hours.

ESCALATION OF TREATMENT: LIGATION AND EMBOLIZATION

Ligation

- SPA.
  - Most common, performed endoscopically.
- Been shown to reduce inpatient stay, increase patient satisfaction, and reduce costs.
  - One-year success rate between 70% to 100%.[5]
  - Must ligate both the SPA and the posterior septal branches.
- Maxillary artery
  - More challenging approach through canine fossa.
  - Electrocautery of posterior maxillary wall before removal.
  - Must ligate internal maxillary artery and ensure descending palatine and SPA are hemostatic.
  - Recurrence rate of 10% to 15%.[6]
  - Complication rate of 25% to 30%.[6]
  - Complicated by dental or nasolacrimal duct injury, facial and gum numbness.
- External Carotid Artery
  - Risk of injury to hypoglossal and vagus nerves.
  - Lower success rate.
  - More often indicated in traumatic or postsurgical epistaxis when there is nasal or ethmoid bony injury, which leads to bleeding beyond the SPA distribution.
- Anterior and Posterior Ethmoid Arteries
  - May be required in patients after internal maxillary artery ligation or SPA ligation who are still bleeding.
  - Lynch incision.
  - Fronto-ethmoid suture line.
  - 24 to 12 to 6 rule. Applies to medial wall of orbit.
    - Represents average distance in mm from anterior lacrimal crest to the anterior ethmoidal foramen, to the posterior ethmoid foramen, and finally the optic canal.

ANGIOGRAPHY AND EMBOLIZATION

- Helps to identify the location of bleeding.
- The success rate is 90%, minor complication rate is 18% to 45%, and major complication rate is up to 2%.[7]
- Only able to embolize external carotid artery and its branches.
- Accidental embolization of posterior and anterior ethmoid arteries of the ophthalmic division of the internal carotid may result in blindness.

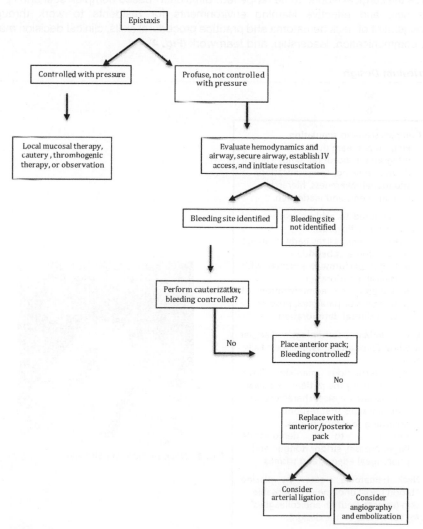

Fig. 3. Algorithm for epistaxis management.

NECK HEMATOMA

An expanding neck hematoma after thyroid surgery is a potentially fatal postoperative complication that requires early detection and immediate response (**Fig. 3**). This rare,

What are the education gaps for an early practitioner?

- Recognition of postoperative neck hematoma and its implications for airway management.
- Use of equipment to manage rapidly expanding hematoma at the bedside (hemostat and/or scissors to open the wound, suction to evacuate clot).
- Postevacuation management knowledge (return to the operating room for definitive management of bleeding, interim management of airway).

yet high-risk clinical scenario can pose many challenges to the junior resident, who is often the first responder. Impending airway compromise must be recognized early and decompression of the hematoma, often at the bedside, is a vital maneuver that requires the surgical wound to be reopened. Simulation-based complex scenarios provide safe and effective learning environments for residents to work through management of neck hematoma and practice procedural skills, clinical decision making, communication, leadership, and teamwork (**Fig. 4**).

Curriculum Design

- Complex scenario simulation.
  - Emphasizes team dynamics.
  - Integrates procedural skills, clinical decision making, communication, situational awareness, hierarchy management, and leadership.
- Easily adapted to achieve learner and educator specific goals:
  - Example: emphasizes early drainage of hematoma at bedside.
    - If not performed, proceed with clinical deterioration.
    - Inappropriate administration of sedatives or paralytics, proceed with clinical deterioration.
- Uses SimMan technology. (Laerdal Medical Corporation, Wappingers Falls, NY)
  - High technology manikin allows programming the patient to display appropriate physical characteristics and vital signs that respond according to interventions.
  - Ability to demonstrate laryngospasm, stridor, tongue and pharyngeal edema, and trismus.
- Neck hematoma created by placing "blood pack" underneath disposable skin (refer to Deutsch and colleagues[8] for full details on the design).
- Refer to scenario details outlined extensively in Deutsch and colleagues.
  - Scenarios can be easily modified and adapted to achieve learner and educator specific goals.

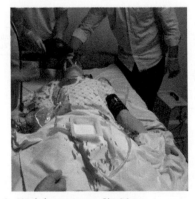

Fig. 4. Neck hematoma SimMan.

Goals for the Early Learner

- Early detection and identification of the high-risk stakes of the clinical situation.
- Immediate communication with senior resident, attending surgeon, anesthesia.
- Effective decompression of hematoma at bedside.
- Safe and efficient airway management strategy.

Learner Curriculum

Pathophysiology and relevant anatomy

- Two potential pathophysiologic mechanisms by which hematoma can produce airway compromise:[9]
  - Direct mechanical compression leading to reduction in cross-sectional area of the airway lumen
  - Development of intrinsic airway edema in response to impaired venous drainage leads to secondary swelling of the supraglottic structures and glottis.
- Hematomas may be either superficial (directly deep to the platysma) or deep (deep to strap muscles/superficial layer of deep cervical fascia).
- Superficial hematomas generally seem to be more impressive in terms of neck swelling.
- Deeper hematomas may be more dangerous.
  - Less easily detected and require less blood accumulation to cause symptoms.
- Rate of hematoma expansion may depend on the mechanism.
  - Venous: slowly expanding.
  - Arterial: rapidly expanding.
- Regardless of the mechanism, the interval between hematoma development and airway obstruction may be surprisingly short.

Presenting signs and symptoms

- Nonspecific symptoms:
  - Change in voice quality, dysphagia, sweating, agitation, and anxiety.
- Physical signs and symptoms:
  - Neck swelling, increased tenderness to palpation, bruising, and oozing from the incision.
  - Jackson–Pratt drains do not prevent hematomas. Drain may demonstrate frankly sanguineous output, possibly no output at all if clotted off.[10]
- Respiratory-specific symptoms:
  - Stridor, hypoxia, dyspnea, tachypnea, and tracheal deviation.

Principals of Successful Management

- Early detection is critical.
- Alert senior resident and attending staff immediately.
- Contact anesthesia to discuss airway management and alert staff in the operating room.
- Patient should be connected to monitors and continuous pulse oximetry.
- Supplemental oxygen and adjunctive airway assist equipment should be available.

Necessary Equipment and Supplies

- Scissors
- Hemostat
- Scalpel
- Suction
- Antiseptic solution

Stabilize the Airway

- While preparing for emergent intubation, decompression of the wound is often a key factor in providing relief from hypoxia and resulting cardiovascular instability.
- Opening of the platysma may not be sufficient.
  - Evacuation of the clot from tight compartment deep to strap muscles and deep fascia may be required.
- Try to maintain sterile technique:
  - Pour antiseptic solution on the incision.
  - Wear sterile gloves if time allows.
  - Use sterile scissors.
- Bleeding after hematoma evacuation can be managed with pressure once airway patency has been achieved.
- Intubation may be very difficult.
- Multiple intubation attempts before opening the wound may aggravate edema, worsening the airway obstruction.
- All airway management options: awake fiberoptic intubation, video-assisted laryngoscopy, traditional direct laryngoscopy, cricothyrotomy, and surgical tracheostomy should be considered.
- Administering sedation and paralytics to patient before intubation may result in loss of airway and create a "cannot ventilate, cannot intubate scenario."
- Patients will require formal neck exploration and hemostasis in the operating room.

SUMMARY

Hemorrhagic emergencies in otolaryngology can present significant challenges to the early practitioner. However, the fundamentals of resuscitation and airway stabilization remain universal to the management of hemorrhage regardless of the scenario in which it presents. The development of procedural skills, clinical decision making, effective communication strategies, and leadership remain critical to ensuring positive patient outcomes. Procedural task trainers and simulation-based complex scenarios provide safe and effective learning environments for young practitioners to build confidence and develop such skills.

Post-Test Questions (Correct answers are in italics)

1. The first step in managing a patient with epistaxis is:
   a. Performing rigid endoscopy.
   b. *Evaluating hemodynamic and airway status.*
   c. Looking for a source of bleeding.
   d. Attempting silver nitrate cautery.
2. Indications for embolization or surgical ligation in the management of epistaxis include which of the following?
   a. Persistent bleeding despite packing.
   b. Nasal anomalies precluding packing.
   c. Failed medical management after 48 to 72 hours.
   d. *All of the above.*
3. You are called to the beside to assess a 42-year-old man 6 hours after uncomplicated total thyroidectomy to evaluate neck swelling. You enter the room to find him tachypneic and with audible stridor. Which of the following actions is most likely to result in immediate respiratory improvement?
   a. Applying oxygen nasal cannula.
   b. Stripping the Jackson–Pratt drains.
   c. *Performing immediate decompression of the wound at bedside.*
   d. Calling anesthesia STAT for rapid sequence intubation.
4. All of the following statements regarding neck hematoma are true *except*:
   a. Intrinsic airway edema develops in response to impaired venous drainage in the neck leading to swelling of the glottis and supraglottis.
   b. Administration of sedation and paralytics before intubation may result in loss of airway.
   c. Change in voice quality, dysphagia, sweating, agitation and anxiety can all be signs of hematoma.
   d. *Jackson–Pratt drains can be used to help prevent neck hematoma.*

SUPPLEMENTARY DATA

Supplementary PDF slides related to this article can be found online at http://www. oto.theclinics.com/.

REFERENCES

1. Malloy KM, Malekzadeh S, Deutsch ES. Simulation-Based ORL emergencies boot camp part 1: curriculum design and airway skills. Laryngoscope 2013; 124(7):1562–5.

2. Villwock JA, Jones K. Recent trends in epistaxis management in the United States: 2008-2010. JAMA Otolaryngol Head Neck Surg 2013;139(12):1279–84.
3. Pettineo CM, Vozenilek JA, Kharasch M, et al. Epistaxis simulator: an innovative design. Simul Healthc 2008;3(4):239–41.
4. Chin CJ, Roth K, Rotenberg BW, et al. Emergencies in otolaryngology-head and neck surgery bootcamp: A novel Canadian experience. Laryngoscope 2014; 124(10):2275–80.
5. Rudmik L, Smith TL. Management of intractable spontaneous epistaxis. Am J Rhinol Allergy 2012;26(1):55–60.
6. Simmen D, Jones N. Epistaxis. In: Cummings CW, Flint PW, editors. Cummings otolaryngology head and neck surgery. Philadelphia: Mosby/Elsevier; 2010. p. 682–94.
7. Sadri M, Midwinter K, Ahmed A, et al. Assessment of safety and efficacy of arterial embolisation in the management of intractable epistaxis. Eur Arch Otorhinolaryngol 2006;263:560–6.
8. Deutsch ES, Malloy KM, Malekzadeh S. Simulation-based otorhinolaryngology emergencies boot camp: Part 3: Complex teamwork scenarios and conclusions. Laryngoscope 2014;124(7):1570–2.
9. Eisele D, Roediger F. In: Cummings CW, Flint PW, editors. Complications of neck surgery. Cummings otolaryngology head and neck surgery. Philadelphia: Mosby/Elsevier; 2010. p. 1726–35.
10. Nambu J, Sugino K, Oishi K, et al. Characteristics of postoperative bleeding after neck surgery. Surgical Science 2013;2013(3):192–5.

SUGGESTED READINGS

The following three articles outline the approach to curriculum design and implementation of a an Otolaryngology Emergencies Boot Camp, designed to provide early trainees with an accelerated introduction to the essential skills needed for successful clinical management of common emergencies in otolaryngology. The objectives of Boot Camp are to teach learners to recognize and triage typical otolaryngology emergencies, perform basic emergency management skills, and communicate effectively with a team. The articles outline the approach to curriculum implementation, design and construction of skills stations and task trainers, and how to effectively use simulation to guide medical decision making in complex clinical scenarios.

Deutsch ES, Malloy KM, Malekzadeh S. Simulation-based otorhinolaryngology emergencies boot camp: part 3: complex teamwork scenarios and conclusions. Laryngoscope 2014;124(7):1570–2.

Malekzadeh S, Deutsch ES, Malloy KM. Simulation-based oral emergencies boot camp part 2: Special skills using task trainers. Laryngoscope 2013;124(7): 1566–9.

Malloy KM, Malekzadeh S, Deutsch ES. Simulation-based ORL emergencies boot camp part 1: curriculum design and airway skills. Laryngoscope 2013;124(7): 1562–5.

Simulation Training for Vascular Emergencies in Endoscopic Sinus and Skull Base Surgery

Rowan Valentine, MBBS, FRACS, PhD*, Vikram Padhye, MBBS, PhD,
Peter-John Wormald, MD

KEYWORDS

- Carotid artery injury • Hemostasis • Endoscopic • Transsphenoidal • Simulation

KEY LEARNING POINTS

At the end of this article, the reader will:

- Be able to identify the major sources of morbidity when internal carotid artery (ICA) injury occurs.
- Be able to describe the ICA vascular catastrophe model.
- Be able to describe the key endoscopic surgical techniques to control the surgical field during an ICA injury.
- Be able to outline the surgical techniques to achieve hemostasis during endoscopic carotid artery injury.
- Be able to describe the late complications following carotid artery injury and how may they be avoided.
- Know if training in vascular emergencies can improve patient outcomes.

Disclosures and conflict of interest: Dr P.-J. Wormald receives royalties from Medtronic ENT for instruments designed and is a consultant for Neilmed Pharmaceuticals. Dr R. Valentine has nothing to disclose.
Department of Surgery, Otorhinolaryngology, Head and Neck Surgery, The Queen Elizabeth Hospital, University of Adelaide, 28 Woodville Road, Woodville, Adelaide, South Australia 5011, Australia
* Corresponding author.
E-mail address: rowan.valentine@gmail.com

Otolaryngol Clin N Am 49 (2016) 877–887
http://dx.doi.org/10.1016/j.otc.2016.02.013
0030-6665/16/$ – see front matter © 2016 Elsevier Inc. All rights reserved.

oto.theclinics.com

INTRODUCTION

> **Why is endoscopic simulated training for vascular complications required?**
>
> - There is a paradigm shift from external approaches to endonasal.
> - Endoscopic approaches are becoming the standard of care for resection of pituitary tumors.
> - Endoscopic resections are common, increasing the chance of experiencing a vascular emergency.
> - Increasingly advanced surgical pathologies are endoscopically resected.
> - Research into internal carotid artery (ICA) rupture management is required.

The last 20 years has seen a paradigm shift from traditional external approaches to the skull base to a completely endoscopic endonasal approach, made possible with the advent of improved technological developments, surgical instrumentation, and an improved understanding of the endoscopic endonasal anatomy. The advantages of endoscopic techniques over traditional external approaches include improved visualization, reduce hospital admission times, avoiding minimal sacrifice of intervening structures, and avoiding external skin incisions.[1]

Transsphenoidal pituitary surgery is common and has an incidence of ICA rupture rate of approximately 1.1%. Ciric and colleagues[2] used a postal questionnaire survey, involving more than 900 neurosurgeons, inquiring about their complication profile. Surgeons who had performed in excess of 500 transsphenoidal pituitary approaches had a 50% chance of being in the situation where they had to manage the carotid artery catastrophe. This finding implies that the increased subspecialization of endonasal skull base surgery is associated with a greater chance of experiencing a carotid artery injury (ie, subspecialty surgeons need to be geared up to manage an ICA injury). More advanced surgical resections center on the management of the ICA and, hence, have a greater chance of ICA injury. Endoscopic resections of craniopharyngiomas, clival chordomas, and chondrosarcomas have an ICA rupture rate of between 5% and 9%.[3–5] The increasing use of endoscopic approaches to the skull base increases the risk of encountering potential vascular injuries; it is essential that the specialist endoscopic skull base surgeon has appropriate training, not only in endonasal skull base anatomy and the avoidance of complications but also in managing a carotid artery catastrophe.

SIMULATION TRAINING

> **What is surgical simulation?**
>
> - Definition
> - Goals of simulation
> - Types of simulation (bench models, cadavers, virtual reality simulators, and live animals)

A simulator is defined as a device or model that is used to train people by imitating the situations that they will need to deal with. It allows users to gain experience and to observe and interact with the simulation via realistic visual, auditory, or tactile cues.[6] The main goals of surgical simulation is for research and development, to develop and teach surgical skill acquisition and excellence, and to transfer the learned techniques to the body of patients in the operating room.[7]

There are a range of different types of surgical simulators, each with their own advantages and disadvantages. Bench models are easily portable and cheap and require no specific supervision but are the least realistic and inanimate. Cadavers are the most anatomically accurate and have high fidelity but are expensive with limited availability of material and are not suitable for vascular injury. Virtual reality surgical simulators are reusable and anatomically accurate, with immediate objective feedback; but the sense of realism varies greater and may also appear inanimate. Animal models have played an important role in surgical education and training and have been used in the medical field since 384 BC. Live animals have a high level of fidelity and offer the most realistic experience with regard to major vascular injuries and tissue hemostasis. The main disadvantages include anatomic differences, high costs, and special facilities are required. There are also ethical dilemmas and animal welfare laws, which need to be addressed sensitively and appropriately.

SIMULATION OF VASCULAR INJURY FOR ENDOSCOPIC SINUS AND SKULL BASE SURGERY

What are the important aspects of an endoscopic model for vascular injury?

- Reproducible, validated model
- Standard instrumentation only required
- Recreates potential surgical scenarios (narrow nasal cavity, bony coverage, injury types)
- High-flow/high-pressure vascular injuries and high-flow/low-pressure vascular injuries
- Recovery model, allowing investigation into short-term and long-term complications
- Large animal models

If simulated training in vascular injuries is to be effective, then the surgical environment needs to be recreated. Surgeons need to be immediately familiar with the surgical environment and instruments that they will be using to control the vascular event. The utilization of standard instrumentation is ideal. The acquisition of surgical skills is impeded if using new unfamiliar instrumentation is required and, hence, unrealistic during the pressures of a major vascular event.

Vascular injuries take on a range of configurations. Each scenario may have a challenging unique set of circumstances. The ideal animal model needs to recreate these challenges and circumstances. The endoscopic vascular injury occurs down a narrow nasal corridor where even a small amount of blood may immediately disorientate the surgeon and disrupt the surgical field. Surgical exposure to the site of vascular injury may range from limited (ie, during sphenoidotomy, during endoscopic sinus surgery) to wide surgical access, such as during an expanded endonasal resection. Simulation needs to be able to recreate both these different circumstances.

The type of vascular injury may also vary in configuration depending on the surgical instrument that has caused the injury. Padhye and colleagues[8] investigated various hemostatic techniques in a range of injury configurations. Injury types investigated included a 3-mm punch injury, a 4-mm linear injury, and a 4-mm stellate injury. This study identified that the linear injury type was associated with the greatest volume of blood loss and the longest time to achieving hemostasis.

Challenging surgical scenarios may occur within high-flow/low-pressure vessels, such as during cavernous sinus bleeding, or within high-flow/high-pressure vessels, such as the carotid artery. High-flow/low-pressure scenarios are considered easier to control during the endoscopic approaches as the surgical field is less threatened. It makes it easier for the surgical team to visualize the defect and act accordingly. However, high-flow/high-pressure injuries are much more challenging because of the pulsatile nature of the blood stream, making visualization of the injury site much more difficult. Rapid exsanguination from an ICA rupture may occur, which will change the vascular event rapidly from a high-flow/high-pressure scenario to the high-flow/low-pressure scenario. Thus, rapid active resuscitation is important during ICA vascular injury simulation to maintain high-flow/high-pressure characteristics.

Short-term and long-term complications following vascular injury are well known and include secondary bleed, pseudoaneurysm formation, and vascular occlusion. Minimizing morbidity following a carotid artery injury relies firstly on achieving hemostasis but secondarily on maintaining vascular patency.[9] Simulating vascular injuries for the purpose of ongoing research and development requires ongoing assessment of the injury site over time to allow analysis of the occurrence of these complications and minimizing these to determine the best management algorithm.

Simulating the clinical scenario has shown to improve skill acquisition, particularly when the environment is simulated.[10] The use of anesthetic machines, monitoring equipment and pressure bag resuscitation and the ability to monitor blood pressure and pulse parameters immediately recreates the familiarity of a working operating room. Perhaps most importantly, live animal surgery creates an environment of life or death placing the trainee under immediate pressure. Large animals are ideal in vascular catastrophe simulation as they have a similar blood volume to humans, have similar blood pressure and pulse characteristics, and are robust.

THE SHEEP MODEL OF INTERNAL CAROTID ARTERY INJURY

- Large sheep used, ICA of similar caliber to humans
- General anesthesia, allowing spontaneous ventilation
- Sheep positioned supine
  - Midline incision
  - Carotids identified bilaterally
  - Jugular vein rapid infuser port
- A Sinus Model encapsulates ICA into the sphenoid sinus
- Standard endoscopic sinus surgery/skull base instrumentation
- Rapid resuscitation with warmed saline

All sheep are weighed, with weight greater than 20 kg, as this size mimics the caliber of the ICA in humans. Preoperative coagulation profiling and full blood count is performed. All sheep are starved 12 to 18 hours before surgery. Induction of general anesthesia is performed via injection with sodium thiopentone (19 mg/kg body weight) into the left jugular vein. Endotracheal intubation then follows with anesthesia maintain by inhalation of 1.5% to 2.0% isoflurane, to a depth that allows spontaneous ventilation. A depth on anesthesia that allows spontaneous ventilation minimizes the concentration of anesthetic required and minimizes the corresponding hypotension.

The sheep are positioned on their backs, and a midline neck incision is performed from the thyroid cartilage to the base of the neck and extended down to the superficial layer of the deep cervical fascia. This fascia is incised, and dissection is continued to the anterior tracheal wall. The visceral fascia is then dissected from the lateral tracheal walls to reveal the right carotid sheath. The carotid artery is then dissected free for a length of 15 cm from the angle of the mandible to the base of the neck. The left carotid artery is also identified as described earlier. The left carotid artery is then cannulated to allow for continuous invasive arterial pressure monitoring. The left internal jugular vein is then cannulated with a rapid infusion catheter exchange set to allow for rapid fluid resuscitation.

The Sinus Model Otorhino Neuro Trainer (SIMONT, Prodelphus, Brazil) simulates the endoscopic environment so that the carotid injuries can be managed with the anatomic limitations seen in the human nasal vestibule, nasal cavity, and sphenoid sinus (**Fig. 1**). This model is an anatomically accurate reconstruction of the nasal cavity and paranasal sinuses. A patented silicon material recreates the colors, consistency, and elasticity of the nasal mucosa and paranasal sinus boney architecture. Routine sinus and skull base surgical instrumentation is used and provides the realistic tissue resistance encountered during endonasal surgery. Bilateral large sphenoidotomies and partial middle turbinectomies are performed. A specially designed detachable posterior sphenoid sinus wall allows the placement of the freely dissected carotid artery within the sphenoid sinus. A plastic cover is placed over the vessel that mimics the thin boney covering over the carotid artery. Four fasteners allow this vessel to be held within the model and prevent blood leaking around the back and the model, allowing blood to run out through the nares of the model. Absence of carotid compression on entry and exit of the carotid artery is confirmed visually and by observing no change in the mean arterial pressure between the left and right carotid arteries. The model is

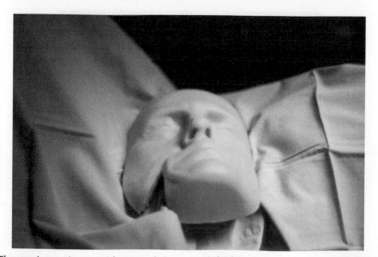

Fig. 1. The endoscopic carotid artery injury model placed into position and fixed to the operating table.

fixed to the operating table and onto the neck of the sheep to prevent displacement during intervention.

Using a 0° rigid endoscope, a standard skull base bur can be used to drill away the plastic plate, simulating the thin boney covering of the carotid siphon within the sphenoid sinus (**Fig. 2**). The Hajek punch can then be used to expose the carotid artery creating a boney window, revealing the pulsatile carotid artery (**Fig. 3**). This window allows for the variable boney exposure that maybe experienced during an unanticipated vascular event. An 11-blade scalpel can be used to create an approximately 4-mm longitudinal incision through the anterior wall of the carotid artery (**Fig. 4**). Immediately, rapid bleeding occurs obstructing the surgical view instantaneously (**Fig. 5**).

Simultaneous fluid resuscitation with warmed normal saline is commenced at approximately 200 mL/min. Rapid resuscitation with a pressure bag continues in order to achieve a mean arterial pressure of the preinjury level. Aggressive simultaneous fluid resuscitation ensures the maintenance of a high-flow, high-pressure vascular injury model. A thermal blanket is used to ensure a constant temperature and prevent the adverse affects of hypothermia on the coagulation cascade.[11]

CONTROLLING THE SURGICAL FIELD

- Optimization of visualization is the basis of management.
- The 2-surgeon technique is paramount.
- Use an endoscope down the contralateral side to the heavy bleeding; a lens cleaning system is a valuable adjunct.
- Use 2 large-bore suction devices, one to direct blood flow while the other manipulates nasoseptal flap out of field.
- Hover the suction on the injury site.

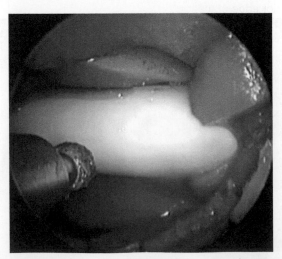

Fig. 2. The plastic shield is drilled with a diamond bur to thin the covering overlying the vessel.

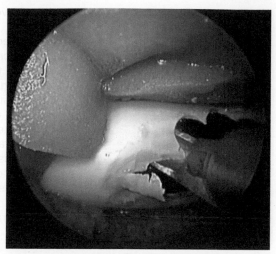

Fig. 3. The Hajek punch is used to expose the carotid vessel.

As in open surgeries, management of the endoscopic bleeding field is centered on the optimization of visualization. This visualization allows surgeons to not only see the injury site but also make decisions in regard to appropriate hemostatic techniques. The major arterial bleeding scenario is made more difficult in endoscopic surgery because of the limited access and the potential for regular loss of vision and soiling of the endoscope, the so-called red out. Through the use of the sheep model, Valentine and Wormald[11,12] were able to simulate a total of 42 carotid and 25 venous injuries in the endoscopic environment and describe critical steps to their control as outlined.

Using a team-based approach to the management is essential. The 2-surgeon technique permits one surgeon to navigate the endoscope while the other can dissect. It can also allow for more instruments to be used through the nasal cavity at a time. Pulsatile bleeding favors one side of the nasal cavity over the other. As a result, vision is best gained by placing the endoscope down the contralateral side to the bleeding and using the posterior edge of the nasal septum as a shield for the endoscope tip.

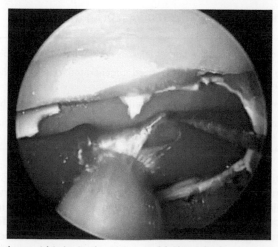

Fig. 4. The exposed carotid is incised with an 11-blade scalpel.

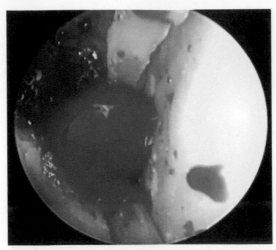

Fig. 5. Pulsatile high-flow/high-pressure vascular injury.

An endoscopic lens cleaning system is also a valuable asset. Despite the endoscope down the contralateral side, it is still susceptible to frequent soiling. Removing the endoscope from the nasal cavity in order clean it can also result in surgeons losing their bearings and position of instruments in the surgical field. A foot-controlled lens cleaning system allows for continuous vision of instrumentation and injury site.

Another key factor is the size and positioning of suction. In particular, the caliber of sucker is an important determinant of how quickly blood can be evacuated from the field. A size 12 French or larger is reliable in this setting. A second suction device is also recommended to manipulate a nasoseptal flap, which is commonly harvested in operations of the skull base and has the potential to obscure the field. Suction may be introduced down the contralateral side of the nose to the endoscope, thereby directing the flow of blood away from the tip and hovered over the site of injury. These recommendations give the surgical team the best chance of maintaining visualization.[12]

HEMOSTATIC TECHNIQUES IN SIMULATED VASCULAR INJURY

- A variety of hemostats have been trialed in the simulated endoscopic setting.
- Flow-able hemostatic matrix, oxidized regenerated cellulose, and bipolar cautery are not advocated.
- Crushed muscle patch is an easily accessible, effective, and reliable hemostat.
- Direct vessel closure techniques can reduce the risk of pseudoaneurysm and maintain normal carotid integrity long-term.

Optimal visualization is one component of the overall management. Success of definitive control is influenced largely by the hemostatic technique used, and simulation has been integral in allowing a variety of hemostats to be prospectively trialed.

Valentine and colleagues[13] performed the first scientific trial of different hemostats in the carotid bleeding setting. In this trial, use of a flow-able hemostatic matrix or oxidized regenerated cellulose resulted in a failure of primary hemostasis. Chitosan gel was effective in 50% of cases initially but failed to maintain hemostasis for the entire duration of the procedure. In contrast, a crushed muscle patch and U-clip anastomotic device (Medtronic, Jacksonville, FL) were both able to gain and maintain hemostasis in 100% of cases. Since this trial, however the, U-clip has ceased production.

Padhye and colleagues[8] followed up this work with a study that looked at different hemostats and their effectiveness on different injury types. Both short-term outcomes as well as long-term complications were evaluated. This trial found that use of a bipolar cautery, which had been previously described in the literature,[14] was difficult to advocate because of the mixed results in obtaining hemostasis. By contrast a crushed muscle patch and aneurysm clip was able to gain primary hemostasis in 100% of cases regardless of injury type. Crushed muscle had a low risk of destabilization and pseudoaneurysm and was the only hemostat associated with a 100% rate of long-term carotid patency. The aneurysm clip had no incidence of pseudoaneurysm, and long-term preservation of blood flow depended on its placement.

In addition to the U-clip and aneurysm clip, Padhye and colleagues[15] have now performed a simulation trial on another direct vessel closure device, the Anastoclip (LeMaitre, Burlington, MA). This device was able to gain primary hemostasis in 100% of cases and had a very low risk of pseudoaneurysm when compared with other techniques.

VASCULAR SIMULATION TRAINING IMPROVING OUTCOMES

- Poorly managed inadvertent ICA injury risks exsanguination and long-term morbidity.
- International vascular injuries workshops are available.
- Vascular simulation training prevents morbidity and mortality as well as reducing surgeon anxiety around an event.[16]

Inadvertent ICA injury can place a patient's life at imminent risk; even despite management, complications, such as pseudoaneurysm and carotico-cavernous fistula, may eventuate. Pseudoaneurysms have a reported incidence of up to 60% after ICA injury and if rupture may have fatal consequences.[17] Valentine and Wormald's[17] review of the current literature discovered 89 cases of published ICA injury, with a reported mortality rate of 15% and a permanent morbidity rate of 26%.

Padhye and colleagues[16] recently reviewed the value of vascular injury training. In this retrospective series, cases of major endoscopic arterial hemorrhage managed by previously endoscopically vascular trained surgeons were reviewed. A total of 9 cases were reported, 8 were ICA injuries and 1 was a basilar artery injury. In each instance, an autologous free crushed muscle graft was used on the injury site to gain successful primary hemostasis. After initial intervention, there were 2 cases of carotid stenosis or occlusion and 1 pseudoaneurysm. In each instance, the patient underwent successful endovascular intervention and made otherwise unremarkable recoveries. As a result, in this small series, with the utilization of a muscle patch, there was a 0% mortality rate and a 0% rate of morbidity.

SUMMARY

Endonasal skull base approaches are becoming increasingly common, and specialist endonasal skull base surgeons need to be familiar with the techniques required to manage a major vascular injury. Live large animal surgical simulation replicates the challenging endoscopic surgical management of a high-flow/high-pressure vascular injury. Simulated endoscopic ICA training has allowed the development of the surgical techniques required to control the surgical field, along with the identification of methods and technologies to achieve rapid hemostasis. Simulated training can improve surgical skill in controlling vascular catastrophes, resulting in better outcomes for patients.

Post-Test Questions (Correct answers are in italics)

1. Which of the following is not important in controlling the surgical field?
   a. *Suction tip placed directly below endoscope*
   b. Placing the endoscope in the nostril without the jet stream of blood
   c. Suction tip placed into contralateral nostril to endoscope
   d. Guiding vascular stream away from tip of endoscope
2. What hemostatic techniques are reliable and rapidly available in today's operating room?
   a. Floseal
   b. Surgicel
   c. U-clip anastomotic device
   d. *Autologous crushed muscle patch*
3. During ongoing intraoperative hemorrhage despite attempted hemostasis, which technique is not useful for determining adequate contralateral cerebral ICA blood flow?
   a. Xenon computed tomography
   b. Single-photon emission computed tomography imaging
   c. *Balloon occlusion test*
   d. Transcranial Doppler
4. What type of vascular closure technique has the lowest risk of pseudoaneurysm formation?
   a. *Direct vascular wall closure*
   b. Autologous crushed muscle patch
   c. Floseal
   d. Surgicel

SUPPLEMENTARY DATA

Supplementary PDF slides related to this article can be found online at http://www.oto.theclinics.com/.

REFERENCES

1. Casler JD, Doolittle AM, Mair EA. Endoscopic surgery of the anterior skull base. Laryngoscope 2005;115(1):16–24.

2. Ciric I, Ragin A, Baumgartner C, et al. Complications of transsphenoidal surgery: results of a national survey, review of the literature, and personal experience. Neurosurgery 1997;40(2):225–36 [discussion: 236–7].

3. Couldwell WT, Weiss MH, Rabb C, et al. Variations on the standard transsphenoidal approach to the sellar region, with emphasis on the extended approaches and parasellar approaches: surgical experience in 105 cases. Neurosurgery 2004;55(3):539–47 [discussion: 547–50].

4. Frank G, Sciarretta V, Calbucci F, et al. The endoscopic transnasal transsphenoidal approach for the treatment of cranial base chordomas and chondrosarcomas. Neurosurgery 2006;59(1 Suppl 1):ONS50-7 [discussion: ONS50-7].
5. Gardner PA, Kassam AB, Snyderman CH, et al. Outcomes following endoscopic, expanded endonasal resection of suprasellar craniopharyngiomas: a case series. J Neurosurg 2008;109(1):6-16.
6. Rosen JM, Long SA, McGrath DM, et al. Simulation in plastic surgery training and education: the path forward. Plast Reconstr Surg 2009;123(2):729-38 [discussion: 739-40].
7. Davies J, Khatib M, Bello F. Open surgical simulation-a review. J Surg Educ 2013; 70(5):618-27.
8. Padhye V, Valentine R, Paramasivan S, et al. Early and late complications of endoscopic hemostatic techniques following different carotid artery injury characteristics. Int Forum Allergy Rhinol 2014;4(8):651-7.
9. Raymond J, Hardy J, Czepko R, et al. Arterial injuries in transsphenoidal surgery for pituitary adenoma; the role of angiography and endovascular treatment. AJNR Am J Neuroradiol 1997;18(4):655-65.
10. Stefanidis D, Sevdalis N, Paige J, et al. Simulation in surgery: what's needed next? Ann Surg 2015;261(5):846-53.
11. Valentine R, Wormald PJ. A vascular catastrophe during endonasal surgery: an endoscopic sheep model. Skull Base 2011;21(2):109-14.
12. Valentine R, Wormald PJ. Controlling the surgical field during a large endoscopic vascular injury. Laryngoscope 2011;121(3):562-6.
13. Valentine R, Boase S, Jervis-Bardy J, et al. The efficacy of hemostatic techniques in the sheep model of carotid artery injury. Int Forum Allergy Rhinol 2011;1(2): 118-22.
14. Kassam A, Snyderman CH, Carrau RL, et al. Endoneurosurgical hemostasis techniques: lessons learned from 400 cases. Neurosurg Focus 2005;19(1):E7.
15. Padhye V, Murphy J, Bassiouni A, et al. Endoscopic direct vessel closure in carotid artery injury. Int Forum Allergy Rhinol 2015;5(3):253-7.
16. Padhye V, Valentine R, Sacks R, et al. Coping with catastrophe: the value of endoscopic vascular injury training. Int Forum Allergy Rhinol 2015;5(3):247-52.
17. Valentine R, Wormald PJ. Carotid artery injury after endonasal surgery. Otolaryngol Clin North Am 2011;44(5):1059-79.

SUGGESTED READINGS

Davies J, Khatib M, Bello F. Open surgical simulation a review. J Surg Educ 2013; 70(5):618-27.
Rosen JM, Long SA, McGrath DM, et al. Simulation in plastic surgery training and education: the path forward. Plast Reconstr Surg 2009;123(2):729-38 [discussion: 739-40].
Stefanidis D, Sevdalis N, Paige J, et al. Simulation in surgery: what's needed next? Ann Surg 2015;261(5):846-53.

Index

Note: Page numbers of article titles are in **boldface** type.

Otolaryngol Clin N Am 49 (2016) 889–898
http://dx.doi.org/10.1016/S0030-6665(16)30041-X
0030-6665/16/$ – see front matter

oto.theclinics.com

Moving?

Make sure your subscription moves with you!

To notify us of your new address, find your **Clinics Account Number** (located on your mailing label above your name), and contact customer service at:

Email: journalscustomerservice-usa@elsevier.com

800-654-2452 (subscribers in the U.S. & Canada)
314-447-8871 (subscribers outside of the U.S. & Canada)

Fax number: 314-447-8029

Elsevier Health Sciences Division
Subscription Customer Service
3251 Riverport Lane
Maryland Heights, MO 63043

*To ensure uninterrupted delivery of your subscription, please notify us at least 4 weeks in advance of move.

Printed and bound by CPI Group (UK) Ltd, Croydon, CR0 4YY

03/10/2024

01040492-0011